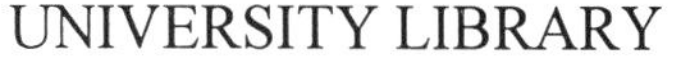

THE NEW LONGEVITY DIET

THE NEW LONGEVITY DIET

How to

·Stay Young

·Stay Healthy

·Stay Slim

by Eating the Foods You Love

DR. HENRY MALLEK, F.A.C.N.

G. P. PUTNAM'S SONS
NEW YORK

The recipes contained in this book are to be followed exactly as written. Neither the publisher nor the author is responsible for an individual reader's health or allergy needs that may require medical supervision.

Every effort has been made to ensure that the information contained in this book is complete and accurate. However, neither the publisher nor the author is engaged in rendering professional advice or services to the individual reader. The ideas, procedures, and suggestions contained in this book are not substitutes for consulting with your physician. You should seek medical supervision for all matters regarding your health.

Neither the author nor the publisher shall be liable or responsible for any loss or damage allegedly arising from any information or suggestion in this book including, without limitation, for any adverse reactions to the recipes contained in this book.

G. P. Putnam's Sons
Publishers Since 1838
a member of
Penguin Putnam Inc.
375 Hudson Street
New York, New York 10014

Published simultaneously in Canada

Library of Congress Cataloging-in-Publication Data
Mallek, Henry.
The new longevity diet : how to stay young, stay healthy, stay
slim by eating the foods you love / by Henry Mallek.
p. cm.
Includes bibliographical references.
ISBN 0-399-14628-8
1. Longevity—Nutritional aspects. 2. Aging—Nutritional
aspects. 3. Nutrition. I. Title.

RA784.M2945 2000 00-055371
613.2—dc21

Printed in the United States of America

1 3 5 7 9 10 8 6 4 2

This book is printed on acid-free paper. ♾

Book design by Tanya Maiboroda

ACKNOWLEDGMENTS

My deepest gratitude to Laura Blake Peterson of the Curtis Brown Literary Agency for her interest in the program that became *The New Longevity Diet*. Her perceptive suggestions were invaluable for developing the book's proposal.

To Jeremy Katz, senior editor at Penguin Putnam, whom I am greatly indebted to for his enthusiasm, encouragement, and guidance. His constructive comments regarding the technical and scientific aspects of the book such as the Longevity Nutrient Chart and the Recommended Longevity Allowances were essential for their presentation. It is impossible to enumerate the many ways his advice and consultation, not to mention his editing skills, greatly enriched the form and content of *The New Longevity Diet*. Thank you, Jeremy.

CONTENTS

THE NEW LONGEVITY DIET

1

HOW LONG DO YOU WANT TO LIVE?

Introduction to the Nutrition of Longevity and the Power of Food

How long do you expect to live—70 years? 80? Do you think that it would be too optimistic to predict you could live a full century?

What if someone came along and told you that if you ate the right amount of foods that are present in the supermarket, you could live to be 120 years old?

You would probably say that person was dreaming, that estimating so high a human life span must be based on wishful thinking. But the potential to live twice as long as our ancestors and up to 40 years longer than the current life expectancy is not unreal. In fact, it is based on scientific evidence—research that shows that our diet is more key to our longevity than we thought.

We are all aware of recommended dietary allowance (RDA) listings that appear on the sides of the packaging of food and snacks. They tell us our recommended daily totals of carbohydrates, fats, protein, vitamins, and minerals we should ingest. Logically, then, the amounts listed should be all we need to stay fit, trim, and healthy. So why are so many Americans overweight and unhealthy? Poor exercise and eating habits have a great deal to do with our country's obesity problem, but more significant is the lack of proper nutrition.

Our RDA charts are failing us.

In addition to the commonly known vitamins and minerals—vitamins C, D, and E, iron, and calcium, to name a few—cited and listed on food packaging, there are many powerful substances in food that were discovered recently and continue to be discovered and researched by scientists. I call them the *longevity nutrients*. These substances—not the same as those more familiar vitamins and minerals—hold the key for achieving new levels of health and slowing down the aging process. Acting differently to improve the body's response to stress, enhance its physiology, and activate and strengthen the immune system, longevity nutrients, when consumed regularly, can ultimately prevent heart disease, cancer, arthritis, and many other chronic diseases. As gerontologists all agree, if you eliminate these life-shortening diseases, you have a much better chance of having a truly long life.

While some of these nutrients have been known about since the early 1900s, they were poorly researched and their benefits were mistakenly seen as harmful effects. Phytates, one group of the longevity nutrients, were called antinutrients because they bind certain minerals in foods and limit their absorption into the body. What was recently discovered is that phytates don't bind just any minerals, they bind minerals that are harmful to the body. Protease inhibitors—another on this list of new nutrients—were considered harmful because they inhibit digestive enzymes. However, recent findings show this inhibition to be small and insignificant. More important, protease inhibitors—found mostly in grains we eat every day—are invaluable anticarcinogens.

As the world has advanced, the human body has failed to evolve to meet the demands of modern society. Advertising would lead you to believe that supplements and megavitamins are the way to arm ourselves. The answer lies not in unnatural, manmade sources, but in the foods we love. Imagine eating delicious food in filling quantities and having, as effects, longer, healthier lives as well as weight loss.

The New Longevity Diet is not some super-diet that would have you eating only one food group—like some that push only proteins or carbohydrates—while neglecting your body's need of the others. It is a well-balanced plan that gives your body what it needs to function at its optimum levels. The best part? No starvation, no bland unchanging menus, no sacrifices. In fact, when you read the list of the longevity nutrients included in *The New Longevity Diet*, the names may seem unfamiliar at first, but you will soon realize that they are present in commonly eaten foods, but your diet, like most people's, is inadequate in many of them—and this program will show you how to correct this.

Most exciting, a diet rich in the longevity nutrients will bring your weight down to where it ought to be—without supplements, diets, drugs, or denial.

This book introduces the longevity nutrients, explains their natural benefits, and reveals what foods contain them. Producing benefits for people of all ages, their discovery will revolutionize the field of nutrition. Everyone who wants to boost their health—not just maintain it—to live longer and more active lives, and to achieve ideal weight, can learn how to use these nutrients and form comprehensive programs to achieve their goals.

By using the longevity nutrients consciously, you can create your own eating plan for the 21st century.

Successful Aging or Getting Better with Age

Often, when people think of aging, a reflex may send them dashing off to the health food store to pick up a bottle of the latest antiaging substance their favorite celebrity touted on television. There is no magic pill for aging. The formula for successfully combating the toll aging takes on our bodies and minds is right under our noses in the foods available at the supermarket or health food store (one aisle over from the miracle pills)—on display and easy to reach. Our world, abundant with its own supplies and resources, makes it easy for us to prevent aging and disease because all the substances we need are contained in wholesome foods, available to most everyone.

The New Longevity Diet simply involves eating the right amounts of these wholesome, tasty foods to boost our bodies' immune, digestive, respiratory, nervous, reproductive, circulatory, endocrine, muscular, skeletal, and skin systems, allowing everything to run smoothly.

If you think about living to the ripe old age of 120, it may not sound appealing, especially if you suffer from what we typically think of as inevitable infirmities of aging. You don't have to look too far to see the effects of aging and disease on your friends, family, and neighbors. In fact, when you look in a mirror, you may be disturbed by what time has done to you! Like it or not, everyone ages. However, because we know more about aging than we ever have before, we can maximize our potential to live as we are designed to, to attain our full life span: a happy, healthy 120 years!

Along the way to this milepost, you will meet diseases interested in interrupting this life span for you, and conquering them will require your active and full participation. This is where the longevity nutrients come in. Longevity nutrients introduce, even into an aging body, a youthful physiology. Because these nutrients also prevent chronic diseases (such as cancer, heart disease, and arthritis), and even improve mood and thought processes, antiaging effects are just one of their benefits.

It would hardly be ideal if people lived to 120 and were not able to achieve their full potential: prevention of aging is not going to do people any good unless they are healthy, happy, and content. Gerontologists—who study the scientific phenomena of aging—characterize several different components of successful aging:

1. avoiding disease and disability
2. being able to maintain physical activity and proper mind function
3. interacting with others or good social contact

Successful aging is impossible if even one of these components is missing.

Enter the longevity nutrients. Making sure you set yourself up to achieve the most out of these three areas is what the *New Longevity Diet* program does best. As you read on, you'll learn how to choose your aging style—old and sick or young and vibrant.

We all have the ability to make the *New Longevity Diet* part of our eating plans, just as we have made other health-conscious efforts in our lives—quitting smoking, limiting exposure to harmful UV rays, exercise, and cutting back on calories. It may sound like too much work, like too much to *do* all of the time but the truth is, you are already on the path, and with this program you will witness the powerful effects nutrition has on aging.

The Longevity Nutrients: Long-Lost Factors in the Antiaging Equation

Most people are familiar enough with common vitamins and minerals. Nutritionists and general practitioners rarely see people with deficiencies of these compounds. Long gone are the days when scurvy—a condition caused by lack of vitamin C—and anemia—due to lack of the mineral iron—plague the masses. However, vitamin and mineral deficiency—like most everything else in nature—has evolved. Today, Americans unwittingly suffer from longevity nutrient starvation.

The longevity nutrients are not the same as typical vitamins and minerals; they are more complex and have a broader range of functions. Each of these compounds has several specific antiaging effects on all body systems, such as our heart, kidneys, skin, and digestive system, to name a few. Each interacts with our organs and systems to prevent them from aging. Common vitamins and minerals—although essential for health—do not have the scope of effects encompassed by these nutrients.

So what are these wonderful longevity nutrients? Take a look at the following list. How many substances do you recognize? While the names may sound foreign and strange to your ear, you should find the effects pleasantly familiar. Don't be surprised if only one or two of these—at most—exotic-sounding words are familiar to you. Without knowing the positive role these nutrients play as antiaging substances, they tend to be harder for us to recognize because they, until now, have not been prescribed as necessary parts of our diet. Their specialized chemical structures make it impossible to classify them into vitamins and minerals the same way other nutrients of our diet may be classified, but they are as important as vitamin C or calcium.

Nucleotides—If you think this term sounds something like DNA, you are absolutely right. Nucleotides are found in food and in our cells' DNA. DNA is made up of nucleic acids, which are in turn composed of nucleotides. These nucleotides are precursors for the cells' DNA, especially in the cells of our immune and digestive systems—when we ingest them.

Saponins—These are found in foods like beans and tofu. Saponins help prevent age-related immune system decline by stimulating certain immune system cells. Saponins also help lower cholesterol and prevent cancer. Cultures with saponin-rich diets—like the Japanese—have been enjoying the benefits for centuries. Perhaps this is why the Japanese tend to have longer life spans than Americans who generally have saponin-poor diets.

Phytates—These are found both inside and outside our cells. You've probably heard of antioxidants, such as vitamin E, embraced as antiaging substances. You can add phytates to this list, but realize that this antioxidant works in a different way: it controls the effects of iron. Iron—in excessive amounts—can lead to the development of harmful free radicals or reactive oxygen species (ROS). ROS are essentially a breeding ground for encouraging and advancing the aging process, so nutrients that get in the way of ROS are relevant and exciting to learn as much about as we can. (For a complete introduction to ROS, see chapter 2, lesson 6, on pages 24–39.)

Protease inhibitors—The next time you eat a potato, keep in mind you are ingesting a substantial supply of the longevity nutrients. Protease inhibitors or substances induced by them find malfunctioning cells in the body. Once there, protease inhibitors interact with the cells' DNA to regulate and stop the cells from malfunctioning. Chromosomes are prone to abnormal changes. Protease inhibitors prevent this from happening. Without these protease inhibitors, cells are more likely to age and become malignant (a diseased growth).

Glutamine—This is a building block of protein. Muscles need glutamine to function properly. It is also an important nutrient for immune system cells, providing the energy they need to carry out their antiaging functions in the body. Another antiaging role of this longevity nutrient is to maintain the supply of specific antioxidants made in our body.

Exorphins—It may be hard to believe that commonly eaten protein foods are a source of several antiaging substances. One group of exorphins have pluripotent—the way you might think of "multipurpose super strength"—antiaging factors. Carnosine, for example, is a pluripotent antiaging factor since it not only protects proteins and DNA, but it also prevents a whole encyclopedia of different molecules from succumbing to various aging effects in several of the body's organs.

Pyrroloquinoline quinone (PQQ)—Only discovered in 1979, PQQ is particularly important because it helps compensate for age-related decreases in activity of certain critical enzymes. Since humans and most animals don't have the capacity to synthesize or make this nutrient, the sole source for getting PQQ is from foods recommended by this program.

Arginine—This nutrient stimulates and releases two very important substances in the body affected by aging: human growth hormone (HGH) and nitric oxide (NO). (Later, I'll explain the role of HGH and NO in aging.) Arginine-rich foods help smooth out the aging process.

Inulin and oligofructose—These have antiaging functions far apart from the others. They navigate through certain bacteria in the colon. Specifically, inulin and oligofructose change bacteria in the colon to produce certain substances called short fatty chain acids (SCFAs). SCFAs remain in the colon to increase the ability of the immune system's function, facilitate DNA repair, and protect proteins from aging. Jerusalem artichokes and dandelion greens are two of the limited food sources for inulin and oligofructose.

Taurine—Compared to some of the more recently discovered longevity nutrients, taurine is an old-timer—it has been known about for approximately 150 years—but how it discourages the aging process is still not completely known. It is found in practically every cell in the body, with high levels in the brain, where its antiaging functions include those of an antioxidant and stabilizer of cell membranes. It is a critical substance for heart functions, but taurine levels decrease with age.

Lignans—These come from certain grains and berries and are recent additions to the longevity nutrient list. Lignans modulate our bodies' hormone levels. Hormones are one of the main characters in the aging story, and lignans have a lot to do with how estrogen and testosterone may discourage antiaging effects.

Quercetin—You remember the saying, "An apple a day keeps the doctor away"? Well, this may actually be true! Apples are one of the best sources of quercetin, and we are just beginning to unravel its complexities. A strong antioxidant, quercetin also gives other antioxidants the opportunity to be as powerful as possible, getting rid of any cells that may be aged or malignant. Onions are another good source of quercetin.

Genistein—This nutrient plays many roles in preventing cells from growing *too much*. For example, even though the formation of new blood vessels—angiogenesis—is indispensable for our growth and development, it is *not* indispensable to people who may suffer from diabetes or rheumatoid arthritis. Too many blood vessels make diabetes and arthritis worse. So, genistein—found mostly in soy and soy products—helps put a cap on how much our cells can grow.

Isothiocyanates—These detoxify or disable destructive chemicals in our bodies. You could say that isothiocyanates are mediators. They negotiate their way through the system of enzymes our body already has in place to break down harmful chemicals. Since detoxification happens in our liver, lungs, and skin, isothiocyanates cover a lot of territory.

Carnitine—If wood burns in a fireplace to produce heat, then cells burn fat in a structure called the mitochondria to supply energy. The main role of carnitine is the transportation of fat into the mitochondria for burning. By ensuring adequate carnitine in the diet, we keep our cellular energy supplies high. The mitochondria need carnitine to function effectively—especially in organs like the heart that are prone to having low levels of carnitine.

Phytosterols—These are related to cholesterol, but have a much better reputation. In fact, phytosterols prevent many of cholesterol's bad effects and do a lot to prevent aging in our artery walls. Phytosterols are found in many of our organs, but they are especially important in the liver and skin.

Monoterpenes—These longevity nutrients are not in short supply. Monoterpenes are abundant in citrus fruits, especially the peel or "zest," and certain herbs, spices, and rice bran oil. Somewhat like isothiocyanates, monoterpenes trigger our body's detoxification systems. They also keep our body's growth factors at bay, helping halt and regulate cell changes—changes that if left to flourish on their own, could affect the aging of cells.

Tannins—For years, the Chinese and Japanese have used tannins as folk remedies to treat ulcers and high blood pressure. Research shows tannins not only help repair DNA, but they also help prevent DNA damage. Where many of the longevity nutrients keep ROS (free radicals) from developing in the first place, tannins—in addition to killing bacteria in wounds—actually scour our bodies, looking for ROS that have already developed.

Organosulfur compounds (OCs)—were first used in 1500 B.C. by Egyptian medical doctors. OCs prevent one of the cardinal effects of blood vessel aging by preventing the loss of elasticity of the aorta. They have a strong track record of antioxidant effects, including a reputation for preventing diseases and stunting the development of harmful chemicals in our bodies that accelerate the aging process. Organosulfur compounds come from the allium plant family, which includes garlic and onions.

Glutathione—This substance seems a custom-made antiaging factor essential for our body to thrive. Cells that don't get enough glutathione suffer harm that can't be repaired. Glutathione certainly accommodates a lot of what our bodies need to work right. From making proteins and regulating cell growth, to making sure our immune systems are the strongest they can be, glutathione is another main character in the antiaging story.

Conjugated linoleic acid—You may be surprised that a fat can have antiaging properties. Poorly understood, fat tends to get a bad rap, but conjugated linoleic acid (CLA) is a "good" fat. Ingesting CLA stimulates the immune system, helps reduce weight, and improves our body composition (such as the amounts of fat and muscle that make up our tissues). CLA is especially abundant in certain types of cheeses.

Where All This Fits In

Now that you have been acquainted with the longevity nutrients, you may be wondering what role they play in extending and improving your life. As a nutritional biochemist, who holds a Ph.D. degree in biochemistry and metabolism from the Massachusetts Institute of Technology, I have come to appreciate that *all* the different substances in food—whether chemically complex or simple—are there for a reason. Specifically, knowing that our cells benefit and depend on so many other substances beyond the usual nutrients like vitamins B, C, and E, means we have to find out "who" these substances are, what they do, and what they are saying to our bodies. Only then can we truly begin to get the most out of food.

Here are some of the highlights:

- Proteins do not always break down the way we thought they did, into their constituent amino acids. Some amino acids are absorbed as chains, made up of two or more amino acids. When they enter the body they can become potent antiaging substances.

- Certain substances we thought never entered the body do not only find their way into our body, but are distributed throughout all the organs to produce antiaging effects.
- Intricate effects of all these longevity nutrients on our cells include a window to see how our organs age. This means:
  - even though the brain is very specific in terms of which nutrients it lets in, longevity nutrients are some of the privileged ones, which means they have and take the opportunity to promote antiaging effects in the brain
  - after a meal, longevity nutrients not only circulate in the blood and promote antiaging effects in the heart, but also help the heart deal with stresses it confronts every day
  - the liver depends on longevity nutrients to work in conjunction with the pathways that detoxify thousands of foreign chemicals that enter our bodies each day
  - longevity nutrients interact with the skeleton to help build bone mass and prevent osteoporosis—a condition that weakens bones. It used to be that calcium and vitamin D were the only nutrients important for healthy bone aging
- The ability of the longevity nutrients to change the direction of age-related declines in our body's immune system and hormones is well documented. An enormous body of research shows that, whether it be the skin, kidneys, reproductive glands, or any system of the body, longevity nutrients are ready, willing, and able to prevent aging.

Nutrition is essential to help us grow and develop, and there is every reason to believe that nutrition also holds the key to aging.

Modern Culture and Nutrition

As societies have become busier and more complex, we have tended to turn away from the natural to the artificial, from "slow" foods to fast foods. Food additives and other chemicals allow the opportunity for us to eat a lot of convenient and spoil-free foods. In one respect, we are fortunate to have this alternative to fit our modern lifestyles. On the other hand, this means many of the foods we ingest are not natural.

Our bodies do not know how to deal with foods that developed after we did—what I like to call "high-tech" foods. Our physiology—as far as we can tell—is the same as that of our ancestors 40 or 60,000 years ago. The ways we tamper with our diet—either by taking in large amounts of these high-tech foods, or eating foods containing manufactured substances—is a ticking time bomb. Not only does diet tampering provide a welcome mat for negative health consequences, but it also denies you the chance to maximize your life span.

Nutritionists are trained to tell you how much vitamin C, zinc, and protein you should eat—these calculations are reliable and scientifically based. However, you can turn to the back of any food or candy package and see the recommended dietary allowance (RDA) to find out the same information. But what of all the other substances in food, including the longevity nutrients? Unfortunately, there is no information. Package labels don't list them and nutritionists don't know about them. One of the main purposes of the *New Longevity Diet* described in this book and my research is to fill in that gap and provide such information—*wholly* lacking in books on nutrition and all modern diet plans. In fact, the chart on p. 120 that lists the longevity nutrient content of many common foods and the recommended longevity allowance chart on p. 138 are not available anywhere else.

Incorporating longevity nutrients into your daily eating plan is a way of making science—in its tried and most natural and basic ways—work for you!

A Brief Introduction to Longevity Nutrients and Weight Loss

When obesity is mentioned, one gets the image of someone who ingests far too many fatty foods and does not burn off the extra calories with exercise. Simply put, obesity is a condition that develops when we take in more calories than our body needs to accomplish what it gets done every day. While this is the general and most commonly known definition, obesity is also due to malnutrition. This may be hard to believe, but think of it in this way: a car needs gas, oil, transmission and brake fluid, antifreeze, and other "nutrients" to accomplish its job of getting you from place to place. Your body functions in much the same way. It cannot accomplish its daily tasks without the proper fuel, and it cannot burn calories without help. Obesity, therefore, is not only due to high caloric consumption, but also to low intake of the proper nutrients—longevity nutrients such as lignans, found in grains like whole wheat, and carnosine, found in proteins.

You might be inclined to say our culture makes it easy for obesity to develop. As you will read about in depth in chapter 9, obesity impairs us. It results in too much fat on our body frames and it affects many of our systems, imitating the effects of aging. No doubt, excess weight should be lost. And because longevity nutrients—such as conjugated linoleic acid—work directly and indirectly to prod and move forward the weight loss process in our body, it is relatively easy for anyone to use this program to achieve weight loss and prevent weight gain—*without counting calories and grams of fat or keeping track of all your ins and outs on a spreadsheet.*

This book not only provides you with the list of nutrients, a diet plan, and sample recipes, but it also combines this information with a viable, practical exercise program (Chapter 10).

Disease and Aging Are Not the Same

Until just a few years ago, disease was often confused with aging. Today, we know the two are separate. So much of what we know about aging and disease comes from the Baltimore Longitudinal Study of Aging (BLSA), which recently reached its "middle age" of forty years. This study—taking place in Baltimore in conjunction with Johns Hopkins University and the National Institutes of Health (NIH)—relies on about 2,470 volunteers who come twice yearly to be studied. More than 800 publications of the study prove a critical point: many so-called "age-related" declines in function are attributable to illnesses and *not* to the process of aging. The longevity nutrients are doubly powerful weapons because they provide important help to ward off chronic diseases and, at the same time, discourage the aging process.

Various diseases commonly associated with aging now appear to be due to lifestyle factors or the environment. While it is true that certain ailments such as heart disease and cancer are more common with age, aging is not the *cause.* What it does mean—based on the latest research—is that conditions such as cardiovascular disease or cerebrovascular brain disease can be reduced or reversed if proper measures are taken. True, genes are a powerful regulator of the way our bodies function, but age research is helping to develop an understanding that genetic factors have much less to do with this than we previously thought.

People are living longer, but many myths about aging still persist. Among them are that old age means frailty, decrepitude, and senility. It is true that the likelihood of developing some disorders such as osteoporosis and cataracts increases with age, but the longevity nutrients seek to prevent unsuccessful aging and strive to prevent age-related diseases. With proper nutrition, these conditions can be prevented from occurring at anytime in life (see the next section, The Longevity Nutrients and Disease Prevention).

Diseases differ from person to person. We may avoid certain diseases, but as everyone knows, we are all susceptible to aging. There isn't a species on the planet that will not age. Aging is the *only* condition that affects everyone after the stage of reproduction is over. However, age changes do not compromise self or increase the likelihood of death. No one has ever died of crow's feet, gray hair, or menopause, yet we continue to wonder: "Why are old cells more vulnerable to the pathology of disease while young cells are not?"

The Longevity Nutrients and Disease Prevention

Nutrition is the factor most accountable and critical to helping people live longer. Contrary to popular belief, nutrition is far more important than drugs, supplements, or anything else in determining how successfully you age. Although medications—whether over-the-counter or prescription—may be prescribed for older folks with the best intentions, many drugs contribute to frailty. Certain drugs have to be taken to prevent disease but this has nothing to do with preventing aging. Aging is *not* a disease but a continuum of normal—or at least predictable—functional alterations that occur with time.

Aging is a complex subject with many different components—a striking distinction from some attractive possibility or notion that one drug or supplement will, by itself, prevent aging. In fact, by taking many drugs, you are not only not helping your body but are hurting it by giving it age advancers.

An example of a health-related disease is osteoporosis. In the 1950s, osteoporosis was a minor problem, but over the last few years it has become a severe health issue. It is a disease resulting from bone loss and can be prevented with proper nutrition and exercise. Hormonal deficiencies lead to bone loss, so by ingesting genistein—a longevity nutrient that acts in the same way as estrogen but without the harmful side effects—you can become an active participant in your aging and combat age-related disease. Just think what could happen if we could return the incidence rate of osteoporosis to what it was in the 1950s!

While maximum life expectancy—120 years—has not changed much, our average life expectancy has increased profoundly in the past century. Rising numbers and proportions of older people have also introduced higher numbers of diseases and disabilities. For example, in a study sample of people 59 years of age, one percent has a severe disease or disabling condition, but in the same study of those 88 years of age, this figure rises to thirteen percent.

It becomes obvious that one objective of living longer is to avoid disease, or as has been suggested, to "compress morbidity" into a shorter time span during the later stages of life. Compression of morbidity has been deeply debated ever since Dr. James Fries challenged the assumption that the aging of a population has to be accompanied by an increasing amount of disability and functional impairment. Fries hypothesized that if average age at the onset of disability and chronic disease could be delayed, then the total amount of disability would decrease—rather than increase—in a mature population. His assumed changes in lifestyle and medical care could prevent or postpone age-related morbidity. So ideally, healthy people would survive to an advanced age, with their vigor and functional independence intact, and in effect, disease would be postponed until the last years of life.

Fries's hypothesis has been confirmed over the last 15 to 20 years: people are living longer and are warding off chronic diseases until much later in their lives. As new knowledge of diet and nutrition becomes available, we come closer to transforming Fries's hypothesis into reality. The *New Longevity Diet* is your first step in making Fries's hypothesis *your* reality.

Preventive Gerontology

We must appreciate that more people are living to 100 today than ever before—a number that has increased remarkably even in the last ten years. For the future, this means the number of centenarians will continue to increase—possibly because of all the new developments in disease prevention. This concept of preventive gerontology simply means we can prevent certain diseases and make it possible for anyone to attain maximum life span—a record set by a French woman named Jean Calmonde who died at the age of 122 on August 4, 1997.

In the past, many diseases or conditions associated with aging or thought to be aging in and of itself included hardening of the arteries, cataract formation, arthritis, decreased kidney function, and graying hair. Several other markers of aging included decreased cardiac reserve, dental decay, increased blood pressure, decreased lung function, increased cholesterol, decreased glucose tolerance, and decreased mental acuity. The discovery that these conditions can be prevented by different measures—such as limiting exposure to toxic chemicals and smoking, stopping illicit drug use, increasing exercise, and making dietary changes—is key.

Aging is inescapable, but how you do it is no longer set in stone. Take control of your life cycle. What *The New Longevity Diet* will afford you is the opportunity to be an active participant in your own life.

How to Use the Longevity Nutrient Program

First, the designer style eating plan: design your own eating plan based on all the longevity nutrients or just the ones you need the most. (The questionnaire will tell you where you need the most help.)

In order to make this process easier for you, I've included two unique features:

- A Recommended Longevity Allowances Chart (p. 138) that will tell you how much of each longevity nutrient you should have in your diet per day.
- A comprehensive table containing the *longevity nutrient* content of the most common foods in the U.S. diet.

This plan introduces one nutrient per day into your diet as a way to familiarize yourself with these foods. Once you've gone through all 21 days, you will be able to pick and choose as you see fit, trying to get your recommended allowances per day. See Chapter 7.

The second plan is the menu-style plan. This is the eating system for those of us who like everything to be simple and easy. Also a 21-day program, this plan introduces you to longevity nutrient eating through already designed menus. Just follow the menu and the accompanying recipes to integrate all these foods into your life. After the 21 days are over, you can begin again (the recipes are delicious!) or you can use the base of knowledge you've gained to start going off on your own. See Chapter 8.

Keep in mind that both of these plans are ambitious. I don't expect you to follow every recommendation or make every recipe. Just by doing what's practical for you, you will improve your body's health immensely.

Lastly, there's the 14-Day *Longevity Nutrient* Weight Reduction Program. This program is designed to slowly and safely reduce weight using the unique proportion of certain longevity nutrients. If you are overweight, this is a great plan to start! See Chapter 9.

Exercise has untold benefits for the body and your metabolism. I've designed an exercise program to work with *The New Longevity Diet*. It's easy and absolutely essential to good lifelong health. See Chapter 10.

2

THE SIX LESSONS: HOW AND WHY WE AGE

Knowing something about how cells function is also basic to understanding aging, but that doesn't mean you have to run to the library to read the latest cell physiology journal. In the six "lessons" that follow, you will get a crash course in basic cell physiology. My intent here is to give you some fundamentally necessary background information to better understand aging and convince you—to convince yourself—how using this program fills a currently unmet need.

While I've borrowed extensively from my nutritional biochemistry courses at Georgetown Medical Center, I have planned these lessons to be a piece of cake. In fact, don't be surprised how much of it may already makes sense to you. In the six lessons that follow—Cell Systems, Cell Division, The Cell Wall, DNA, Cellular Aging, and the effects of ROS on all of these, you'll learn all you need to know about cell function, biochemistry, and aging.

Lesson One: Cell Systems

The body is organized into several different systems. The circulatory, nervous, and renal systems are just three of them. These systems are composed of tissues. Tissues in turn, are made up of cells, all similar in structure and function. All cells—no matter what part of the body they come from—have the same basic structure, energy metabolism, and reproductive system.

A typical cell is divided into compartments called organelles. Organelles are walled off from each other by membranes that control what gets in and what goes out of the cell. Just as all cells have the same basic structure, all cells contain the same basic types of organelles, but they differ in how many they have of each type. The number of organelle or compartment types each cell has depends on its purpose and location in our body.

Mitochondria are organelles that burn fuel—fats included—in our cells for energy and are the only organelles, aside from the nucleus, that contain DNA. As many as 1,000 or more mitochondria burn fuel in any of our cells, producing energy the cell needs to run. It should be pointed out here that all of our body's cells—whether in the muscles, brain, or elsewhere—use the same kind of fuels, *all* derived directly from what we eat.

Think for a minute about what you need to navigate your way through the world each day—two cups of coffee in the morning, a muffin, maybe a treat midday, not to mention all of the mechanical and electronic items that clutter your bag or briefcase but "organize" your life. Regardless of whether it's time or simply peace and quiet, how much of it you need depends on what you need and where you are. Different people have different needs.

Cells, too, need special things to function, and different types of cells need different things in varying amounts, including the longevity nutrients: muscle cells require different longevity nutrients—carnitine—than the skin does—isothiocyanates. The longevity nutrients offer to all body tissues and cells antiaging and disease-preventing advantages.

As stated earlier, the different organelles have particular and distinct requirements. The nucleus needs nucleic acids to make DNA. Other compartments—like parts of the cell that get rid of toxins—need antioxidants. Since the mitochondria's job is to make fuel, they need nutrients that help them do this. Specifically, mitochondria need nutrients that help them produce energy and also protect them from toxic ROS that we know are generated in these compartments.

Lesson Two: Cell Division—The Need for Stimulating Company!

Every cell exists as the result of a process called cell division, which ensures a continuous supply of new cells as older ones are lost. In order for tissues to be healthy, healthy cells must continue to produce others. When too few new cells are produced, the consequence, inevitably, is aging and disease.

When it is time for a cell to divide, it goes through a growth phase and makes DNA before it passes through a second phase. This is followed by cell division in a process called mitosis. The result of mitosis is the production of new cells—daughter cells.

Eventually cells stop dividing and become senescent. This means the cells show signs of growing old: the cells lose their ability to proliferate and their ability to make DNA. At this point, the cells have taken on characteristics of old cells.

Aged cells don't respond the same way to stimulation as younger cells do, but recent research reveals that nucleotides, saponins, inulin, and oligofructose are some of the longevity nutrients that can stimulate certain systems of cells in our bodies that decline with age.

THE CELL CYCLE CONTROL SYSTEM

This whole cyclical process—cells dividing to produce new ones and, in turn, dividing again so that more new ones are made—may hold the key to aging. This cyclical process may even hold the key to antiaging. So, it makes sense that the possibility of controlling cell division has fascinated cell physiologists for years. To this end, gerontologists have discovered two universal events about aging: the failure to produce new cells regularly

continued on next page

and replace old ones, and the failure to produce new cells during times of stress.

At once, these two realities become research questions: how do we prevent these failures? If cell division is the answer, then we must ask another question: what regulates cell division? A set of proteins called the *cell cycle control system* regulates cell division and signals the cell when it is time to divide. In order for the cell cycle control system to work, a number of conditions must be met, including the precise copying of DNA in mitosis. Certain enzymes must be present to make sure DNA is copied precisely.

One body function depends on another, which in turn depends upon another. Scientists' search backward through these functions brings us to this point: the cell cycle control system could be at the heart of the aging problem. If its parts aren't synthesized—or made to work together and thrive off of each other's strengths and weaknesses—then the cell's ability to divide is drastically compromised, and aging takes the place of potential growing.

Though precise factors regulating the cell cycle control system continue to be researched, we already know that nutrient intake stimulates this system. And the nutrients they need? The longevity nutrients! Cells in some organs—such as those in the digestive system—divide more quickly than others. This means these cells need more of certain kinds of nutrients than other kinds. Some systems, such as the immune system, need constant stimulation to form new cells. Longevity nutrients are a major source of the stimulation that keeps the cell cycle control system operating. Without them, cells would not be able to regularly replace other cells lost to age nor those lost during times of stress.

Lesson Three: The Cell Wall—The Gatekeeper

Every cell is surrounded by a wall, or membrane, which acts like a gatekeeper, selectively controlling what enters and exits the cell, allowing nutrients to enter only when they are needed, getting rid of waste products when they're not.

Cell membranes are everywhere: the nucleus is enclosed by a cell membrane, and mitochondria are surrounded by cell membranes, as are all the organelles.

Like other parts of the cell, cell membranes show changes with aging. Growth factors that stimulate a young cell may not stimulate an old or senescent cell. When a cell shows no ability to respond properly to a chemical, a signal is sent indicating that the cell has changed in some way, which—taking us full circle now—means that the cell may cease to divide or lose its attachment to other cells in tissue, seriously compromising the ability of the tissue to function.

How can we get growth factors to work in older cells just like they do in younger cells? Many factors—some we know much more about than others—answer the question, but the longevity nutrients could unlock the secret to making old cells act young.

Lesson Four: DNA

The centerpiece of the cell is a round enclosed area called the nucleus. The nucleus contains the chromosomes—threadlike substances made up of DNA—that determine our unique genetic traits. The DNA found in our cells' chromosomes contain a code with all the genetic information needed to run the cells in our body. When cells divide—go through mitosis—they copy the DNA code in the nucleus and pass it on to the new cells. This occurs every time the cells divide. DNA truly controls every single function in our cells.

We all have traits. For instance, while you may have brown eyes, your siblings may have green or hazel eyes. From the color of our eyes and hair to whether or not we can digest milk, traits are different for everyone. Genes are the part of the DNA molecule that control how the specific protein is made. Since every cell in our body makes proteins and requires DNA, without proteins we would not exist. There is not one function inside our entire body that does not involve proteins.

DNA VITALITY AND PROTECTION

DNA, when it is damaged, impacts a cell's genetic fidelity. DNA replication cannot be accomplished, and as a result, normal cell growth is no longer normal. Since damaged DNA shows up as the serious destruction of our

continued on next page

tissues or even in the death of our cells, damaged DNA *must* be fixed. Many scientists think failure to repair DNA is one of the main causes of our deterioration and aging.

One of the many different tools our body has to repair damaged DNA and RNA is called *excision repair.* Excision repair removes damaged parts of the DNA molecule and replaces them with new parts. Excision repair, like other DNA repair systems, needs the longevity nutrients to function adequately.

Any change in proteins may get in the way of the DNA doing its job—to make other proteins for the cells. Some enzymes involved in making proteins also decline with age. Since new longevity nutrients protect the ROS attack on proteins to make sure our cells' DNA can continue its work to make proteins, using the new longevity nutrients is essential.

The subject of proteins takes on even greater significance by introducing the protein found universally in all animal species and attributed a front seat role in the effects of aging—*collagen.* Collagen is the major structural molecule in our skin. Without collagen, our skin would lose its tone. Collagen is found in the walls of blood vessels, where it prevents them from becoming too rigid, and among many other places, collagen is also found in hair. Change in collagen is a very serious problem in aging. In practically all groups of animals—including humans—changes in collagen are shown to occur with age.

One of the processes responsible for collagen changes is called *glycation.* Glycation means that sugar molecules attach to collagen and produce dramatic changes in its structure and function. When this occurs, advanced glycation endproducts (AGEs) form. Then collagen molecules become cross-linked, resulting in rigidity and dysfunction of tissues.

Diabetics usually have a problem with glycation of collagen, since higher sugar levels can be found in the blood of diabetics. As such, the context for the recommendation that people with diabetes strictly control their blood glucose levels is relevant.

Several of the new longevity nutrients help our bodies modulate blood sugar levels and prevent not only hyperglycemia but also hypoglycemia. No one knows why this structural chemical—collagen—changes. But, the best way to prevent collagen from changing—to keep your blood sugar under control to prevent age changes in your body's collagen—is through your diet and using the new longevity nutrients *in* your diet.

DNA makes proteins through another molecule called RNA, which is a large molecule similar to our DNA. RNA makes proteins by copying—a process called transcription—the DNA's blueprint or instructions. This means the RNA transcribes information relevant to how to make protein molecules from the DNA.

Lesson Five: Cellular Aging

Over the last 30 years, scientists have learned a lot about the life span of our cells by studying them in tissue cultures. Studying cells in a laboratory lets scientists get a bird's-eye view of what happens in our body as it progresses through different parts of our life span. Cell culture allows us to learn about *apoptosis*: the death of our cells. Cell death may seem like a harmful thing, but it is simply nature's way of getting rid of old cells.

If our old cells had no way to dispose of themselves, the result would be comparable to never taking the garbage out. The waste would build up, cluttering up your kitchen and, eventually, taking over your entire house.

If your whole house would look like a garbage can, think about what your body would look like—inside and out—if it did not shed itself of old, useless cells! When balanced with mitosis, apoptosis is naturally a part of the life cycle.

WHAT IS CELL AGING?

Whenever gerontologists talk about the subject of aging, they make a distinction between *aging* and *senescence*. Aging is the process in which an organism becomes vulnerable to environmental obstacles, whereas senescence refers to the progressively slow deterioration or changes that start when an organism matures—or grows up—and goes on through its life.

Cellular aging is not measured by calendar time but instead by the number of times a particular type of cell naturally divides. Senescent cells, therefore, continue to live on for a certain amount of time after they have stopped multiplying and dividing. Eventually, they die, and eventually, all the cells in a culture become senescent.

continued on next page

Although senescent cells accumulate in our body as it ages, their role in aging is still mostly unknown. What we *do* know is that senescent cells are not dormant. They affect their tissue's environment in many ways. For example, senescent cells secrete inflammatory substances, degrading the matrix proteins around them. The possibility for even a relatively small number of senescent cells to destroy tissue integrity and function is real.

Lesson Six: Reactive Oxygen Species (ROS)

Free radicals are another term for reactive oxygen species (ROS). Mainstream media tend to give the term "free radical" a lot of wear and tear. ROS is the scientific term, and it's the one I prefer.

ROS are produced by a series of reactions that combine oxygen with a molecule in the cell. The resulting ROS attack other molecules in the cell in a series of reactions called propagation reactions. Propagation reactions that produce ROS can be stopped by neutralizing chemicals. Again, ROS reactions are involved in aging, because with age, unneeded chemicals accumulate in the body's cells. In other words, in ROS reactions, normal molecules are replaced by abnormal molecules.

ROS can be combated with antioxidants. Antioxidants are chemical agents that break the chain reactions that occur in the cells of the body. Common antioxidants include vitamins C and E. What you'll discover with *The New Longevity Diet* is that these two are only the tip of the iceberg—that there are almost infinite other beneficial substances in foods. The longevity nutrients—antioxidants as well, but functioning in much different ways than the usual vitamin antioxidants—offer unique protective effects in *every* tissue of the body whether it be muscles, the kidney, or the brain.

What distinguishes the longevity nutrients' antioxidant functions even further is the responsibility they take for acting in ways besides just "knocking out" ROS or blocking their production in the body's cells. For example, certain minerals increase the production of ROS. The longevity nutrients modulate—or keep in line—the levels of these minerals in our body systems. They also collaborate with various detoxification systems in the cells to limit the production of chemicals that lead to ROS. *The New Longevity Diet* specifically limits your cells' exposure to chemicals that cause ROS, while, at the same time, blocking the production of these toxic substances.

Ingesting more calories than our body needs to accomplish what it gets done every day is another factor that produces ROS. The leaner you are, the lower the levels of ROS are in your body's organs. *The New Longevity Diet* is a 21-day program carefully designed not only to provide you with adequate intakes of the longevity nutrients to prevent aging, but also, for those people who want to, to simultaneously help you achieve weight loss and maximize ideal body composition. For those who are overweight, use of the 14-day longevity nutrient weight-loss program will affect weight loss while at the same time producing the antiaging effects of the longevity nutrients.

At this point, congratulations are in order. You have finished the six lessons of our course in cellular biochemistry and ROS, and the most important lesson to take from this is that the longevity nutrients can help every kind of cell in the body. The longevity nutrients help our bodies' cells by satisfying their individual needs—stimulating growth and division, repairing DNA damage, and attacking ROS—to become our best allies in making sure cells run their business the right way.

By now you should have an appreciation of some facets of aging at the cellular level. It's important to start here because cells are the basic unit of function of every organ in the body. What happens in our cells is key to understanding the aging of our body's organs.

The Longevity Nutrients and Organs: A System That Works Well Together

All the cells in the body are organized in systems, or organs such as the liver, kidneys, and brain. These in turn, are susceptible to whatever changes that aging causes in those cells. So let us pause a moment, before we look at those organs and systems in more depth, to revisit the point of this book: understanding aging, so that we may prevent it. Aging happens for all animal life forms—for all, that is, except the sea anemone, which continually replaces its cells.

Many lower life forms enter a period of *rapid* aging following maturation, or adulthood, after which they enter a period of senescence and die. A mouse has the potential to live for about 2 years, the average horse for about 46 years, your pet dog for about 20 years, and the common housefly for a few weeks. (These maximum life spans were determined by the age of the oldest known survivor from a large population of these animals.) Humans differ from other animal species in that they age *gradually* after reaching adulthood, thus we have the longest potential life span, about 120 years. Such differences in life span have fascinated biochemists to hypothesize why there is so much variation in longevity for different species. What is more, they have sought to explain why we age in the first place.

The current thinking among gerontologists is that "homeostasis failure" best explains aging. Homeostasis failure is an inability of body functions to maintain a healthy "balance." The following sections show how aging affects specific organs and body systems and how the longevity nutrients can help. As you read, remember the concept of homeostasis failure, because it points the way toward achieving maximum life span. The key is to give your body everything it needs to continue maintaining and repairing its cells. By eating foods containing the longevity nutrients, you can help every part of your body adapt to the demands placed on it by time, urging it to repair damaged DNA, replace and discard old proteins, fight toxins, counteract ROS, and reach its full potential life span.

The Brain: The Body's Most Complex Organ

The brain is so complex that even the words we associate with it such as mind, consciousness, and memory are very difficult to define. Such things as passions, desires, and urges emanate from the brain. The very idea of encountering something in our environment and storing it for later recall is an amazing feat that is shared only with certain primates. The brain uses 20 percent of the oxygen we consume every day and, as a result, is prone to the harmful effects of ROS. Nutrients enter the brain through a specialized gate called the blood brain barrier (BBB), which selectively controls what enters and exits the brain. Several age-related diseases of the brain such as Alzheimer's and Parkinson's are due to destruction of various parts of the brain.

ROS attack brain proteins resulting in their damage. There are no molecules that are immune from ROS damage including those containing DNA. DNA damage has great ramifications for all brain cell functions. Although progress is being made, what is most important is that right now we have at our disposal the longevity nutrients that can interact with the brain in many ways to prevent aging and aid in its many essential functions.

Some longevity nutrients for the brain include:

- Protease inhibitors
- Glutathione
- Glutamine
- Phytates

The Cardiovascular System: The Body's Amazing Pump

This system is composed of the heart and blood vessels (arteries, veins, and capillaries). In addition to disease, our hearts and blood vessels manifest distinct aging changes. One of these has to do with aging changes in the collagen and elastin of the arteries resulting in increased stiffness of the arteries: changes which affect the function of the heart. The cause here may be due to the production of ROS and the accumulation of Advanced Glycation Endproducts (AGEs). High blood sugar (hyperglycemia) has been implicated in the developments of AGEs. ROS are also one of the causes of atherosclerosis (hardening of the arteries).

Subtle differences in cardiovascular function between young and old individuals only shows up during times of stress or physical activity. The longevity nutrients can close the gap in heart function during activity. Hypertension, or high blood pressure, is a disease: the same vascular changes that occur in very old people with age occur in younger people with hypertension. These changes are so similar that hypertension has been referred to as "accelerated aging." They include high blood pressure, thickened walls of the aorta, enlargement of the left ventricle, and prolonged heart contraction. Those with hypertension can take a very important antiaging step by having their hypertension diagnosed and treated by their physician.

Some longevity nutrients for the heart and blood vessels include:

- Carnitine
- Taurine
- Tannins

The Immune System: Our Body's Umbrella

Our bodies are bombarded by any number of bacteria, viruses, pollutants, and other toxins. No matter what part of us is threatened, the skin, lungs or kidneys, for example, only one system can protect us—the immune system. The immune system plays a critical role in aging but in order to carry out this function it requires the longevity nutrients. The successful initiation of an immune response to antigens depends on several cell types, such as lymphocytes, macrophages, and natural killer (NK) cells. Aging affects the immune system as shown by a decrease in the ability to form antibodies and a delay in reactions to antigens encountered earlier in life. Although the total number of immune cells may not fall with age, there is failure to regulate cell production in the face of infection as one gets older.

Diet and nutrition affect the immune system; those lacking certain nutrients have more problems with infection than those with an adequate diet. On the other hand, obesity decreases antibody production and the number of immune cells. Immunosenescence can be significantly curtailed by ingesting the longevity nutrients. The immune system is like a citadel astride key trade routes; it is the most important defense organ of our body and one which must work properly all the time to ensure our survival.

Some longevity nutrients involved in the immune system include:

- Nucleotides
- Saponins
- Glutamine

The Skin: The Body's Cover

The part of ourselves that most readily shows our age is the skin. The skin ages in two ways: intrinsically (by itself) and by photoaging, which is caused by continued exposure to the sun. Photoaged skin has irregular pigmentations with deep lines and a leathery consistency. Intrinsically aged skin is usually smooth and unblemished, but has a loss of elasticity. The skin is divided into an epidermis or upper layer, and under it the dermis. Collagen and elastin are the main structural proteins of the dermis. Collagen provides strength to the skin and with loss, skin loses it resilience. Elastin gives skin its pliability. Excessive sun exposure causes changes in elastin resulting in "crows' feet" around the eyes.

As we grow older the blood vessels of the dermis decrease, which affects the delivery of nutrients to the skin and its ability to halt aging. The skin is a formidable barrier to toxic substances. It has a very competent immune system, which is affected by aging. There is progressive loss of DNA cells in skin with age. The cells from a young person's skin divide for a longer time than the cells taken from an older person. On a sunny day light is absorbed by the skin, which activates certain molecules such as ROS, which can cause damage to skin cells and is a factor in aging.

Some longevity nutrients for skin aging:

- Carnosine
- Phytates

Muscle: I Want to Go There

Muscle and its cells are different from others in the body. Muscles have fibers and the cells inside these fibers are specialized because of two proteins, actin and myosin, which affect muscle contraction. Loss of muscle mass with age causes sarcopenia resulting in reduced activity, increased vulnerability to injury, and metabolic effects involving other body systems. Protein, the most important structural chemical in muscle, decreases with age probably as a result of ROSs. Several hormones such as estrogen, testosterone, growth hormone (GH), and insulinlike growth factor (IGF-1) maintain muscle mass. Age-related decreases in these hormones result in loss of muscle.

No matter where a muscle is located, whether in the limbs, the heart, or the digestive system, age-related declines can occur. The functional integrity of muscles is linked to maintenance of adequate repair processes. The older one gets, the slower the rate of muscle synthesis. The longevity nutrient program provides nutrients that help to reverse muscle aging and is well-balanced in amino acids for muscle protein synthesis. In addition, losing weight as directed by the program increases GH and IGF-1 levels.

Some longevity nutrients involved in muscle:

- PQQ
- Glutamine
- CLA

Kidneys: The Body's Purifiers

Most people are familiar with the function of the kidneys: ridding the body of waste that comes from the metabolism of foods and also from harmful chemicals that enter the body. The job of balancing fluid intake and excretion is also delegated to the kidneys. In this way the kidneys provide the proper environment for every cell in the body to function normally. The kidneys purify the total blood volume of an individual 60 times a day! These functions of the kidney are carried out by specialized filtering devices called glomeruli. Each kidney has about a million glomeruli, but they decrease as we age. The kidneys are susceptible to the development of AGEs in the walls of the glomeruli. This affects the ability of the glomeruli to filter blood and remove toxic substances. When AGEs form in the walls of blood vessels, they may interfere with the effects of nitric oxide (NO) in changing blood flow through the arteries of the kidneys. This also may affect the ability of the kidneys to filter blood.

Not unexpectedly, the kidneys are an important site for ROS attack. In the kidney, the glomeruli can come under ROS attack interfering with blood filtration. The result is an accumulation of toxic substances. Thankfully the kidney is endowed with a number of antioxidant systems that can counteract the effect of these ROSs. Many of these include the longevity nutrients. Diet plays a role in kidney function; a very high-protein diet stresses the filtering units resulting in their deterioration. Because of the constant filtering of the blood every day, the kidneys are in constant contact with nutrients. These include the longevity nutrients, which are always available to prevent aging and disease.

Some important longevity nutrients for the kidney:

- Arginine
- Taurine
- Tannins

Bone: Framework for the Body

If you look at the small handful of articles published on bone and osteoporosis before 1980 you will see only a scattering of research reports. However, over the last two decades an explosion of osteoporosis studies have been published. This condition has gone from neglected disease to journalistic stardom with hundreds of articles published every year. This research has taught us a lot about nutrition and the requirements of bone-building nutrients, such as calcium, vitamin D, and the longevity nutrients. Osteoporosis is not a manifestation of aging. It is a disease and can be treated.

Osteoporosis is a decrease in bone mass, which usually has its inception at age 50. Starting then, we lose approximately .5 percent to 1.0 percent bone per year! Several different hormones and growth factors play a role in bone physiology. These include vitamin D, GH, estrogen, and the longevity nutrients. One new development is that men are also affected by osteoporosis. In fact, men have more problems with bone fractures than women! Unlike women, reduced levels of the male hormone, testosterone, are involved here. For both men and women, exercise plays an important role in bone structure and density.

Some important longevity nutrients for bone include:

- Genistein
- Daidzein
- Arginine
- Taurine

The Liver: Nutrient Guardian for the Body

If ever there was an organ that played a central role in the body's metabolism, the liver would be a unanimous choice. A typical normal meal contains carbohydrates, fats, proteins, minerals, vitamins, and the longevity nutrients. In addition, thousands of toxic substances and bacteria are part of a meal. If you ever wondered where these substances ended up, the liver is where. The liver is also a reservoir for glucose, where it is stored as a substance called glycogen. The uptake and release of glucose from glycogen is under the control of insulin and another hormone called glucagon. Adequate function of these hormones depends on antioxidants such as the longevity nutrients.

The liver makes proteins for export to other organs, a process dependent on DNA and RNA. One of the most important functions of the liver is to detoxify and neutralize harmful chemicals that enter the body every day, such as pesticides, carcinogens, and drugs that we have taken. This system of enzymes rids the body of thousands of toxic chemicals, which enter it every day through the digestive system, lungs, and skin. Some of the aging problems of the liver include inability to detoxify large amounts of toxic substances and the accumulation of old proteins and other aged molecules.

Longevity nutrients involved in liver function include:

- Carnosine
- Isothiocyanates
- Nucleotides
- Saponins
- Glutathione

Lungs: The Breath of Life

The lungs, part of the respiratory system, play a major role in our body's nutrition. How can this be, since no foods or beverages are assimilated here? If you thought about oxygen, you have found another puzzle piece for your body's wizardry. We often think of essential nutrients as vitamins and minerals. But not only is oxygen the most important of these, it is more essential. Oxygen is a "nutrient gas." The respiratory system includes the lungs and the passageways of air from the mouth and nose to the lungs. All these passages not only permit the entry of oxygen and exit of carbon dioxide, but they also intercept and eliminate unwanted substances inhaled with oxygen. Important here is the immune system with such cells as phagocytes and lymphocytes ridding the lungs of offending agents, clearing cellular debris, and repairing injury. Important in this defense is a chemical lining the lungs called surfactant, which contains longevity nutrients that act as antioxidants blocking the formation of ROS.

The exchanges of gases in the lungs occur in cells called the alveoli, which enlarge with age. Elastin and collagen are the main structural lung proteins. Changes in elastin that occur with age affect the ability of the lungs to contract. As a result of aging, elastin breaks down, releasing particles that cause the production of ROSs. The structures that make it possible for the lungs to inhale and exhale are the chest and its respiratory muscles. Aging of these muscles is similar to what happens to muscles in other areas of the body.

Some longevity nutrients important in lung function include:

- Glutathione
- Protease inhibitors
- Monoterpenes

Hormones in Aging

Life would be impossible without hormones. A hormone is a substance synthesized in one organ and transferred to another organ to effect a change in some metabolic process. With this in mind, some hormones, because of their wide-reaching effects, have been implicated in the aging process.

Several different groups of organs synthesize and produce hormones. These groups of hormones show definite changes with aging. Probably the most commonly known are the hormonal changes that occur in women at the time of menopause. We now know there are similar changes that occur with aging in men, called andropause. The third type of change involves a certain gland—the adrenal gland. Aging changes in this gland occur during adrenopause. Finally there is somatopause, which involves age changes in growth hormone (GH).

Somatopause

This story starts with a hormone, growth hormone (GH), made in a gland next to the brain called the anterior pituitary gland. Its importance in childhood growth has long been established but its role in adult life has not been explored until recently. It is now clear that this hormone has significant effects on many aspects of an adult's carbohydrate, fat, and protein metabolism. GH secretion peaks in most people around age 20 and then declines until it reaches a plateau in the sixth decade of life. GH is responsible for many changes that occur with age. For example, GH metabolism is why muscle mass falls progressively after age 40 while total body fat does just the opposite. These unhealthy changes in body composition are accompanied by increased insulin levels, which lead to insulin resistance.

Doctors have tried various ways to stimulate secretion of this hormone. One method involved giving GH to elderly people, which resulted in increased bone density and beneficial effects on muscle mass and strength. However, GH supplements cause certain problems and when people stop taking them the positive effects of the hormones stop immediately. A more natural way to achieve optimum GH levels is by using the longevity nutrient program, which uses nutrition, exercise, and diet to improve hormone secretion.

Some longevity nutrients important for the somatopause:

- Arginine
- Taurine

The Andropause

Women have their menopause and men have their andropause. Although these terms have the same suffix they are different, not only because of the hormones involved, but also the way these hormones change with age. The main hormone implicated in the andropause is testosterone, which belongs to a group of hormones called androgens. Testosterone is made in the testes and is produced under the direction of signals that come from the anterior pituitary part of the brain, which, as you remember, also controls the secretion of GH. As a man ages, he can expect declines in the amount of testosterone secreted. This may result in loss of bone and muscle mass along with increased fat deposition. This hormone may also be involved in brain function; some deterioration in memory and cognitive functions has been correlated to low levels of this hormone.

Ever since a French physiologist in 1889 announced he had devised a rejuvenating therapy for the mind and body by injecting himself with testosterone extracts, a fascination with the use of testosterone took hold and has endured. Since this discovery numerous studies have been conducted regarding testosterone's effects on muscle and other functions in elderly men. Although such studies revealed increased muscle strength, certain problems such as retention of fluids and cardiovascular disease were observed. As a result, additional studies are needed to confirm long-term safe uses of testosterone. Faced with the current lack of data concerning the safety and health benefits of testosterone therapy, the best choice for men who are experiencing andropause is to use the longevity nutrient program to lose abdominal fat and prevent the effects of testosterone decline on the body.

Some longevity nutrients important for the andropause:

- Taurine
- Phytosterols
- Saponins

The Adrenopause

Like the andropause the adrenopause involves glands whose actions are controlled by the pituitary gland. In this case it is instead the adrenal glands that are involved in an axis—the hypothalamic-pituitary-adrenal axis (HPA). Two adrenal glands are found one on top of each kidney. They secrete several hormones including the glucocorticoids and the adrenal androgens, which include dehydroepiandrosterone (DHEA). The glucocorticoids—which include cortisol and corticosterone—have far-reaching effects on metabolism. They are extraordinarily responsive to stress, at which time they cause the breakdown and release of amino acids, fats, and glucose.

We survive as humans by maintaining a complex and harmonious equilibrium with our environment, a process called homeostasis. Stress threatens homeostasis. The ability to adapt to stressful situations is regulated by the HPA axis. Stress has a direct effect on the HPA axis, resulting in the outpouring of cortisol from the adrenal glands, helping the body to adapt to the stress. Although this response is required to combat stress, problems arise when the HPA axis continues to function after the stress. Such long-term activation of the HPA axis has been implicated in aging and certain diseases. Use of the longevity nutrients along with weight reduction and exercise help this problem during the adrenopause.

Longevity nutrients involved in the adrenopause include:

- Genistein
- Phytosterols
- Carnitines

The Menopause

Probably more people are aware of the hormone changes during the menopause than any other endocrine condition. Of all the hormone changes during aging, those during the menopause are most rapid. In contrast, the andropause in men goes on almost indefinitely. The menopause affects women around age 50, at which time cycling estradiol (estrogen) production is reduced and replaced by very low estradiol levels. Until a few years ago the prevailing view was that menopause resulted from exhaustion of estrogen production from the ovaries. Like the andropause and the somatopause, the most recent thinking is that age-related changes in the central nervous system affect the hypothalamus-pituitary axis, which stimulates and controls estrogen production in the ovaries.

Taking estrogen and progestins delays the development of atherosclerosis, bone loss, and cognitive impairment. These hormones have, however, been associated with increased risk of cancer. Estrogen acts in the body by way of receptors on the surface of cells wherever these cells may be. However, other effects of estrogen in addition to surface cell changes occur because of its behavior as an antioxidant as well. In fact, the estrogen molecule has characteristics that specifically let it behave this way, creating important consequences not only in terms of addressing menopause symptoms but also for aging. One way estrogen acts as an antioxidant is by preventing oxidation of low density lipoproteins (LDL), which leads to atherosclerosis. Several longevity nutrients imitate estrogen's effects.

Some longevity nutrients important for the menopause include:

- Genistein
- Daidzein

The Aging Joint

Most of us, depending upon our age, have experienced painful joints. For some people, it is an occasional problem associated with excessive exercise but for the majority of elderly people, painful joints are a chronic debilitating condition that eventually may require surgery. Each joint is an exquisitely well-oiled part of machinery in our body. Tissues such as tendons, muscles, bones, cartilage, and blood vessels play an important part in joint structure and function. One of the most important tissues in a joint is cartilage. Cartilage is a distinct tissue even though its molecules are similar to those of bone. Three changes in joints affect how they function throughout the lifespan. The first change is osetoarthritis (OA), an inflammatory joint disease. Next is degeneration, which comes from excessive use of joints. The final change is aging joints, which produces distinct changes. One sign of joint aging is disruption of the organized matrix of joint molecules leading to decreased tensile strength and joint stiffness.

Bone and muscle are important structural components of the joint. Use of the longevity nutrients for these tissues obviously would be expected to help joints. Other tissues in the joint are tendons, which are made of collagen and elastin. Aging changes in collagen and elastin come about from the production of Advanced Glycation Endproducts (AGEs), compromising joint function. The joint distinguishes itself in another way because unlike other organs the joint is not served by a large vessel. This means nutrients must enter it in alternative ways via blood vessels that emanate from the bone, or by way of the synovial fluid, which fills the joint space and provides nutrients to all the joint tissues. Optimum transfer of nutrients through the synovial fluid occurs only when pressure is relieved from the joint.

Some longevity nutrients important for the joints include:

- Carnosine
- Lignans
- Glutamine

The Digestive System: Where Antiaging Really Starts

Nutritionists have long appreciated the role of digestion in promoting and maintaining good health. This appreciation deepens with each new discovery about the digestive system. For example, nutritionists now know that the digestive system does much more than simply admit calories into the body. It actively chooses which and how much of the compounds in food to admit into the body and which to discard. Because of this, nutritionists now recognize that the digestive system, long underappreciated in discussions of longevity, is an important player for a long and healthy life. The digestive system consists of the mouth, esophagus, stomach, small intestine, and colon.

Fats, carbohydrates, and protein are broken down into their constituent parts by the grinding actions of the stomach and the enzymes of the intestines. The key anatomical structure that allows the intestines to digest and absorb nutrients from a meal are the villi, which project into the intestines. The villi are very dynamic, producing thousands of cells each day, which carry out the digestive process in the intestines. These cells also regulate the process of assimilation—allowing nutrients alone to enter the body. Longevity nutrients stimulate the cells in the villi, thus enhancing their function and retarding the aging process. The intestinal tract is endowed with a potent immune system called the Gut Associated Lymphoid Tissue (GALT). This guards against all the toxic substances and bacteria, which enter the digestive tract with each meal and snack.

Some longevity nutrients important for digestive function include:

- Glutamine
- Phytate
- Nucleotides

3

WHERE ARE THE LONGEVITY NUTRIENTS?

This purpose of this program is to help readers add in those long-missing factors in the antiaging equation: the longevity nutrients. The list of substances that qualify for longevity nutrient status is quite extensive and grows by leaps and bounds as new information is accumulated about them. Quite possibly, new longevity nutrients will be added to this list in the future, but incorporating the 21 that follow into your diet will go a long way to giving you a long life.

We Have Come a Long Way, but We Still Have a Long Way to Go

How long do you expect to live? Your expectations should exceed those of your ancestors, and quite reasonably so. Today, individuals are living longer and more actively than ever before. In ancient Rome, people lived for about 30 years. In America, by the turn of the 20th century, the average human life expectancy had risen to just 47 years. At that time, a lucky few—an estimated 25 percent of Americans—lived to be age 65.

Now, as the 21st century begins, 70 percent of the population reaches this age, and many even surpass it. Most men can expect to live until they are 72 years old and most women until they are 78. Even more astounding is the fact that record numbers of people have reached the 100-year mark: currently, more than 36,000 centenarians reside in the United States.

What has caused this recent and rapid increase in life expectancy? Although advances in medical treatments have contributed, one cannot ignore the astounding effect that lifestyle changes have had on potential longevity. Primary among these lifestyle changes are changes in nutritional habits. Think back to your family's eating habits when you were a child, or leaf through a cookbook published decades ago. It becomes clear that cooking with fats, salt, and sugar was more acceptable then than it is now. People did not realize the difference between *saturated* and *unsaturated* fats—lard was an all-too-common cooking ingredient. Now, many consumers can even distinguish between *monounsaturated* and *polyunsaturated* fats.

Through the years, nutritionists have greatly expanded their understanding of the roles played by vitamins, minerals, carbohydrates, protein, and fats in health maintenance and in disease treatment and prevention. Dissemination of this information has aided the general population in making daily diet choices. As a result, most people have learned how to choose foods carefully. They ensure that their diets contain enough vitamins, for example, and exclude harmful or unnecessary amounts of other substances.

Despite these advances, however, our bodies *still* do not achieve the maximum benefits food can provide. Even if nutrition-conscious eaters refer to the recommended dietary allowances (RDAs) of vitamins, protein, and minerals, or build their meals from the food pyramid, they may miss out on some critical nutrients. This occurs because these long-trusted guidelines are not based on and fail to include recent research regarding the longevity nutrients. The current plans simply do not take them into account.

This plan does.

Discovery of the longevity nutrients will take us farther on this journey toward optimum health and longer life. If current nutritional knowledge has allowed us to add 30 years to our lives, imagine how many we can hope to add in decades to come.

We Are What We Eat

It should come as no surprise that the definition of what is essential to our diet is always expanding, considering that the average meal contains thousands of different chemicals! Only recently have these chemicals—ones humans have eaten for thousands of years—been studied for their effects on health and aging.

At the turn of the 20th century, doctors little understood vitamins and minerals. Many even doubted the need for these substances now considered indispensable. Rather, they thought all foods contained elements that could easily be converted into chemicals that make up the body, thereby serving all its needs. To doctors years ago, it did not make any difference what people ate.

Today, everyone knows the importance of eating foods that contain certain vitamins and minerals, because the body cannot make them on its own. Nutritionists have also discovered that although the body may be able to synthesize some of these essential chemicals on its own, it cannot always make enough of them. Besides genetic makeup, no other factor is more important in determining health and longevity than nutrition. Therefore, controlling one's diet is extremely important because, quite simply, every molecule in the human body ultimately comes from the foods one eats. Food factors critically into the way the body's cells function and age.

One way to control diet is to follow nutrition guidelines. These targets, set by scientists and printed on food labels, advise what is essential to the diet. Over the years, these guidelines have instructed that essential nutrients, when eaten daily in the proper amounts, will give you what you need in terms of proper dietary intake.

But the truth is that these guidelines are outdated. While they'll keep you from developing scurvy or beriberi, the current nutritional guidelines don't do much for improving longevity. With knowledge of the latest in nutrition science people can finally take advantage of the abundant times in which we live. Instead of eating solely to prevent deficiencies, people can begin to eat in order to achieve optimum health and maximum longevity.

Turning a Negative into a Positive

For many years, some of the longevity nutrients were believed to be substances called *antinutrients*, because scientists couldn't yet see their positive effects. They were blamed for having a number of negative powers, such as interfering with digestion, reducing the absorption of other nutrients, and inhibiting the growth process.

But one of the most significant research developments over the past few years has been the finding that antinutrients hold great promise as antiaging substances. Hundreds of studies concluded that antinutrients, rather than inhibiting body processes, actually enhance our physiology in numerous and unique ways. They play an important role in the fight against aging and chronic diseases.

For example, one group of longevity nutrients, called phytates, was classified as antinutrients because they bound certain minerals in foods, thereby limiting their digestion and absorption by the body. But today, this effect is considered beneficial, because phytates bind minerals that are not only harmful to the body but which are also implicated in the aging process.

Another group of longevity nutrients that were once thought to be antinutrients, protease inhibitors, are found in certain grains. Protease inhibitors were once considered to be harmful because they inhibited digestive enzymes. This effect is no longer considered significant, and a positive power of protease inhibitors has been uncovered: these food constituents are potent, long-lasting anticarcinogens. That is, they fight cancerous agents in the body and produce remarkable antiaging effects.

For years, nutritionists were slow to realize the health benefits of the longevity nutrients. It's no wonder, considering their bad reputation as anti-nutrients! Today, however, with the advent of new research methods and a better understanding of how the body works, a clearer picture of longevity nutrients' diverse roles has emerged. Compared to the typical vitamin and mineral (for example, vitamin E or zinc) the longevity nutrients have many more and wider-ranging effects. We now understand that their wide-ranging effects are essential to keeping the body in balance.

New Roles for Old Nutrients

Some of the longevity nutrients were discovered years ago but were passed over by medical research. Flavonoids were discovered back in the 1930s by the same person who uncovered the vital role of vitamin C. What attracted Professor Szent-Gyorgyi when he discovered flavonoids was the role they played in prolonging the lives of laboratory animals. Not too much was done with this finding because aging research was not popular in the 1930s when scientists were far more interested in discovering vitamins.

Carnosine is another example of a nutrient that was nearly ignored for decades after its discovery. This longevity nutrient was discovered by Russian scientists in 1900. Over the next 75 years, only a handful of papers were published concerning the effects of carnosine. Although it was known even then that muscles have large amounts of carnosine, its role in this tissue was not appreciated until the antioxidant theory was proposed a few years ago. Today, carnosine's function as an antioxidant in muscle is being investigated in relation to aging and preservation of muscle mass.

Science continually discovers that the longevity nutrients have new effects, many of them life-lengthening. Case in point are phytosterols, which have been known for years to have beneficial effects on the body's metabolism of cholesterol. However, new research has shown in the last few years that they have important effects on the regulation of cell growth: an important finding for the prevention of both aging and cancer.

Many longevity nutrients such as tannins have been ingested unknowingly for thousands of years. The history of tea—a tannin-containing drink—as a beverage can be traced back to around 2700 B.C. when it was consumed by the emperors of China. Within the last few years, detailed research and epidemiological studies of tea drinkers have shown them to have a low risk of heart disease, stroke, and several types of cancer. Tea also has an antioxidant role, which is attributed to tannins. Some studies, in fact, have shown that these antioxidants are more powerful than vitamin C, one of the body's most prevalent antioxidants.

Arginine was isolated and named in 1886. For many years after its discovery, its sole function was thought to reside in the kidneys where it is involved in the detoxification of ammonia. What we know now about this longevity nutrient would certainly surprise its discoverer. Today, we know that arginine improves the function of the senescent immune system, retards the growth of cancer, and enhances the body's healing capacity. It also boosts the production of many hormones and is a precursor for substances that stimulate growth. Although its original function of ammonia detoxification is still one of its most important, we now see arginine playing many other, equally important, functions in the body.

On the other hand, some longevity nutrients really are new. Pyrroloquinoline quinone (PQQ) is one such nutrient that was first discovered to exist in lower life-forms in 1979. Since that date, a number of papers have been published showing its presence in the tissues of other animals and humans. PQQ plays a number of different roles in various enzymes systems, many of which are still being investigated in terms of aging.

The advent and use of the longevity nutrients reminds one of the history of the microwave oven, which, while discovered back in the 1950s, did not become popular until many decades after its discovery. The microwave had to wait for our lifestyles to need it. Many of the longevity nutrients were discovered years ago but ignored. Because of our quick-fix and high-tech eating habits, they have become conspicuous by their absence.

Universal Presence

Not only are the longevity nutrients diverse in their antiaging and disease-preventing effects, but they are also widely distributed in different foods. In fact, it's hard to think of a food that does not have at least one longevity nutrient. Not only are the longevity nutrients dispersed throughout the food chain, but they are present in the different parts of a fruit, vegetable, or protein source. The peel of an orange or lemon may hold the key to preventing the aging process! Different parts of the onion may contain more of the same substance that has been shown to prevent age-related diseases. The outer layer of the wheat kernel or bran was often considered to be only a source of fiber but now is known to have longevity nutrients that have very positive effects on the body's metabolism. Artichokes have substances in them that our bodies can't digest but that our colon bacteria thrive on. Even the old standby, milk—practically everyone's first food—has a very powerful substance that plays a healthful role in modulating the ways we function.

Where Are the Longevity Nutrients?

At first sight, when confronted with all the longevity nutrients, one can easily get intimidated and confused. But rest assured that these exotic-sounding substances are present in the foods you know well. *The New Longevity Diet* may ask you to add some foods or change your dietary proportions around, but you won't encounter what nutritionists call "menu shock." Practically everyone has heard of vitamin C or vitamin D, but the chances are pretty good that they may never have heard of nucleotides, monoterpenes, or phytates. It becomes an awful lot to absorb.

Keep in mind that you already ingest a great variety of foods. We have access to so many foods, many more than our ancestors. And amid the choices we routinely make at the grocery store lies the secret to a much longer, healthier life.

Food Families

As we look at the total nutrition picture, it's helpful to divide up the universe of foods into some simple and sensible families.

- Cereal Family—Often, when we talk about cereals, we are thinking only of wheat. There are, however, many others, including rice, corn, oats, and rye. Barley, millet, and sorghum are not a part of the typical American diet, but they are important staples in other countries. Longevity nutrients that come from this family include phytates, lignans, and protease inhibitors.

- Citrus Family—This includes grapefruit, kumquats, lemons, limes, oranges, tangelos, tangerines, and citrons. Not only do the flesh and juice of these foods contain important antiaging substances, but the peel does as well. This family is the principal source of the longevity nutrient monoterpenes.
- Composite Family—Here are the lettuces (leaf and romaine), endive, escarole, chicory, dandelion greens, artichokes and the spice tarragon. Often thought of as a source of vitamins and fiber, these vegetables offer the longevity nutrients inulin and oligofructose.
- Fungus Family—Mushrooms, morels, truffles, and yeast belong here. Longevity nutrients present in this family include the nucleotides.
- Beet Family—Besides beets, this family contains the vegetables chard, spinach, and quinoa. Spinach is a longevity nutrient–seeker's delight as it provides several longevity nutrients. Quinoa, a food staple of the Peruvian people, is also an excellent source of longevity nutrients.
- Gourd Family—This group contains melons such as cantaloupe, honeydew, Persian melon, muskmelon, pumpkin, and watermelon. The squash, zucchini, and cucumber are also included, and these make excellent sources of the longevity nutrient glutathione.
- Grape Family—This family consists of fruits that grow on vines. Raisins are included here. Longevity nutrients derived from this group include the tannins.
- Heath Family—Various berries such as the blueberry, cranberry, lingonberry, and teaberry belong to this family. These and many more are excellent sources of longevity nutrients, one prominent example being lignans.
- Laurel Family–This is an unusually diverse group of foods, including avocados, bay leaves, cinnamon, and sassafras. The avocado is a moderate source of the longevity nutrient glutathione.
- Legume Family—This family includes soybeans and peanuts in one group, and legumes such as beans, lentils, and peas in another group. These foods play a substantial role in the longevity nutrient program because several longevity nutrients, including phytoestrogens and saponins, are found here. Saponins dominate this group of foods.

- Lily Family—So named by botanists, this family contains onions, chives, asparagus, garlic, leeks, scallions, and shallots. In addition to other longevity nutrients, this family contains the organosulfur compounds.
- Maize Family—Really this includes only one food: corn. By virtue of its bran and other components, though, corn contains a number of different longevity nutrients such as phytates and protease inhibitors.
- Mint Family—In addition to mint, spearmint, and peppermint, this family includes thyme, sage, rosemary, oregano, and marjoram. The mint family is a good source of monoterpene and phytosterols.
- Mulberry Family—Figs are included here. Although other members of this family exist, not much is known concerning the amount and types of longevity nutrients they contain, with the exception of tannins.
- Mustard Family—The vegetables in this family include broccoli, brussels sprouts, cabbage, cauliflower, collards, horseradish, kale, kohlrabi, mustard, radishes, turnips, and watercress. These contain a very important longevity nutrient, isothiocyanates.
- Parsley Family—In addition to parsley, this family contains a number of other herbs and spices, such as caraway, coriander, cumin, dill, and fennel. The principal foods in this family are carrots, celery, and celeriac, each of which contains several longevity nutrients, such as lignans and pyrroloquinoline quinone (PQQ).
- Plantain Family—Included here are the banana and plantain, and both foods contain the longevity nutrient tannins, inulin, oligofructose, and glutathione.
- Plum Family—Apricots, cherries, nectarines, peaches, persimmons, and plums all belong here. Phytosterols are found in many of these foods, while persimmons are a good source of tannins.
- Potato or Nightshade Family—Besides the potato, this family contains eggplant, green peppers, red peppers, chilies, and tomatoes. Protease inhibitors are an important longevity nutrient found in potatoes, and PQQ is found in moderate levels in green peppers.
- Rose Family—One subgroup contains the apple, pear, and quince; the other includes blackberries, raspberries, boysenberries, and

strawberries. Apples are an important source of quercetin, and this longevity nutrient can be found in the juice and cider of this fruit in addition to its flesh. The quince is a large yellow apple, also a good source, and is eaten in parts of Asia. Blackberries and strawberries are high in tannins.

- Nut Family—Walnuts, pecans, cashews, and brazil nuts are each classified as separate subfamilies. Large amounts of arginine are found in most of these, as well as lesser levels of phytates.
- Tea Family—Tea provides the longevity nutrients tannins and PQQ.
- Chocolate Family—Included here are cocoa and the kola bean, which are high in the longevity nutrient arginine.

Some longevity nutrients are found in protein foods, which are classified into the following families:

- Meat Family—Included here are beef, lamb, pork, rabbit, and wild game. The longevity nutrient carnitine is found in these foods.
- Poultry Family—Chicken, turkey, partridge, quail, pheasant, and goose belong here. Chicken and turkey are very high in the longevity nutrient taurine.
- Fish Family—Hundreds of different species exist, including both fresh and saltwater varieties. These contain significant levels of the longevity nutrients glutamine, arginine, and taurine.
- Seafood Family—This group includes the crab, shrimp, scallop, crayfish, lobster, clam, oyster, mussel, octopus, periwinkle, and squid. The longevity nutrient nucleotides are found in several of these foods.
- Dairy Family—Cheese, milk, and yogurt are all members of this family. The longevity nutrient conjugated linoleic acid (CLA) is found in most of these foods.

As you can see, the longevity nutrients are readily available in a wide range of foods for anyone to gain their healthful effects. And they have always been there, even though no one paid much attention to them. So instead of looking for some new drug or chemical to retard aging, look to nature. These appetizing foods offer a far more effective way to deal with aging and achieve the maximum life span.

The Best Source of the Longevity Nutrients: Food versus Supplements

At the present time, supplements containing most longevity nutrients are not available. Even if they did exist in pill form, scientists doubt whether they would as effectively improve the body's physiology and prevent aging. By far, the best way we know to take advantage of the longevity nutrients' healthful properties is to eat them in their natural state.

One of the reasons to opt for natural food sources over supplements is that each longevity nutrient is actually made up of several different compounds. For example, saponins, those immune system boosters, are composed of many different substances. Each substance may differ in potency, depending upon the food source. Since we do not yet know which saponin substances are more effective, it makes sense to eat foods containing all of them.

Another reason for favoring food sources is that foods contain other substances that activate the longevity nutrients' effects. You may have heard about studies done with vitamins which have come to similar conclusions: other chemicals in foods trigger and maximize vitamins' benefits. When animals were fed a synthetic diet containing all the necessary vitamins, minerals, and macronutrients, they developed more diseases than animals fed natural foods. This outcome was not caused by chemicals in the synthetic diet, but rather by the lack of longevity nutrients in unnatural sources. Until more information is gleaned about the longevity nutrients and their interactions with other food substances, we should go for the comprehensive, natural foods approach.

We now have indisputable evidence that eating foods containing longevity nutrients prevents disease and the aging process in humans. In a recent, large-scale study of diet and food consumption by people in the United States, it was shown that individuals whose diet was diverse and contained high levels of the longevity nutrients lived longer and suffered less from disease than those who ate a small number of foods devoid of the longevity nutrients. Quite explicitly, the more meager the intake of longevity nutrients, the shorter the life expectancy and the greater the incidence of disease.

With so many studies pointing to their importance, it appears critical to increase one's intake of the longevity nutrients. There is no better way to accomplish this than by following the longevity nutrient program. If one or more of the major food sources is missing, say fruits or vegetables or grains, the longevity nutrients are missing as well. If we want to ensure optimum function of our bodies' vital systems, and if we want to roll back the years and prevent the aging process, we must restore longevity nutrients—those missing factors in the antiaging equation—and the best way to do that is by following this program.

4

THE LONGEVITY NUTRIENT GALLERY

You use and benefit from things *every* day, but you don't need to know how they work in order to use them, right? You just let them "do their thing," so to speak. Our bodies are like that. In fact, they're pretty good at being maintenance free *if* they have what they need to do it. We take many of these fine-tuned mechanisms for granted, remaining ignorant of them until something goes wrong. But, unlike your heater or air-conditioner, refrigerator or electricity, your body is a little harder to ignore. Your body *depends* on you to notice it. Your body *depends on you* to know what it needs!

To stop your body from breaking down means prevention. It means management. It means *preventing* disease and *preventing* aging and managing your own aging process to the best extent possible.

As you know, aging is not a onetime event. It is a

process, and since every organ in our body works in a different way, this means aging does its work in a different way on each organ. As inconvenient and as complicated as it may sound, each of our organs requires *different* antiaging factors. But, inconvenient and complicated-sounding tasks are the longevity nutrients' specialty! No *one* panacea or magic zap deals with *all* the different ways our body ages. To deal with this reality, our body needs a *set* of antiaging compounds—the longevity nutrients.

The longevity nutrients are unique because they are so versatile. There is not much point to preventing aging in our liver while ignoring what aging is doing to our kidneys, skeleton, or joints. If you do that, the only thing you'll gain is a healthy liver when you die young. The longevity nutrients deal with *all* of our body's organs. Not *one* organ in our body can afford to be deprived of attention. Longevity nutrients are capable of providing this type of attention.

People often ask how long it takes for longevity nutrients to reverse the aging process. My answer depends on which longevity nutrient we are talking about. Some nutrients take longer than others to produce benefits and show effects. Since each nutrient has unique composition, characteristics, and tasks, our body adjusts differently to each nutrient's intake. For example, inulin and oligofructose don't get to work immediately. It takes time for them to build up the right type of colon bacteria to produce the relevant antiaging factors. At the other extreme, glutathione distributes itself at once throughout our body's various systems.

As a general rule, before you have completed the 21-day *New Longevity Diet,* a majority of the compounds will have started to exert antiaging and antidisease effects on your body.

Looking for Answers

Longevity nutrients achieve extraordinary health benefits by interacting with our body's metabolism—how it breaks down particles and what it does with them—certain areas of which become dysfunctional as we age. As you keep reading, you'll see how longevity nutrients actually reverse deteriorating changes in our body: they support our immune system, limit the development of ROS, modulate the growth of individual cells, and impact many other aspects of aging. Remember, aging is a complex process, and major gaps still exist in our understanding of it. However, we have learned enough about the longevity nutrients to make scientifically based recommendations for their use as antiaging substances.

As scientists continue to look for answers to how and why we age, they have learned to distinguish aging from disease. They separate the aging process itself from conditions such as Alzheimer's disease or osteoporosis. Aging and disease may cross paths, but they are distinct things. The longevity nutrients work their magic on both processes. Longevity nutrients not only reverse the aging process but prevent major organ diseases, *regardless of age.*

The Longevity Nutrient Gallery

Now that you know how cells function and how aging affects different organs, it is time to delve into how the longevity nutrients work to prevent aging and optimize health.

1. Nucleotides: Parts of the DNA Building Kit

Are you happy with how your DNA is built? Do you know you can undertake DNA renovations with just your diet as a tool? An important biochemical advancement made in the past five years has changed the way nutritionists look at the parts of food.

Scientists used to think that the body's cells had to make all the parts of the DNA molecule themselves with no help. Now, we know more. We know many DNA parts can be found *preformed* in our diet. Our food is like a DNA building kit that provides structural components of DNA to enhance and regulate its production.

Nucleotides are the key substances in DNA production. Actually, six different nucleotides exist, which link together to make up the DNA molecule. The DNA's linked arrangement forms the famous "double helix configuration," you are probably familiar with. The arrangement of our DNA also spells out our genetic code. While DNA grants us our individuality, it also provides the blueprint for manufacturing *all* our body's chemicals.

Each of our body's cells houses a six-foot-long DNA molecule, and this molecule is reproduced more than a trillion times during a person's lifetime. Each time one of these cells divides and multiplies, it *must* produce new DNA. Nucleotides are necessary for this to happen. In fact, only *one* replication of all the cells in our body requires 10,000,000,000,000—ten trillion—nucleotides. Different body tissues require different amounts of nucleotides depending on their cell production rate. Cells that divide fast—like those in the blood or digestive tract—need more DNA than those that divide slowly, such as those in the brain. In fact, tissues under constant stress—such as the skin—may also need larger amounts of nucleotides to function than if they weren't under constant stress. It's hard not to see why it's so important to have an adequate supply of nucleotides in our diet.

Our immune and digestive systems need nucleotides too—when invading bacteria and viruses challenge our body, our immune system is expected to take a lead role. Our immune system must step up its production of lymphocytes—cells that fight infection. You might have guessed that, in fact, our immune system lymphocytes *definitely* decline as we age. Nucleotides help our body fight lymphocyte decline, but a specific type of nucleotide is required to make this happen. Our body produces only some of these specific nucleotides—our diet supplies the rest.

The cell lining of our intestinal tract is replaced so often—every three to six days—that nucleotides, which make up these cells' DNA, are needed around the clock. The more nucleotides you get from your diet, the less energy your body has to use making them. As a result, you allow your body to concentrate on using its energy to make other important molecules that are part of its daily regimen.

With that in mind, how much of this longevity nutrient do you need exactly? Recent research indicates adults need from 450 to 700 milligrams of nucleotides each day: dietary nucleotides help to fulfill this requirement of the important DNA building blocks.

2. Saponins: They May Look Like Soap, but They Taste a Lot Better!

Saponins get their name from what happens when they are extracted from their source—plants—and mixed with water: they froth and foam on the surface—like soap. The fact that half of a saponin molecule is water insoluble explains this soapy behavior.

Saponins don't enter our body's cells. Instead, they do their work on our cells by attaching to the outsides of our cell walls. This behavior sets saponins apart from other longevity nutrients, which do their work *inside* our cells.

That saponins exist in certain foods is old news, but like many longevity nutrients, the reality of what they do was misunderstood. Saponins, previously tabbed as harmful antinutrients, are, today, showered with praise for their ability to prevent aging and disease. Saponin-rich foods improve our digestive functioning. They help control our appetite and regulate what nutrients our body absorbs. Saponins help regulate how our bodies absorb glucose. This means people who suffer from hypoglycemia—a disturbance in sugar metabolism that can lead to low energy levels and even diabetes—probably realize the greatest benefit from this particular function of saponins. Even more important though, saponins may protect our body from producing too much insulin, eventually preventing aging and serious age-related diseases including hypertension, diabetes, and high blood lipid levels. Controlling and adjusting insulin levels is a pillar of antiaging strategy.

Saponins also sharpen our ability to immunize ourselves against invaders by inhibiting the growth of viruses and aiding in the regulation of abnormal cell growth. There is even evidence that they kill cancer cells. Saponins stimulate our immune system by attaching to receptor sites on the outside of immune cells, turbocharging the immune cell's response. They also help increase the number of lymphocytes in our body, thereby warding off immune decline.

Saponins have effects on lipid metabolism. In other words, eating saponins lowers blood cholesterol. Over a hundred years ago, European diets had high amounts of saponins from oats and a food called "peas"—a mixture of various legumes. People who ate these foods suffered far less from heart disease than people do today. The conventional scientific wisdom held that the fiber in these diets was more responsible than saponins for encouraging a healthy heart, but saponins' cholesterol-binding effect led scientists to consider saponins the more potent factor.

Saponins have a regulatory effect on the intestinal tract as well. Our bodies produce bile—a substance important in regulating the metabolism of cholesterol—but too much of this good thing is associated with the development of colon cancer and other health problems. Fortunately, the amount and chemical makeup of bile depends upon what we eat, and saponins have an amazing tendency to bind and neutralize bile, keeping it well in line.

Compared to typical Asian diets, American and western European diets contain very small amounts of saponins. People in Japan eat about three times more saponins per day than the average U.S. citizen. This hearty amount has been correlated with a longer life span and a lower disease rate in Japan than in the United States. Boosting your saponin intake makes sense.

3. Phytates: Ancient, Life-Extending Compounds

A 2,000-year-old tomb was recently excavated and a cache of seeds was discovered. When these ancient seeds were planted, they germinated just as well as seeds purchased today would grow. How could something be preserved so long and still have the potential to live? The answer is lies in phytates—longevity nutrients with boggling antiaging properties.

Phytates, which are large, complex molecules, are in the cells of every tissue in our body. They used to be considered useless and even harmful because they bind up minerals, making these minerals unavailable for the body to absorb. We now know that the ability to bind up minerals such as copper and iron, when present in excessive and unhealthy amounts, works to our body's benefit. For example, phytates interact with iron, a mineral that takes part in the development of ROS, to prevent aging. Phytates control iron and its capacity to make ROS by binding the mineral and keeping it in its less reactive state. Each phytate molecule can bind as many as six iron atoms at one time and hold onto these atoms indefinitely.

"Iron withholding" is another way phytates mingle with iron, this time to our immune system's benefit. Invading microorganisms and tumor cells need iron to survive inside our bodies. Iron withholding denies iron to these invaders, especially in the liver (a popular place for large amounts of iron), starving them out.

Phytates activate NK (natural killer) cells whose special job is to prevent tumors from developing in our body. NK cells spread throughout the body to quickly kill or eliminate cells that become cancerous or senescent, and phytates are the alarm clock that activates NK cells.

Phytates also have a starring role in our brain. As we age, neuron activity slows down, but phytates keep our neurons active.

Phytic acid—a metabolite of dietary phytates—is a precursor for a molecule called IP6 (or inositol hexaphosphate, if your tongue needs exercise), and nearly every cell in the body needs IP6. IP6 is one of the most important cell function regulators, governing our cells to proliferate and differentiate, and managing the intracellular communication among the cell's membrane, nucleus, and organelles. Senescent cells *encourage* aging because of their limited number of cell divisions, but phytates goose the process back into shape. By eating phytates, you are sharpening the skills of one of the most important regulators of cell differentiation and proliferation, discouraging the aging process. Even though our cells make IP6, eating phytates eases the body's workload—a point we've made about other longevity nutrients.

Studies show phytates may also prevent certain types of cancer. People living in Finland have a much lower incidence of colon cancer than those living in Denmark—even though each country's diet has about the same level of fiber. So what's the answer? Finns eat more phytate-rich foods than the Danes.

How do phytates prevent aging and fight cancer? They maintain normal cell growth rates. Eating more phytates restores normal growth rates to our cells, diminishing accelerated, uncontrolled growth. On the other hand, if our cells lose the ability to divide at all, senescence sets in. Again, phytic acid—part of our cell's regulatory system—keeps senescence at bay.

4. Protease Inhibitors

For many years, these longevity nutrients were blamed for getting in the *way* of the digestive process: protease inhibitors were thought to inhibit digestive enzymes called *proteases*—hence their name. The thinking has changed. Proteases themselves have been fingered as culprits in a number of diseases including hypertension, osteoarthritis, and other chronic degenerative conditions. Moreover, viruses rely on proteases to help them invade our bodies.

Several animal studies conclude diets high in protease inhibitors increase life span dramatically. Why does this happen? Protease inhibitors protect DNA. As humans age, our genes become unstable and lose their ability to accurately reproduce. Protease inhibitors stabilize genes, promoting homeostasis. Protease inhibitors may also help prevent colon, breast, and prostate cancers. Seventh-Day Adventists—who eat a vegetarian diet and consume high levels of protease inhibitors—have a far lower incidence of these common types of cancer and also tend to live longer than the general population.

Scientists are just *beginning* to unravel the antiaging effects of protease inhibitors. Cancer-prevention studies of protease inhibitors are just now in the early stages of understanding how powerful these substances may be. Repairing damaged DNA and stimulating DNA growth can be added to the résumé of protease inhibitors as well.

Although many different foods have a supply of protease inhibitors, we know the most about soybeans. In fact, Japanese people—who consume much more protease inhibitors in their diets than Americans do—have a low incidence of cancer. People in Japan consume 10 grams of protease inhibitors per day, compared to 2.5 grams per day in the United States. Japanese people have the longest life expectancy of all industrialized countries. It's not surprising that a consensus exists among nutritionists that in the U.S., we should consume more protease inhibitors—at least matching the level of the Japanese diet.

5. Glutamine: The Great Anabolic Effector

Until a few years ago, the longevity nutrient glutamine was classified as "nonessential" because our muscles store large amounts of it. It was thought that whenever the body needed more glutamine, it could simply get it from the muscles and release it to other tissues. However, this supply is not unlimited. Recent research shows muscle-stored glutamine is quickly used up during times of mental and physical stress—including during infection and disease. Extremely low levels of glutamine are even life threatening. Nutritionists now understand we must eat enough foods rich in this longevity nutrient to make sure we can tap its benefits.

Glutamine is an amino acid—a building block of proteins. It prevents aging by helping keep cells from deteriorating. Glutamine also helps make antioxidants, synthesize DNA, eliminate ammonia, and prevent age-related muscle breakdown. Because glutamine has to support the production of another longevity nutrient called glutathione, we need enough glutamine to keep up our stores while having ample amounts on hand to support the production of glutathione.

Glutamine imposes a range of effects on our immune system. An aging immune system functions well until it is challenged by an infection. That's when glutamine steps up to share the burden, jump-starting the immune system to help it. It is an energy source for our intestinal and immune system cells as well as a precursor for DNA synthesis.

Glutamine also detoxifies and regulates our bodies' toxic ammonia levels. This nutrient collects ammonia and brings it to the kidneys for elimination. Glutamine eliminates ammonia from the brain, and other brain functions depend on glutamine. Inadequate intakes of glutamine may precipitate depression, memory loss, and even decreased sex drive.

Lymphocytes are also dependent on glutamine and must take it in

EXORPHINS: A BREAK IN THE LIST AND MORE HELP FROM PROTEINS

Scientists used to think eating protein-rich foods meant protein digested completely into its tiny building blocks: amino acids. New research shows this may not necessarily be the case. Proteins break down only partially into exorphins. Exorphins then enter the bloodstream and prevent aging and disease throughout the body. There are three types of exorphins—caseomorphins, cyclic peptides, and carnosine—only one of which is a full-fledged new nutrient.

Eating carbohydrates and fiber at the expense of protein—advocated by some health experts—may result in deficiencies of fundamental anti-aging substances and may promote life-threatening health problems. People who eat protein deficient diets tend to be lacking in exorphins.

Our brain, muscles, and liver depend on exorphins to do their jobs. In the brain, exorphins change their name to endorphins. Endorphins influence how our brain carries out some of its most critical activities, including pain control, mood elevation, behavior regulation, and appetite control.

For steering what kind of mood we think we are in, think milk. Milk, whether whole or low-fat, contains another group of exorphins called caseomorphins. In addition to preventing certain diseases, caseomorphins benefit mood and sleep. In fact, the custom of drinking milk to help people fall asleep works precisely because caseomorphins affect our brain's "sleep center."

Appetite control depends on cyclic peptides—exorphins found in white bread, tuna, and shrimp. Cyclic peptides regulate digestion and are absorbed by the brain for use in appetite control.

every day. When microorganisms invade the body, lymphocytes immediately draw on muscle stores of glutamine—stores that must be replenished.

Our skin needs glutamine to stay healthy and young. Fibroblasts—essential to skin cells—depend on glutamine to keep tissue strong and supple. Fibroblasts malfunction with age, one of the causes of both intrinsic and photoaged skin. Since glutamine is the principal nutrient for fibroblasts, getting enough of this longevity nutrient to our skin is a priority.

6. Carnosine: The Pluripotent Antiaging New Longevity Nutrient

First identified about a century ago, carnosine is made up of two amino acids. Despite its simple molecular structure, carnosine seems to go above and beyond its call of duty to combat particular aging effects—in a different way than any of the other longevity nutrients.

It is beyond the scope of this book to describe the biochemical ramifications of how two simple amino acids could prevent aging. But suffice it to say that when carnosine is added to mature and senescent cells in a cell dish, they change into juvenile cells. When such cells are administered carnosine, they divide many more times than they normally would *without* the carnosine. Substances with this effect are *rare.*

Carnosine also discourages another two hallmarks of aging, protein carbonyl groups and collagen cross links, from developing and forming. In so doing, carnosine alleviates one major aging problem—healthy cells taking on the characteristics of old cells. Okay, what does this *really* mean to you and your body? It means you get to keep tissue that stays in shape. Carnosine gets rid of negative protein molecules so that our body remains capable of keeping its connective tissue from aging.

Carnosine labors in our brain too, helping it to do its metabolic work. Studies show carnosine protects our brain when it gets less blood than it needs and protects our brain when it is injured or inflamed by inhibiting ROS damage.

So, how do we keep our carnosine levels up? Not only can we get plenty of it from the foods we choose for our diets, but studies show people who exercise have higher levels of carnosine in their bodies than people who do not. Carnosine levels taper off when we experience stress, and since some stressors simply cannot be avoided, adequate diet and exercise are the best and most reliable places to find and maintain our body's supply of carnosine.

7. Pyrroloquinoline Quinone (PQQ): The Vitamin Imitator

Even nutritionists have trouble pronouncing this longevity nutrient—we just call it PQQ. PQQ combines some of the most potent properties of the B vitamins and vitamin C. We used to think PQQ helped only animals, but now it is considered essential to humans. This longevity nutrient sharpens our cells' ability to make energy, synthesizes tissues, and prevents mood disturbances. PQQ presents itself to our adrenal glands, cardiovascular system, eyes, liver, muscles, pancreas, skin, and spleen. Moreover, PQQ helps our immune system make sure certain cells—such as neutrophils—function effectively.

As an antioxidant, PQQ leaves no room for doubt. Our liver constantly encounters toxic chemicals. The liver's job is to detoxify these chemicals, but its ability to keep up can become overwhelmed. Enter PQQ. PQQ helps relieve our liver when it is overburdened. PQQ protects the liver when it can't work as hard as it needs to work.

In fact, as an antioxidant, PQQ is generous. PQQ not only helps combat ROS on its own, it also teams up with other antioxidants to make sure they stay around in adequate doses. For example, as you have learned, many antioxidants depend on glutathione. This means our glutathione system gets overloaded. Since so many antioxidants need glutathione to perform their own job, incoming ROS can easily challenge the glutathione system. PQQ protects the glutathione system against overwork.

Our adrenal glands especially depend on PQQ. Adrenal glands—we have one above each kidney—are essential to how our body reacts to stress. What makes your heart beat faster? What makes your skin develop goose bumps when you sense danger or when you approach a potentially stressful situation, such as speaking in public? Hormones from your adrenal glands. This response system depends on PQQ. PQQ may also prevent overreaction of this stress response.

Our skin depends on PQQ too. PQQ retains our skin's tone. Without enough PQQ, aging skin loses its fibrous texture and ability to heal after trauma.

PQQ, an unusual vitamin and an antiaging substance, has not yet told its full story. With research areas overflowing with new information—especially in terms of the extent to which PQQ interacts with our brain to prevent damage and control ROS—it only makes sense to stay tuned.

8. Arginine: Our Fountain of Youth

Arginine, once thought of as just another amino acid with no special function, has been found to affect nearly every part of our bodies. A cationic molecule—a small chemical with a positive charge—arginine reduces the charge of other molecules in our body, doing all its work through other molecules. As a result, arginine stimulates the release of hormones our body needs. It also combats stressors, neutralizes and eliminates toxic chemicals, and makes sure our immune system works right.

Arginine stimulates the synthesis and release of growth hormone (GH)—a critical factor in retaining adequate bone and muscle, keeping skin young, and improving heart and kidney function. Growth hormone regulates our body composition—how much of it is made up of muscle and fat, for example. As we age, we secrete less GH; some people lose as much as 14 percent GH every decade they age.

Arginine is also crucial to the production of nitric oxide (NO). Nitric oxide is another recent discovery. The scientific community considered nitric oxide so profound that it designated nitric oxide "Molecule of the Year" in 1994. Though we have only known about nitric oxide for a relatively short time, it is one of the oldest chemicals found in living systems. The horseshoe crab—whose metabolic system has gone unchanged for more than 50 million years—has NO in its body in exactly the same form as we do. What can NO do for humans? Nitric oxide regulates our brain's learning and memory processes. It also regulates our cardiovascular system's blood vessel operation, and the male reproductive system's ability to produce sperm. Without arginine, NO would not be produced, and none of these functions would be possible.

Arginine levels decrease with age. As a result, NO levels decrease with age too. Since NO interacts with so many other aspects of our aging process, keeping its levels up is a critical antiaging strategy. For example, nitric oxide, through its modulation by arginine, helps prevent stiffness and rigidity in blood vessels, and recent studies show consuming arginine-*rich* foods reduces the risk of heart disease.

Another effect of aging is the body's loss of its ability to heal wounds. Arginine stimulates our skin to produce connective tissue so that healing is faster and more complete. Arginine also encourages immune cell production.

9. Inulin and Oligofructose: Never Neglect Your Colon!

Inulin and oligofructose are carbohydrates, and the powerful work they assume with our colon easily qualifies them for the longevity nutrient list. Although you probably don't make a special effort to give your colon much thought (in fact, you may specifically avoid thinking of it), you know something about how central your colon is to your life.

The bacteria in your colon hold the job of finishing our digestion, making an end product called short chain fatty acids (SCFAs). The colon's bacteria are anaerobic bacteria that thrive without oxygen. Although they don't need oxygen, they do require specific types of fiber to do their job: resistant starch and oligosaccharides.

When we ingest these types of carbohydrates (fiber), this means we are giving the bacteria what it needs. We are providing the bacteria's food source and building up their reserves.

At the end product of all of this diligent bacterial effort, SCFAs affect the body locally and system wide. Locally, SCFAs provide the colon with its food source. By feeding the colon, SCFAs work with the DNA to influence how the colon's cells grow and differentiate. SCFAs also leave the colon and our blood transports them to various organs in the body. There, SCFAs spread their wealth into the muscles, as a unique energy source, the liver to inhibit cholesterol production, and into the kidneys, heart, and brain.

While our colon depends on its bacteria to digest fiber, the *type* of nutrients we ingest affects the quality of the bacteria. Eating more of the appropriate types of carbohydrates (such as inulin and oligofructose) encourages the growth of beneficial bacteria (such as bifidobacteria and lactobacilli) while discouraging the proliferation of harmful bacteria—such as *C. perfringens* and *E. coli*. Inulin and oligofructose restore good bacteria—especially bifidobacteria—to high and healthy levels. As a result, SCFAs levels are increased to, in turn, release their antiaging benefits: facilitating DNA repair, helping cells fix proteins, and sharpening our immune system.

Inulin and oligofructose come in limited amounts and are only in certain foods. One of these foods is the Jerusalem artichoke—one of the oldest cultivated crops in the New World.

10. The Mysteries of Taurine

The longevity nutrient and amino acid taurine was first discovered in an ox (Latin name: "taurus"). At that point, taurine earned the distinction as the only amino acid to have its own sign of the zodiac. Taurine stands out for another reason too: it does not combine with other amino acids to form protein. Instead, taurine is usually found roaming free inside our body's cells. As a result, taurine has raised extraordinary curiosity among scientists about its relationship to health and aging.

We have more taurine in our body's cells than any other amino acid—most of it in our heart, brain, liver, kidney, and muscles. As with other longevity nutrients, our body can make taurine, mainly in our liver and brain, but, only in limited quantities. The body can't make enough to completely satisfy its needs.

Until the 1970s, taurine was mostly just a passing curiosity. Researchers took interest when they noticed a taurine deficiency among cats. Cats do not have the necessary enzymes to produce taurine and taurine deficiency is a life-threatening problem for them. Cat food manufacturers now include taurine in their products.

Taurine's relationship to cats—established more than 20 years ago now—set the stage for finding more about what it does in humans. And scientists still think it has not completely revealed its potential. To begin with, taurine is a potent antioxidant, even standing in for other antioxidants in their absence. The male reproductive system has no other naturally occurring antioxidant except taurine. By preventing testosterone decline, specifically during andropause, taurine improves how the muscles, bones, and other organs endure.

Taurine also interacts with our immune system. It is the major amino acid in the immune cells, known as neutrophils. When we take taurine in through our diet, its levels increase in our body to give neutrophils more staying power to battle infection and clear away bacteria.

Taurine lends itself to our heart too, as both an antioxidant and a regulator of calcium levels. As an antioxidant to our heart and lungs, taurine protects our body from toxic effects imposed by a number of substances—such as ozone—we inhale every day. The heart depends on calcium to regulate its muscle contraction. If, for some reason, calcium encounters a problem doing this and its levels fall, taurine is on call to step in and help regulate our heart muscle contraction. Taurine's protective effect here is different from what you may expect: taurine doesn't change or modify the low calcium levels. Instead, taurine works with what it finds, compensating for low calcium levels, rather than changing the actual levels.

When our body systems experience stress-induced changes—such as our heart's calcium levels—taurine becomes somewhat of a troublemaker from stress's point of view. It antagonizes these stress-induced changes by producing *other* changes that let our body get back to its work—but taurine does all this without reestablishing homeostasis. What taurine establishes, instead, is called *enantiostasis*. This explains taurine's protective feature: protecting the heart from negative effects of calcium imbalance, rather than trying to change calcium levels back to normal. By working like this, it makes its intent obvious: to protect the heart and give the heart time to get back its necessary calcium levels or to repair its system back to normal cardiac function.

Taurine protects our body from ROS differently than other antioxidants like glutathione. Antioxidants such as glutathione trap or scavenge ROS to restore homeostasis. Taurine takes a different approach. In its enantiostatic way, taurine reduces ROS toxicity by targeting and modifying their negative effects, rather than targeting the ROS themselves.

In vegetarian diets, taurine is low. People living in Third World countries may tend to have more illness from toxic chemicals than people living in other parts of the world due to their low dietary taurine intake.

Our brain contains taurine, and the amount it has decreases as we age. Since our brain depends on protection from toxic agents, preventing low taurine levels is a priority. While we humans make taurine in our livers, we still have surprisingly low levels of the enzymes we need to make it.

11. Tannins: Ancient Compounds with New Age-Prevention Roles

Tannins have been used for centuries to tan leather. Tanning is a process that lightens the leather's color by binding the proteins that make it dark. Although tanning leather has little to do with human health and the prevention of aging, protein-binding properties have a lot to do with these things.

As you are used to by now, tannins—like most *longevity nutrients*—have more complex, chemical names: epigallocatechin-3-gallate (EGCG) and epigallocatechin (EGC), but I'll refer to these substances simply as *tannins.*

Tannins cause an astringent taste sensation. Green apples, cider, red wine, and tea all have astringent tastes. The way some foods look—their appearance—is the clue to their *tannin* content. Beans that are red, black, or bronze contain higher tannin levels than white beans. Red onions contain more tannins than white onions. But tannins are more than superficial—their benefit reaches far beyond flavor and appearance.

For ages, tannins have been used to remedy various ailments. They are the active chemical in many Chinese and Japanese folk medicines, some of which even include the highly tannic rhubarb, used to treat inflammation, high blood pressure, ulcers, and kidney problems. Raspberries, or tea made from their leaves, have a long history in the treatment of ulcers and throat inflammation. For many years, tannins have also been known to kill bacteria and viral organisms in wounds.

Today, acquired immune deficiency syndrome (AIDS) researchers are looking at tannins' effects on the ability of viruses to replicate. Because tannins easily combine with enzymes that make the HIV virus—the virus that causes AIDS—tannins show the potential to control the HIV virus from growing.

Tannins also block the formation of cancer-causing agents, eliminate toxic agents from the blood, and limit enzymes that raise blood pressure. Tannins also fight ROS—not by blocking their development the way other longevity nutrients do, but by scavenging for ROS after they have already formed.

Finally, tannins help prevent a common cause of aging: DNA mutation—when a cell gets wrong directions and ends up doing the wrong thing because its DNA is damaged. Nucleic acids—which make up DNA—are susceptible to ROS. As a result, altered—or damaged—DNA is often copied in that altered condition. When this happens, the DNA cannot be transferred to other cells. Apply this reality to the cells in your whole body, and you can see how far this malfunction extends itself—especially since it is impossible to overstate the value of our DNA. So, even in small amounts, tannins—these obliging longevity nutrients—spur enzymes to repair our bodies' DNA.

As you know, ROS are oxidants. One way to understand how ROS affect our body is to consider oxidative stress. Oxidative stress is an imbalance in the oxidant (ROS)/antioxidant status of a cell. If there are not enough antioxidants in the cell to counteract the oxidant stress imposed on the cell, then the cell becomes imbalanced. An imbalance means too many oxidants—or ROS—and not enough antioxidants. The ideal situation is obvious: every cell would have enough antioxidants to counteract the number of oxidants—oxidants that inject oxidative damage to exceptionally important cell molecules: DNA, protein and fats, or lipids.

With this in mind, you also know that several diseases such as cancer, heart disease, and inflammatory diseases, including arthritis, are associated with and are probably caused by a poor oxidant/antioxidant balance. We now think aging causes this *same* imbalance.

Studies in the United States and China reveal the extent to which high tannin consumption results in a highly favorable oxidant/antioxidant balance.

We know smokers have a higher oxidant level. They produce more ROS than nonsmokers. Studies that look at smokers and nonsmokers show that smokers with high tea intake *still* achieve a favorable oxidant/antioxidant balance, even though they smoke. And of course, smoking is only one example of a condition that promotes oxidative stress. Tannins reduce oxidative stress no matter what causes it. Tannins may also protect our body's cells from harm caused by nitrates—obnoxious chemical substances found in commonly eaten fruits and vegetables and sometimes used as food preservatives.

Even though tea is consumed as three beverages—green, black, and oolong—all tea comes from green tea. Green tea contains the highest levels of tannins. Black tea—which is actually fermented green tea—contains two substances derived from tannins: theaflavins and thearubigins. Oolong tea—also fermented—has the least amount of tannins and other chemicals from green tea.

Tannins are among other poorly characterized compounds; they assume so many potential functions we are still entirely unclear what they are all about. This means tannins and many other complex compounds provoke investigators all over the world to continue scrutinizing them intensely, specifically because how these compounds *fully* relate to aging and disease prevention has not been figured out yet. With that in mind, you'll meet all the tannin-containing foods in chapter 7.

12. Monoterpenes: New Longevity Nutrients with a Knockout Punch

As we age, the likelihood that our cells change from normal to malignant increases. The more our bodies can control this process, the better we make our chances to remain healthy and realize our maximum life span. Since monoterpenes control cell growth and prevent the spread of malignancy, these longevity nutrients are invaluable.

Other longevity nutrients control cell growth, but monoterpenes are unique in the way they do this. While cholesterol is a chemical with essential functions, it is best known for the harmful things it does. Cells make cholesterol from very simple chemicals. One of these simple chemicals is farnesyl—a substance that regulates and promotes cell growth. Monoterpenes purposefully look for and selectively knock out farnesyl, but *only in malignant or pre-malignant* cells. The result? These malignant or pre-malignant cells are prevented from growing and reproducing.

Many monoterpenes are derived from a precursor—d-limonene, found in the peels of citrus fruits. Other monoterpenes include carveol, carvone, menthol, spearmint, and perillyl alcohol. Because of its pleasant fragrance, d-limonene is often added to cosmetics, soaps, and cleaning products. While we don't know if any fragrance enters our body, it certainly would be a creative way to obtain this longevity nutrient. Monoterpenes begin working the moment they are ingested. At once, monoterpenes assimilate into our body and transport themselves to various organs. But because monoterpenes metabolize so fast, they must be constantly replenished.

Monoterpenes not only stop the formation and progression of cancer cells, but they can also slow down malignant tumors that have already developed. Monoterpenes prevent carcinogens and other toxic chemicals from interacting with DNA, making it as hard as possible for them to promote cancer.

Finally, since monoterpenes interact with messenger or signal proteins that promote cell death they are invaluable to the prevention of aging.

13. Conjugated Linoleic Acid: One of Milk's Finest Longevity Nutrients

In recent years, you may have heard a lot about essential fatty acids—healthy substances found mostly in vegetable oils. Conjugated linoleic acid (CLA) is one of these essential fatty acids. Fats are lipids, and lipids are extremely versatile molecules involved in thousands of different metabolic functions. More than simply a calorie source for our body's energy, lipids help our brain cells function and enable the digestive tract to assimilate fat-soluble vitamins (A, D, E, and K).

Studies show that CLA may have extraordinary parts to play in regulation of cell division and growth, improving how our immune system works, and optimizing our body composition—all of which help with the reach to live longer and healthier.

CLA was discovered in 1991—to the surprise of many nutritionists—in the extracts of cooked meat. Other foods have CLA, but finding CLA in cooked meats was totally unexpected. It didn't seem to make sense, based on what we knew about what happens to meat during the cooking process. When meats are cooked—especially well cooked—they produce cancer-causing substances called heterocyclic amines. CLA, on the other hand, was found to be a potent anticarcinogen. But, unlike other anticarcinogens tested in lab studies, CLA was actually found in the body after foods with CLA were ingested.

CLA's powerful anticancer feature halts the initiation of tumors and their progression and growth. Our cells' walls are built with lipids, and CLA is found in our cells' walls. As already pointed out, the cell wall is part of the cell that exchanges information with other cells. CLA's presence in the cellular membranes means it's in a position to influence how the messenger chemicals that control cell death and tumor development are allowed to express themselves during the aging process.

CLA is a paradoxical molecule. It is both an antioxidant and an ROS! How can this be? CLA exists in an uncharged state. It can use its oxidative power to kill cancer cells. But this same uncharged state lets CLA function as a scavenger of ROS. CLA prevents cell damage from ROS, and at the same time, gets rid of any of our body's malfunctioning cells. Amazing.

Tests on laboratory animals show CLA works to benefit two types of body tissue that regulate body composition: fat and muscle. Ingesting CLA stimulates fat cells, but CLA also stimulates muscle cells to take *up* the fats. The result? A well-regulated body composition.

Milk and milk products are excellent sources of CLA. They are proven to raise body levels of CLA. Studies in Finland show milk consumption corresponds to a reduced risk of getting breast cancer. Studies with women who belong to the Hare Krishna religious group—who traditionally drink a lot of milk—have shown reduced cancer risks and tend to live longer than other groups of the population as well. Beef and lamb are also excellent sources of CLA.

14. Glutathione: Potent Multipurpose Longevity Nutrient

Glutathione, a longevity nutrient made up of three amino acids, is concentrated in our liver, lungs, and kidneys. These three organs, the toxic clearinghouse of our body, are brimming with glutathione to help them get rid of unwanted chemicals.

Homeostasis, the balance of all our body's functions, depends on glutathione to keep the proper balance between the number of toxic agents that enter our body and the number of toxic agents our body disposes of. When homeostasis is upset, aging is the result.

Glutathione is found in two parts of our cells: cytoplasm and mitochondria. In the cytoplasm, glutathione is a roving antioxidant. In the mitochondria, which holds about 10 percent of our glutathione, glutathione stays put and protects the mitochondria from ROS attack. In addition to detoxification, glutathione protects our body against carcinogens and helps maintain proper protein structure.

Glutathione's link to the aging process is definite. Proof from studies of glutathione levels in species ranging from mosquitoes to humans show an age-related decline: the older we get the more glutathione we lose.

Glutathione's versatility pinpoints our rising vulnerability to certain conditions as we age. The older we get, the more we expose ourselves to the possibility of developing an unhealthy or threatening condition. This vulnerability may be due to impairment of systems in our body that rely on glutathione—systems such as DNA repair, enzymes, and detoxification processes in our liver and immune systems.

Most tissues where glutathione is found keep it inside their cells. However, in the lungs, it is found in the cells' lining fluids called surfactant. Our eyes' lenses are particularly vulnerable to ROS attack because they are constantly exposed to sunlight, and light activates ROS production. With age, not only do glutathione levels decrease in our eyes' lenses, but, for people who develop cataracts in one or both of their eye's lenses, glutathione drops off even more.

Glutathione acts in the brain as a major neuroprotective substance. Even though the blood-brain barrier (BBB) is a key screen for what is allowed to get into our brain, toxicants, viruses, and other harmful substances often bypass the gate. Studies are beginning to reveal that glutathione works in areas of the brain especially vulnerable to toxic substances, protecting this vital organ from damage.

Levels of glutathione decrease with age, but we can replenish our supply of glutathione by eating glutathione-rich foods. Your body is depending on you to keep glutathione levels in the optimum antiaging range.

15. Organosulfur Compounds: Zest For Life

Some foods advertise their antiaging powers with a potent smell. Such is true of organosulfur compounds, the longevity nutrient discovered in a food group called the allium family. Allium family goods—onions, shallots, scallions, leeks, garlic, and chives—have been linked to low incidence of common cancers. People in countries bordering the Mediterranean Sea, who eat a lot of foods from the allium family, show reduced risks for developing colon and breast cancers. People in other parts of the world who share this reduced risk also show results of OCs' protective work. A good example are the populations of Poland, Italy, and the state of Georgia where Vidalia onions are grown.

In addition to helping other chemicals —such as glutathione—do their work, OCs shield our body from ROS damage and prevent carcinogenic nitrate compounds from forming. OCs fight harmful bacteria too. When you add onion or garlic to a menu, you are not only spicing up your life but extending it as well.

16. Lignans: A Hormone and an Antihormone at the Same Time

It's been about 20 years since the first lignans—one called enterolactone and the other enterodiol—were detected in humans. Since then, four more types of lignans have been discovered, and nutritionists think there are probably more. Lignans are present at exceptionally high levels in our body. They follow a cyclical pattern, similar to the hormones of the menstrual cycle, and it was this cyclical pattern that first alerted nutritionists to the fact that these longevity nutrients had similar effects to female sex hormones.

When first discovered, lignans were thought to be like estrogens. But further studies led scientists to conclude that lignans have more of an antiestrogen effect. This lends to a regulatory effect that keeps estrogen levels in check. High levels of estrogen have been linked to cancer, especially breast cancer, and keeping estrogen in the normal range mitigates its harmful effects on the body.

Lignans do not leave males out of the picture. In fact, lignans take care of the older male body. Lignans put the brakes on how male hormones are allowed to influence cell growth in the prostate. Lignans may not only be responsible for helping prevent prostate cancer, but also for lessening its susceptibility to the effects of aging.

17. Flavonoids

Flavonoids—a relatively new group of longevity nutrients—were actually discovered in 1936 by the same person who discovered vitamin C. Unlike vitamin C, however, flavonoids were not appreciated as important nutrients until about 15 years ago.

More than 4,000 different flavonoids exist, and this great variety of flavonoids is responsible for much of our food's taste, fragrance, texture, and astringency. And that's just the window dressing. Flavonoids also fight bacteria and viruses, reduce inflammation, block the effects of ROS, prevent blood clots, and work with various systems in the liver involved in detoxification.

Over the years, much attention has been paid to flavonoids' role in preventing heart disease and cancer. This function has given rise to the so-called "French paradox," a popular research subject. People who live in southern France experience a very low incidence of cardiovascular heart disease—even though they smoke and consume a high-fat diet. Medical researchers think the flavonoids in red wine, which people in southern France routinely drink, is the reason for their good health. A similar study in the Netherlands also showed coronary heart disease was much lower in elderly males who maintained a certain intake of flavonoids although their diet showed a much longer list of flavonoids sources: tea, onions, apples, and—again—red wine. In the United States, more than 30 percent of all deaths are caused by heart disease, and it has been estimated that the average American eats only about 170 milligrams of flavonoids per day, minuscule by French or Dutch standards.

As antioxidants, flavonoids suppress the oxidation of low density lipoproteins (LDLs or bad cholesterol) that creates cholesterol buildup in our arteries. Flavonoids also control the harmful oxidant effects of iron. In fact, in many cases, flavonoids are better antioxidants than vitamins C and E. However, they are rendered even more effective when eaten with vitamins C and E and with other known antioxidants.

QUERCETIN: A KEY FLAVONOID

The longevity nutrient quercetin belongs to a family of flavonoids called flavonols. One of the most common substances in this family, quercetin can help you achieve maximum life span in several ways. It protects LDL from oxidation, fights viruses, and prevents many types of cancer.

One of the most convincing arguments for quercetin's health benefits comes from the Netherlands. The dietary histories of thousands of people were studied to determine the effects of diet on heart disease development. This life-threatening problem was shown to be inversely related to the intake of flavonoids—and in particular, quercetin. In other words, people who consumed high quercetin levels were less likely to get heart disease.

How does this longevity nutrient achieve its benefits? The answer lies in its antioxidant role; quercetin scavenges ROS, binds harmful minerals, and prevents oxidation of LDL. Quercetin also targets cancerous and aged cells for elimination from the body.

One of the most important antiaging effects of quercetin is on our DNA. Damage to DNA such as "single strand breaks"—in which DNA is literally broken up—occurs with age and may have a range of causes. Quercetin, which has been shown to enter cells, inhibits strand breakage.

Quercetin has an important effect on inflammatory conditions, aiming to achieve a balanced response rather than an imbalanced one. Some inflammation is an important body defense, but too much can be debilitating.

You raise quercetin levels in the body by eating foods that contain it; a recent study showed that subjects who ate onions had detectable levels of quercetin in their blood for a full 48 hours afterward.

Research continues to look at our body's absorption rate of this these longevity nutrients, but in the meantime, we know the flavonoid-rich foods included in this program should be included in your diet.

We still have a long way to go to determine the effects of all the different flavonoids present in foods. At this point, only a relatively small number of flavonoids have been investigated, but results so far are encouraging. One flavonoid found in spices—such as thyme—prevents the glycation of proteins that usually comes with age, and other flavonoids in grapefruits help the liver eliminate toxins and break down medications.

18. Isoflavonoids: Genistein and Daidzein

Isoflavonoids: More Plant Hormones for Both Men and Women

Isoflavonoids belong to a group of flavonoids called phytoestrogens (plant estrogens), which are so named because they act in a similar fashion to the female hormone.

This family of plant chemicals includes many different substances, only some of which have been studied. Better known members of this family are genistein, daidzein, equol, coumestrol, and lignans.

Chemicals that act like estrogens are found in many different types of foods. Isoflavonoids, however, behave as both estrogens and *anti-estrogens* at the same time (remember lignans). In Japan, women suffer a much lower incidence of premenstrual syndrome (PMS), when compared with women living in the United States. They also experience a lower incidence of breast cancer. Phytoestrogens—including isoflavonoids—are the reason for this difference and are present in the various soybean foods consumed by Japanese women. Even though phytoestrogens are not as potent as women's own estrogen, high estrogen blood levels do result from such a diet. In fact, the estrogen blood levels in Japanese women who consume soybeans is much higher than the levels produced by their own bodies.

The irony here is that isoflavonoids stimulate the body like a hormone, yet they decrease the incidence of diseases caused by high hormone levels. We do not fully understand how these longevity nutrients accomplish this, but they do nonetheless. Combined with exercise and adequate calcium intake, isoflavonoids prevent bone loss and promote bone density in both men and women.

Phytoestrogens present science with a perplexing situation. Estrogen is an anabolic stimulatory hormone, associated with an increased risk of breast cancer, while, on the other hand, phytoestrogens correlate with a decreased incidence of breast cancer.

The isoflavonoid story does not apply only to women. Men whose diet is rich in animal fat are at higher risk of developing prostate cancer than those whose diet is rich in isoflavonoids. Vegetarians prove this—they exhibit low incidence of this disease. The same irony is at play here: prostate cancer is caused by high levels of hormones associated with a high-fat diet. But estrogen treatment of prostate cancer is one therapy that has brought success over the years. Adding phytoestrogens to a man's diet influences the metabolism of the prostate gland in the same way that estrogen therapy does. They also inhibit the conversion of the male hormone testosterone to the more harmful dihydrotestosterone.

In other words, a diet high in isoflavonoids changes the hormone mix in the body—improving health and preventing aging. Isoflavonoids—those helpful phytoestrogens—have much to offer people of both genders and all ages.

Genistein and Daidzein

These two isoflavonoids are mainly found in soybeans. Although historically they have been classified as phytoestrogens, genistein and daidzein have made antiaging effects apparent. One of these effects is to inhibit abnormal cell growth and proliferation. The group of proteins, called protein tyrosine kinases (PTK), are involved in abnormal growth of cells. Given the millions of cells in our body, it is understandable that some will become abnormal, but both genistein and daidzein are involved in regulating PTK expression in cells, regulating proliferation of cells.

Both of these compounds regulate blood vessel growth, which takes place with age. Blood vessel growth is called angiogenesis, and although it may seem like a good idea for the body to carry out this process, it is actually a hallmark of several diseases such as cancer, diabetes, and rheumatoid arthritis. Think of it in this way: if a tumor did not have access to a blood supply, it could not grow. Arthritis is a case in point: the inflammation in arthritis would stop because blood could not deliver inflammatory cells to it.

Genistein controls the growth of those endothelial cells involved in a proliferating artery. By doing this, genistein does not allow angiogenesis to take place, while leaving blood vessel maintenance undis-

COUMESTANS

The last group of estrogen-like longevity nutrients are the coumestans. They operate the same ways as the other plant hormones, mimicking the actions of estrogen with none of the negative side effects. But coumestans are as much as 15 times stronger in their estrogenic activity.

Of all the phytoestrogens, we know the least about coumestans, but they are currently being studied to learn more about their effects on the body. Regular consumption of them eases menopause symptoms, and recent research also suggests a role for them in the prevention of aging. Eating foods with coumestans provides another natural way to improve the body's estrogen status and access to its health benefits. I haven't included comments in this program, but look out for more information on them as research goes forward.

turbed. Genistein guards against the proliferation of blood vessel cells but also the proliferation of many cells that happen to be growing out of control.

Ingesting genistein and daidzein results in their accumulation not only in the blood, but in the liver, lungs, and kidney—where the highest levels are found. Moderate amounts are also found in the heart, muscle, and spleen, with the lowest amounts found in the brain and the male reproductive organs. In these various organs, genistein is a key antioxidant. Ingestion of these longevity nutrients halts the decline of the immune system with age (immunosenescence). Daidzein, in particular, has a stimulatory effect on lymphocytes and cytokines of our immune systems.

19. Isothiocyanates: Toxin Zappers

Isothiocyanates come from a food family called cruciferous vegetables, which includes broccoli, cabbage, and brussels sprouts. Isothiocyanates are chemopreventors. They work against the harmful chemicals that enter the body from the outside and the especially toxic ones produced as a result of metabolism. Found in several tissues including the lungs, breast, esophagus, liver, small intestine, colon, and bladder, isothiocyanates protect these delicate organs from damage by xenobiotics—toxic foreign chemicals that enter tissues.

Isothiocyanates affect chemoprevention by working with the sophisticated detoxification system called the cytochrome P-450 system—an essential part of our liver function. Because this detoxification system gets rid of xenobiotics, it is sometimes called the xenobiotic metabolizing system (XME).

The cytochrome P-450 system is extraordinarily sophisticated and is made up of two phases. Phase I has a set of enzymes that modify xenobiotics for combination with neutralizing chemicals. The actual combination and elimination of the toxin is the provenance of Phase II.

Although this may sound like a neat way to get rid of xenobiotics, it unfortunately does not always work to the advantage of your health. Sometimes the Phase I system, in the process of modifying xenobiotics, converts the xenobiotic into a *more* harmful chemical! Isothiocyanates modulate and depress the Phase I system so that xenobiotics don't become more harmful.

20. Carnitine

The longevity nutrient carnitine plays an integral role in the body's ability to make energy. Carnitine transports the fats to be burned by the mitochondria for generating energy. It should be no surprise, then, that areas of the body that require the most energy—the heart, muscles, brain, and kidneys—contain the highest amounts of carnitine. In addition to providing fuel, carnitine protects mitochondria by fighting the ROSs or free radical and DNA damage that usually come with aging.

Our body has the capacity to produce its own carnitine—a process requiring dietary proteins, vitamins, and minerals. Chances are, if you are emphasizing carbohydrates at the expense of protein, your body is not producing the most carnitine it has the potential to produce. But even if it were, our body alone is *still* not an adequate source of carnitine. Sufficient levels must be achieved by eating carnitine-rich foods. A study in which student volunteers were placed on a carnitine-deficient diet for 28 days helped establish this piece of knowledge. Over that time, they showed a 42 percent decline in their carnitine levels. When they increased their carnitine consumption at the end of the study, their levels increased to normal.

The repercussions of carnitine deficiency can be serious. Angina—the heart condition characterized by chest pains—is caused by the heart not receiving enough energy. Decreased carnitine levels in the brain have also been implicated in Alzheimer's disease. Extending its reach even further, carnitine deficiency has been connected to chronic fatigue syndrome. Recent investigations by scientists in the United Kingdom have shown that 70 percent of people with chronic fatigue syndrome have abnormal mitochondria and low blood levels of carnitine. With adequate carnitine intake, a significant number of these patients improve and enjoy higher levels of energy.

Carnitine also has an effect on how mitochondria ages. The total number of mitochondria in our cells seems to decline with age, making it harder for our organs to do their job. Carnitine levels also decline with age. It may be that by boosting carnitine levels we can repopulate our cells with mitochondria, while reinvigorating the ones we already have. There is much more to be learned about carnitine, considering all that we know about carnitine and some ideas that we just suspect. Ingesting foods with carnitine makes an awful lot of sense as an antiaging strategy.

21. Phytosterols: Cholesterol's Distant Cousin

Phytosterols, the plant version of cholesterol, occupy the last but not the best position in this list of longevity nutrients. At least 44 different phytosterols exist, but to date, most interest has focused on three of these: sitosterol, campesterol, and stigmasterol.

In the 1950s, scientists discovered that cholesterol levels in patients whose diets were supplemented with phytosterols decreased by as much as 20 percent. Not only were LDL levels reduced, but good cholesterol (HDL) levels were raised significantly. Around the world, diets rich in phytosterols are linked with low incidence of heart disease. A 1991 study showed that people in Japan, who consume about 373 milligrams of this longevity nutrient per day, experience lower incidences of heart disease than people in western countries such as Britain, where daily intake reaches only about 167 milligrams per day. Some populations consume even more phytosterols: the Tarahumara people of Mexico ingest more than 400 milligrams per day through a diet favoring beans and corn. In fact, for centuries, this group has been noted for their physical fitness and tradition of long-distance running.

How do plant sterols achieve these benefits? They interact with cells that line our blood vessels, preventing blood clots. This function prevents hardening of the arteries as well. Phytosterols also help prevent colon cancer by blocking the absorption of bad cholesterol, curbing the growth of harmful bacteria, and interacting with DNA to prevent gene abnormalities. Moreover, they stimulate our immune system by promoting the proliferation of lymphocytes. Phytosterols also have the ability to selectively locate and eliminate tumor cells by interacting with certain chemical pathways that control tumor cell growth. This effect extends well beyond our digestive tract cells, since even small amounts of these substances are found throughout the body. Phytosterols are even sent to the skin, spleen, liver, and lungs to prevent aging in these tissues. When you consider how easily bad cholesterol can invade your body and how precious phytosterol intake is, you cannot help but want to improve your diet. About 40 percent of the bad cholesterol you eat is absorbed into your body, but only about 5 percent of dietary phytosterols make it into your cells. Fortunately, a little bit goes a long way.

5

HOW TO LIVE TO BE 120 BY EATING THE RIGHT FOODS

The New Longevity Diet *Questionnaire*

The longevity nutrients' effects are manifold, affecting every system of the body, and it is of utmost importance to eat defined levels of these substances every day. But how can you make sure you are eating enough of the right foods? How can you learn the lifelong nutritional habits that open doors to maximum health and longevity? *The New Longevity Diet* is a comprehensive method designed to help you change your diet so that you may benefit from all the antiaging, disease-preventing powers of these remarkable compounds.

The *New Longevity Diet* program asks you to take a total of six steps which will allow you to identify the strengths and weaknesses of your current diet and help you begin to make necessary, positive changes:

Program Guideline

1. Check off the foods you eat in the food frequency questionnaire and score your diet using the scoring key on page 94.
2. Use your score to determine your overall longevity nutrient "fitness" by adding all of your scores from each food category. Compare this value with the optimum Overall Longevity Nutrient Quotient.
3. Compare your scores for each food category with the optimum level for each one. Determine whether you are at the optimum level, you are deficient, you are in need of improvement, or you have a poor intake.
4. To get an idea of which longevity nutrient you are deficient in for each food category, look at the scoring key on page 94, paying attention to the primary and secondary nutrients.
5. Follow the 21-day plan by designing your own eating program by choosing one of the longevity nutrients each day, paying special attention to the nutrients you are most deficient in.
6. Follow the 21-day menu plan, which provides all the food choices you need daily for each longevity nutrient, paying special attention to the nutrients you are most deficient in.

Note: If you suspect that you are significantly overweight, turn to Chapter 9 to determine your ideal weight. Then, use *The New Longevity Diet* weight loss program to achieve your goal weight. After you have reached that milestone, it's time to follow the steps above.

Designer-Style Eating Versus Menu-Style Eating

Everyone has different likes when it comes to a nutrition program—everyone has an individual eating style. Some people don't want to have to think about food; they hate planning their own meals and prefer programs that just tell them exactly what to eat and when to eat it with a complete menu. Many of my patients who prefer this method say it makes life better because they can carry their menus to the supermarket and do the shopping for the whole phase all at once. I call these patients "menu style."

Others hate being so regimented. They prefer to design their own menus, following the guidelines of *The New Longevity Diet* so that their meals will suit their day-to-day preferences. For some, it's not just the question of taste; many of my patients have common health concerns such as high cholesterol, high blood pressure, or allergies that necessitate their being able to personalize their menus. Regardless whether it's a question of palate or health, I call these patients "designer style."

Still, others are somewhere in between. They start out preferring specific menu plans but after a while, they want a little variety. As a result, they switch to the designer-style plan.

As different as these two styles are, they are equally valid. For this reason, *The New Longevity Diet* suits both styles.

For menu style people, I have provided specific day-to-day and meal-by-meal menus for you to follow. These menus are varied and are never boring. Accompanying this section are recipes for most of the entrees of each day.

For designer-style people, I have included lists of foods containing exact amounts of each longevity nutrient. There is also a list of the ideal amount of each longevity nutrient that you need per day.

For those who enjoy the benefits of both styles, they can easily pick and choose between the two approaches.

The New Longevity Diet will never ask you to ingest foods you don't like or find aversive. The complete longevity nutrient list on pages 120–137 as well as the 21-Day longevity nutrient recipe program (chapter 8) ensure your not having to eat any of the foods you dislike. You can build a diet and menu out of only the foods you prefer to eat and still reap the full benefits of the program!

The New Longevity Diet Questionnaire Instructions

By filling out the questionnaire before you start the program, you will not only determine the adequacy of your present diet in the longevity nutrients, you will discover what you must do to change it. Do not be daunted by the project, though. I have seen people even with the lowest scores significantly change their longevity nutrient intake without any problems.

The food frequency questionnaire is designed to provide objective information about how often you presently eat the longevity nutrients. At first sight, this kind of questionnaire may seem to be an inadequate way to determine information about one's whole diet. On the contrary, this method has been proven quite accurate in terms of what it can tell you. So it serves as a great starting point from which to embark on the *Longevity Diet* program.

The questionnaire contains seven categories of commonly eaten foods and is designed to check your consumption of these foods over the last six months. For most people, checking their diet for this duration of time is an accurate measure of their longevity nutrient intake over the last two years. For each food, there is a frequency of eating this food and a score that gives it a certain power for the amounts and types of longevity nutrients. The questionnaire is done by circling the frequency and adding it to the longevity nutrient points. By adding together the frequency and longevity nutrient points for all the foods in a section, you can arrive at a score that indicates how adequate your present diet is in longevity nutrients for this category. Your score will tell you if your diet is optimum, needs improvement, is deficient, or is poor. Certain foods are seasonal foods, and if that food is not available, follow the scoring as indicated.

The result is your personalized New Longevity Nutrient Quotient (see chart below).

The Most Frequently Asked Questions About the Questionnaire.

1. What happens if I like and eat a food that is not on the questionnaire?

Most of the foods in the questionnaire are commonly eaten by practically everyone and I've never had a patient who couldn't fill out the questionnaire to get meaningful information about their longevity nutrient intake.

2. Why aren't all the foods normally eaten listed on the questionnaire?

The questionnaire is carefully designed to represent foods with optimum longevity nutrients. In this way, it is a vehicle to measure and rate your current longevity nutrient intake.

3. I just determined my score and it is very low. Can I change my diet so that I can get enough of the longevity nutrients?

You certainly can. In fact, the longevity nutrient program was devised so that people with the lowest scores can significantly improve their longevity nutrient intake and all their antiaging effects. People with the largest new longevity nutrient deficits can change their diets to gain the age-preventing, disease-fighting benefits of these.

4. I take vitamin and mineral supplements. How do they relate to the questionnaire?

The questionnaire does not bother with supplements because they do not contain longevity nutrients, and therefore are not a factor in determining longevity nutrient levels.

5. I'm not sure if my intake of a certain vegetable is once per week or only monthly. Is this important?

Try to be accurate. Most people are able to be accurate about their frequency of consumption, but if you need help, ask your spouse, a family member, or a friend if they can help you.

The New Longevity Nutrient Questionnaire is designed to show you the adequacy of your longevity nutrients for each of the major food groups and to point you in the direction to making the right choices to correct your longevity nutrient intake. To answer this questionnaire circle the frequency of each food in your diet. Add this frequency to the corresponding number of Longevity Nutrient Points. If you choose "N" for almost never, do not add any New Nutrient Points to the total column for that food. When you are finished add all the numbers in the "Total" column to find your Longevity Nutrient Intake level for that food group.

Sample Questionnaire

Food	Frequency	Longevity Nutrient Points	Total
grape or grape juice	N, 0, (1), 2, 3, 4, 5	1	**2**
peach	(N), 0, 1, 2, 3, 4, 5	2	**0**
apple, apple juice, or cider	N, 0, (1), 2, 3, 4, 5	2	**3**
banana	N, 0, (1), 2, 3, 4, 5	2	**3**
papaya	N, (0), 1, 2, 3, 4, 5	1	**1**
berries or berry juice	N, 0, 1, 2, (3), 4, 5	2	**5**
orange or orange juice	N, 0, 1, 2, 3, (4), 5	2	**6**
grapefruit or grapefruit juice	(N), 0, 1, 2, 3, 4, 5	2	**0**
lemon or lime beverages or foods	N, 0, (1), 2, 3, 4, 5	2	**3**
pear or pear juice	N, (0), 1, 2, 3, 4, 5	3	**3**
plum	N, 0, (1), 2, 3, 4, 5	2	**3**
tomato or tomato juice	N, 0, 1, (2), 3, 4, 5	3	**5**
avocado	N, 0, 1, (2), 3, 4, 5	1	**3**

Remember, if you circle "N," do NOT add the Longevity Nutrient Points!

Frequency:

Total Fruit and Fruit Juice Points = 37

N = almost never

0 = 2–3 times per month

1 = once per week

2 = twice per week

3 = three times per week

4 = four times per week

5 = five or more times per week

New Nutrient Questionnaire

Vegetables	Frequency	Longevity Nutrient Points	Total
leeks or scallions	N, 0, 1, 2, 3, 4, 5	2	
lettuce	N, 0, 1, 2, 3, 4, 5	2	
cauliflower	N, 0, 1, 2, 3, 4, 5	4	
carrots	N, 0, 1, 2, 3, 4, 5	3	
mushrooms	N, 0, 1, 2, 3, 4, 5	3	
spinach	N, 0, 1, 2, 3, 4, 5	4	
asparagus	N, 0, 1, 2, 3, 4, 5	4	
potato	N, 0, 1, 2, 3, 4, 5	4	
sweet potato	N, 0, 1, 2, 3, 4, 5	1	
corn	N, 0, 1, 2, 3, 4, 5	3	
broccoli	N, 0, 1, 2, 3, 4, 5	3	
onions or shallots	N, 0, 1, 2, 3, 4, 5	3	
brussels sprouts	N, 0, 1, 2, 3, 4, 5	3	
garlic	N, 0, 1, 2, 3, 4, 5	3	
cabbage	N, 0, 1, 2, 3, 4, 5	4	
celery	N, 0, 1, 2, 3, 4, 5	2	
artichoke	N, 0, 1, 2, 3, 4, 5	1	

Frequency:

N = almost never

0 = 2–3 times per month

1 = once per week

2 = twice per week

3 = three times per week

4 = four times per week

5 = five or more times per week

Total Vegetable Points ______

84+ Optimum

67–83 Needs Improvement

50–66 Deficient

49– Poor

KEEP IN MIND:

Think about the use of vegetables based upon the season. Depending on where you live, you may eat certain vegetables over others at different times of the year. If this is the case, determine the new optimum by subtracting the Longevity Nutrient Points for that vegetable from the current optimum.

New Nutrient Questionnaire

Fruits or Fruit Juices	Frequency	Longevity Nutrient Points	Total
grape* or grape juice	N, 0, 1, 2, 3, 4, 5	1	
peach*	N, 0, 1, 2, 3, 4, 5	2	
apple or apple juice	N, 0, 1, 2, 3, 4, 5	2	
banana	N, 0, 1, 2, 3, 4, 5	2	
papaya	N, 0, 1, 2, 3, 4, 5	1	
berries*† or berry juice	N, 0, 1, 2, 3, 4, 5	2	
orange or orange juice	N, 0, 1, 2, 3, 4, 5	2	
grapefruit or grapefruit juice	N, 0, 1, 2, 3, 4, 5	2	
lemon or lime beverages or foods	N, 0, 1, 2, 3, 4, 5	1	
pear	N, 0, 1, 2, 3, 4, 5	3	
plum*	N, 0, 1, 2, 3, 4, 5	2	
tomato or tomato juice	N, 0, 1, 2, 3, 4, 5	3	
avocado	N, 0, 1, 2, 3, 4, 5	1	

Frequency:

N = almost never

0 = 2–3 times per month

1 = once per week

2 = twice per week

3 = three times per week

4 = four times per week

5 = five or more times per week

Total fruits/juice points = ______

46+ Optimum

37–45 Needs Improvement

28–36 Deficient

27– Poor

* indicates a seasonal fruit; if that fruit is not available at this time of year, the optimum is lower (40 or above).

† includes strawberries, blueberries, raspberries, and blackberries

KEEP IN MIND:

Don't forget fruits and berries used in desserts or condiments. The small amounts in these foods have significant levels of longevity nutrients.

New Nutrient Questionnaire

Dairy Products	Frequency	Longevity Nutrient Points	Total
Parmesan cheese	N, 0, 1, 2, 3, 4, 5	2	
Gruyere cheese	N, 0, 1, 2, 3, 4, 5	2	
milk (skim, lowfat, or whole)	N, 0, 1, 2, 3, 4, 5	2	
Provolone cheese	N, 0, 1, 2, 3, 4, 5	1	
ice cream	N, 0, 1, 2, 3, 4, 5	1	
Colby cheese	N, 0, 1, 2, 3, 4, 5	2	
Ricotta cheese	N, 0, 1, 2, 3, 4, 5	2	
Muenster cheese	N, 0, 1, 2, 3, 4, 5	2	
Mozzarella cheese	N, 0, 1, 2, 3, 4, 5	2	
Cheddar cheese	N, 0, 1, 2, 3, 4, 5	2	
Swiss cheese	N, 0, 1, 2, 3, 4, 5	1	
Blue cheese	N, 0, 1, 2, 3, 4, 5	2	
American processed cheese	N, 0, 1, 2, 3, 4, 5	2	
cottage cheese	N, 0, 1, 2, 3, 4, 5	3	
Cream cheese	N, 0, 1, 2, 3, 4, 5	2	
Romano cheese	N, 0, 1, 2, 3, 4, 5	2	
Gouda cheese	N, 0, 1, 2, 3, 4, 5	2	
yogurt	N, 0, 1, 2, 3, 4, 5	1	

Frequency:

N = almost never

0 = 2–3 times per month

1 = once per week

2 = twice per week

3 = three times per week

4 = four times per week

5 = five or more times per week

Total dairy points= ______

45+ Optimum

36–44 Needs Improvement

27–35 Deficient

26– Poor

KEEP IN MIND:

Remember to include any foods that contain dairy products, such as pizza, milk added to beverages, and desserts with cream.

New Nutrient Questionnaire

Nuts and Seeds	Frequency	Longevity Nutrient Points	Total
pumpkin, sesame, or sunflower seeds	N, 0, 1, 2, 3, 4, 5	1	
almond	N, 0, 1, 2, 3, 4, 5	3	
cashew	N, 0, 1, 2, 3, 4, 5	3	
pecan	N, 0, 1, 2, 3, 4, 5	2	
pistachio	N, 0, 1, 2, 3, 4, 5	2	
walnut	N, 0, 1, 2, 3, 4, 5	1	

Frequency:

N = almost never

0 = 2–3 times per month

1 = once per week

2 = twice per week

3 = three times per week

4 = four times per week

5 = five or more times per week

Total Nut/Seeds points ______

16+ Optimum

13–15 Needs Improvement

10–12 Deficient

9– Poor

KEEP IN MIND:

Remember to include any foods that contain nuts or seeds, such as pastries and candy. Whether by themselves or eaten as part of a food, they count as a serving.

New Nutrient Questionnaire

Grains, Pastas, and Cereals	Frequency	Longevity Nutrient Points	Total
wheat, whole-wheat, or cracked bread	N, 0, 1, 2, 3, 4, 5	4	
rye or pumpernickel bread	N, 0, 1, 2, 3, 4, 5	3	
Italian or French bread	N, 0, 1, 2, 3, 4, 5	1	
pita bread	N, 0, 1, 2, 3, 4, 5	1	
muffin	N, 0, 1, 2, 3, 4, 5	2	
pasta	N, 0, 1, 2, 3, 4, 5	1	
rice cereal	N, 0, 1, 2, 3, 4, 5	1	
bagel	N, 0, 1, 2, 3, 4, 5	2	
corn bread	N, 0, 1, 2, 3, 4, 5	1	
bran breads or cereals (high fiber)	N, 0, 1, 2, 3, 4, 5	3	
white rice	N, 0, 1, 2, 3, 4, 5	4	
pancakes	N, 0, 1, 2, 3, 4, 5	1	
rolls, biscuits, or buns	N, 0, 1, 2, 3, 4, 5	2	
oats	N, 0, 1, 2, 3, 4, 5	3	
saltine, Ritz, or Wheat Thins crackers	N, 0, 1, 2, 3, 4, 5	1	
wheat cereal (i.e., Wheaties)	N, 0, 1, 2, 3, 4, 5	3	
granola	N, 0, 1, 2, 3, 4, 5	2	

Frequency:

N = almost never

0 = 2–3 times per month

1 = once per week

2 = twice per week

3 = three times per week

4 = four times per week

5 = five or more times per week

Total grains, etc. points ______

70+ Optimum

56–69 Needs Improvement

42–55 Deficient

41 – Poor

KEEP IN MIND:

There are hundreds of foods that make up cereals, breads, and other grain products. Consult the Longevity Nutrient Chart if you are confused about this group of foods.

New Nutrient Questionnaire

Meats/Fish/Seafood and Beans	Frequency	Longevity Nutrient Points	Total
turkey	N, 0, 1, 2, 3, 4, 5	5	
chicken	N, 0, 1, 2, 3, 4, 5	4	
beef	N, 0, 1, 2, 3, 4, 5	4	
lamb	N, 0, 1, 2, 3, 4, 5	2	
veal	N, 0, 1, 2, 3, 4, 5	4	
pork	N, 0, 1, 2, 3, 4, 5	5	
fish	N, 0, 1, 2, 3, 4, 5	3	
seafood	N, 0, 1, 2, 3, 4, 5	3	
soy foods (tofu, soy bacon, soy yogurt, etc.)	N, 0, 1, 2, 3, 4, 5	4	
green peas or beans	N, 0, 1, 2, 3, 4, 5	3	
dried beans	N, 0, 1, 2, 3, 4, 5	3	
peanuts	N, 0, 1, 2, 3, 4, 5	4	

Frequency:

N = almost never

0 = 2–3 times per month

1 = once per week

2 = twice per week

3 = three times per week

4 = four times per week

5 = five or more times per week

Total meat points ______

55+ Optimum

44–54 Needs Improvement

33–43 Deficient

32– Poor

KEEP IN MIND:

If you are not familiar with the different types of beans, read the section on saponins. Also, if you regularly eat wild game such as venison, check the beef category. For pheasant or partridge, check the chicken category.

New Nutrient Questionnaire

Beverages	Frequency	Longevity Nutrient Points	Total
red wine	N, 0, 1, 2, 3, 4, 5	3	
oolong tea	N, 0, 1, 2, 3, 4, 5	1	
green tea	N, 0, 1, 2, 3, 4, 5	3	
black tea	N, 0, 1, 2, 3, 4, 5	2	

Frequency:

N = almost never

0 = 2–3 times per month

1 = once per week

2 = twice per week

3 = three times per week

4 = four times per week

5 = five or more times per week

Total beverage points ______

20+ Optimum

16–19 Needs Improvement

12–15 Deficient

11– Poor

KEEP IN MIND:

Do not include herbal teas, but do include any black or green teas that are flavored or have condiments added to them.

Your Overall Longevity Nutrient Quotient

Optimum Score	Needs Improvement	Deficient	Poor
336+	269–335	202–268	201–

Your Specific Longevity Nutrient Quotient

Vegetables:

Optimum: 84

Needs Improvement: 67–83

Deficient: 50–66

Poor: 49–

If you scored less than the optimum for *Vegetables,* concentrate on

Primary: **phytosterols, guercetin,** and **glutathione**

Secondary: **PQQ, OCs,** and **isothiocyanates**

Your Specific Longevity Nutrient Quotient

Fruits and Fruit Juices:

Optimum: 46+

Needs Improvement: 37–45

Deficient: 28–36

Poor: 27–

If you scored less than the optimum for *Fruits and Fruit Juices,* concentrate on

Primary: **monoterpenes, CLA,** and **phytosterols**

Secondary: **guercetin** and **tannins**

Your Specific Longevity Nutrient Quotient

Dairy Products:

Optimum: 45+

Needs Improvement: 36–44

Deficient: 27–35

Poor: 26–

If you scored less than the optimum for *Dairy Products,* concentrate on **CLA, glutamine,** and **arginine.**

Your Specific Longevity Nutrient Quotient

Nuts and Seeds:
Optimum: 16+
Needs Improvement: 13–15
Deficient: 10–12
Poor: 9–

If you scored less than the optimum for *Nuts and Seeds,* concentrate on
Primary: **arginine** and **phytates**
Secondary: **phytosterols** and **protease inhibitors**

Your Specific Longevity Nutrient Quotient

Grains, Pastas, and Cereals:
Optimum: 70+
Needs Improvement: 56–69
Deficient: 42–55
Poor: 41–

If you scored less than the optimum for *Grains, Pastas, and Cereals,* concentrate on **glutamine, arginine, lignans,** and **phytates.**

Your Specific Longevity Nutrient Quotient

Meats, Fish, Seafood, and Beans:
Optimum: 55+
Needs Improvement: 44–54
Deficient: 33–43
Poor: 32–

If you scored less than the optimum for *Meats, Fish, Seafood, and Beans,* concentrate on
Primary: **nucleotides, arginine, saponins,** and **carnitine**
Secondary: **taurine, exorphins, phytoestrogens,** and **phytates**

Your Specific Longevity Nutrient Quotient

Beverages:
Optimum: 20+
Needs Improvement: 16–19
Deficient: 12–15
Poor: 11 –

If you scored less than the optimum for *Beverages,* concentrate on **PQQ, tannins,** and **quercetin.**

6

WHAT'S WRONG WITH THE WAY AMERICANS EAT?

If twenty people were to answer the question, "What's wrong with the way Americans eat?" they probably would offer twenty different replies. Such differences of opinion lead many Americans to become confused about nutrition, explaining why many do not eat properly. These dietary deficiencies are present in spite of the fact that we have access to more foods and nutritional supplements than any other country in the world. Further, millions of dollars are spent annually on nutrition research in the United States. Despite this knowledge and concern, however, Americans just do not seem to know what or how to eat.

Why is there so much confusion? Blame it on the press, on television health reporters, on physicians not fully trained in the science of nutrition, or on the nutrition community itself. Probably all of the above share responsibility for the puzzlement. A famous professor of nutrition at the Massachusetts Institute of Technology once stated that 99 percent of the population has opinions about nutrition, but only one percent has the facts. Because of this lack of factual knowledge, most people are unsure about the nutritional content of particular foods, or about which foods they should eat or avoid. No matter who is to blame, the American people are eating poorly, getting more obese than ever, suffering from all manner of preventable chronic illnesses, and dying too young.

What do Nutritionists Know About the Way Americans Eat?

Approximately every ten years, nutritionists analyze comprehensive surveys of America's eating habits. The most recent survey was completed in 1991, and the data illustrated that certain dietary trends had changed since the previous survey. First of all, Americans are reducing their high cholesterol levels. Also, children generally are eating better. Almost everyone is eating meat, poultry, and fish, drinking milk, consuming more vegetables and fruits, and nearly everyone consumes a variety of grain products—pasta, pizza, bread, rolls, cereals, and desserts.

The same surveys also show, however, that Americans are ingesting high amounts of caloric sweeteners, such as high fructose corn syrups, and low-calorie soft drinks. Between 1972 and 1992, for example, the consumption of regular and low-calorie soft drinks climbed alarmingly from 26 to 44 gallons per person each year. Additionally, this survey revealed that 35 to 40 percent of the population takes dietary supplements, though this practice is more common in women than in men. The most popular supplements are vitamin and mineral combinations—or megavitamins—single vitamins such as vitamin C, and minerals such as calcium.

At first glance, the survey results may sound like good news: Americans are eating pretty well and are concerned with getting enough vitamins and minerals. On the one hand, this is true. American eating habits have definitely improved since the last study as evidenced by fewer vitamin and mineral deficiencies and, with the exception of too much fat intake, little overconsumption of most nutrients. But is everyone choosing the right foods for a healthy combination of nutrients? Are we gaining every advantage our diet can offer? When you take into consideration research and knowledge gained about the longevity nutrients, the answer is a resounding "No!"

When counseling patients about nutrition-related issues, I check for several factors that I have found to lead to poor nutrition. Only when people understand the following *eight causes of poor eating habits* can they begin to change their diets.

Over my 20-plus years of practice, I've seen the American diet improve. However, the underlying problems that lead to less-than-optimal nutrition have remained stubbornly intractable.

Eight Causes of Poor Eating Habits

CAUSE 1: MISINFORMATION

One of my new patients complained, "First they say that margarine is good for you, and then they say it's bad. Salt used to be bad for you, and now it's not. I don't listen to *them* anymore." The ongoing nutritional debates occurring among health experts often frustrate and confuse people.

Different claims about nutrition abound, but the sad fact is that many are poorly substantiated. Take, for example, caffeine. Many people think caffeine is a harmful substance and that drinking coffee causes health problems. Upon studying the research on caffeine and coffee consumption, however, one is hard put to find a report, in any reputable medical journal, arguing that drinking one or two cups of coffee a day is harmful. Misinformation like this often leads one to eat or avoid the wrong foods, or to give up on trying to follow correct nutritional advice altogether.

Although tremendous strides have been made in expanding the public's basic nutrition knowledge, many areas still cause confusion. People think that vitamins and minerals are the only substances that count in a food, but as you will see, there are much more important components of food than these substances. By gaining a better understanding of nutrition through the *New Longevity Diet*, you can learn to avoid that mire of confusion. You can sidestep the frustration that comes as the media hails a "super food" one day, only to declare the next that it is a food to avoid at all costs.

CAUSE 2: OVER-RELIANCE ON ONE OF THE MAJOR FOOD GROUPS

Most adults have been taught the importance of a well-balanced diet, but many ignore this advice and concentrate on one food group at the expense of the others. Often, this choice is based on the belief that one group is healthier than another. Dieters are probably familiar with this kind of advice: eat either a high-protein or a high-carbohydrate diet in order to lose weight. Eating this way, however, can lead to nutrient imbalances and cause poor nutritional health in some dieters. By including all the food groups in one's diet, a person gains access to a variety of nutrients without the threat of deficiency or imbalance. Using the longevity nutrient questionnaire will provide valuable information regarding your balance of longevity nutrient.

CAUSE 3: EATING FOR THE WRONG REASONS

The human body has a demanding physiology dependent on food. Often, this physiology can get out of sync, especially when one is under stress, depressed, or even elated. This condition often occurs because people rely on food as a way to deal with stresses and emotions. Many eat even when their bodies do not require any nutrients. Such a habit is problematic because people may begin to misuse foods to combat their psychological and emotional problems, instead of using foods to provide nutritional benefits. What results is a situation in which people choose and eat the wrong foods, ones that are harmful to their health.

CAUSE 4: TIME—IT SHOULD BE ON YOUR SIDE

Recent studies have confirmed that Americans have more free time now than they had 40 years ago. At the same time, however, many feel stressed and pressured for time as they cram work, family and home responsibilities, and social activities into their lives. Consequently, many feel that time spent doing "nothing" is wasteful, while investing more time in work is highly esteemed. Unfortunately, not enough Americans value eating time as important. So they tend to de-emphasize it when faced with other activities. They cannot be faulted for wanting to eat as quickly as possible so that they can proceed with the rest of their day. However, when Americans "grab a bite," they often choose foods lacking the adequate nutrient levels one would receive in a carefully and properly prepared meal.

CAUSE 5: LESS RELIANCE ON NATURAL FOODS

How many times did your mother recommend a snack of diet soda and cotton candy? Probably not as frequently as she advised you to eat "carrots to see well" and "fish to make you smarter." The logic is as true today as it was many years ago: the more processed a food, the poorer the nutrient content. Synthetic (man-made) foods do not contain all the different nutritious substances found in natural foods. So, mother's advice has stood the test of time. As more and more studies are conducted, it becomes clearer that natural foods offer a multitude of health benefits never duplicated in synthetic foods. A diet filled with natural foods leads to greater intake of the longevity nutrients.

CAUSE 6: MORE RELIANCE ON SUPPLEMENTS

More Americans are taking vitamin, mineral, and other nutritional supplements than ever before, which may explain why deficiencies of those nutrients are uncommon. While this sounds like good news, upon further investigation one can see the problems that result. First of all, taking supplements provides the body with concentrated amounts of only that supplement—not all the other substances a balanced diet of natural foods can provide. Second, because most people are confused about nutritional data, they have a hard time determining which supplements to take. Finally, supplements provide a set amount of a particular nutrient, regardless of whether that amount is adequate for that individual's dietary needs. More often than not, serious health repercussions could result because too much of some supplements can be dangerous. Because supplements are nonprescription, people often take too much license and misuse or overuse them. I'm not saying supplements are bad—they must be taken with a properly balanced diet, not in place of one.

CAUSE 7: CUTTING BACK ON FATS

Believe it or not, one of the most common factors responsible for poor eating habits is concern over fat and caloric intake. Obviously, excess weight is a health hazard and should be avoided. The desire to stay slim, however, often results in nutritional compromises. Cutting back on fats—which is good—sometimes leads to nutrient deficiencies as whole groups of foods are avoided because they can be considered "bad." But some of these "bad" foods may contain essential longevity nutrients. One must carefully ensure that adequate nutrient levels are consumed during a low-calorie regimen—not an easy feat.

CAUSE 8: SITUATIONS

One should never underestimate the effect of one's surroundings on eating behavior. People often eat differently when they are at a party, on vacation, or at work. Enough of these situational changes in one's life can have a powerfully negative effect on nutrient intake.

Each of these eight factors can negatively affect one's diet, causing imbalances in vitamins, minerals, macronutrients, carbohydrates, protein, and fats. Although current eating behaviors may pose a threat to adequate vitamin and mineral consumption, the real problem is lack of knowledge about the longevity nutrients. These amazing substances hold the keys to a truly balanced diet and the prevention of aging.

7

THE 21-DAY *NEW LONGEVITY DIET* FOR "DESIGNER-STYLE" EATERS

Now that you are better informed about how the longevity nutrients function, it is time to put theory into practice. Read the program's ground rules, then refer to "The 21-Day Guide" for each day's longevity nutrient, a brief explanation of its benefits, and tables revealing its sources. Now you can embark on your own personalized program for optimum health and maximum longevity.

The New Longevity Diet for "designer-style" eaters requires a commitment from you. You're going to have to give serious thought to how you plan your meals and your shopping. But the rewards of this are immense. You'll see your diet filled with foods that once were forbidden, you'll be experiencing a great variety in your eating, and you'll be substantially improving your health as well!

This is a habit-changing program. It's been my experience with my patients that giving people hard-and-fast rules to follow makes it easier to get into a new style of eating. After you've gone through the cycle once, you'll be eating with the longevity nutrients in mind fairly easily. My patients report that they soon begin integrating the longevity nutrients into their diets unconsciously. After the first three weeks, you should feel free to take a looser approach. Try and keep your longevity nutrient levels high, but don't beat yourself up over it. A great way of doing this is simply to make some key longevity nutrient foods part of your regular diet.

So with all of that in mind, read on. It's time to eat for a long and healthy life!

Program Guidelines: The Ground Rules

1. Choose foods from that list that contain the longevity nutrient for that day.
2. Pick two foods containing that longevity nutrient and use them in two different meals/snacks for that day.

So What Does a Serving Look Like?

Since all of the foods recommended in the program are low in fat, you need not be so concerned with serving sizes. However, the following guide helps you determine how much food is meant by a "serving."

Bread, Cereal, Rice, and Pasta

One serving =

- 1 slice of bread
- 1 oz. of ready-to-eat cereal, rice, or pasta
- ½ cup of cooked cereal, rice, or pasta
- 3 or 4 small, plain crackers

Vegetables

One serving =

- 1 cup of raw leafy vegetables
- ½ cup of other vegetables, cooked or chopped raw
- ¾ cup of vegetable juice

Fruits

One serving =

1 medium piece of fruit (for example, apple, banana, orange)
½ cup chopped, cooked, or canned fruit
¾ cup fruit juice

Milk, Yogurt, Cheese

One serving =

1 cup of milk or yogurt
1½ oz. of natural cheese
2 oz. of processed cheese

Meat, Poultry, Fish, Dry Beans, Eggs, and Nuts

One serving =

2–3 oz. of cooked lean meat, poultry, or fish
½ cup of dry beans
1–2 eggs cooked
2 tablespoons of peanut butter

How much is 1 ounce of meat, chicken, fish, or cheese? Refer to this table:

1 oz. of lean meat, poultry, or cheese = the size of a matchbook
3 oz. = the size of a deck of cards
8 oz. = the size of a paperback book

Background Foods

To review, on each day of *The New Longevity Diet,* you will focus on one longevity nutrient. On days in which that nutrient comes from fruits, vegetables, or dairy you should ingest two servings. On days in which the longevity nutrient comes from protein foods, you should eat 1–2 servings of proteins. And on the day in which the longevity nutrient source is a grain, you should eat 2 servings of grains.

Of course, even though one food group provides the emphasized longevity nutrient each day, you must also eat foods from the other groups. The following chart is a handy guide to consult to determine the number of background servings to use with each longevity nutrient:

Longevity Nutrient Type	Longevity Nutrient Serving	Vegetables	Fruits	Grains: Bread, Rice, Cereals, Pasta	Meat, Poultry, Fish, Eggs, Nuts, Beans	Dairy Products: Milk, Yogurt, Cheese
Vegetables	2	3	3	6	2	2
Fruits	2	5	1	6	2	2
Grains: rice, bread, cereals, pasta	2	5	3	4	2	2
Meat, Poultry, Fish, Eggs Nuts, Beans	2	5	3	6	0	2
Dairy Products: Milk, Yogurt, Cheese	2	5	3	6	2	0

The 21-Day Guide to Longevity Nutrient Sources

Any nutritionist will tell you that if you want to increase your body's levels of a vitamin or mineral, you need to know how much of that nutrient is present in the foods or beverages you plan to eat. Although nutrients can be lost during food preparation (or even after food is ingested), if you start off knowing the exact amounts of a nutrient in a food, you have all the data you need to increase its levels in your body.

The promise of *The New Longevity Diet* is that you will be able to raise longevity nutrient levels in your body's various systems just by eating certain foods. This goal is achieved by choosing longevity nutrients from the lists of foods on pages 120–137. One list is provided for each longevity nutrient in those foods. In fact, this is probably the most concise compilation of food levels of these substances that has ever been published.

I am often asked how accurate the longevity nutrient values are. The utmost care has been taken to ensure that not only are the determinations precise, but also that the data are the latest available.

Beginning with nucleotides and ending with the phytosterols, here is the 21-day guide to the longevity nutrients and the common foods in which they can be found. A complete RDA chart for the longevity nutrients can be found at the end of this chapter.

Day #1: Nucleotides

Although the body can make nucleotides itself, we especially benefit from dietary sources. Nucleotides are found in many different foods because food cells contain nucleotides as the building blocks of their own DNA. It is easy to obtain some nucleotides in the diet, but the trick is getting enough. Choose foods with the most concentrated levels, such as certain types of fish, seafood, and beef.

Among grains and vegetables, nucleotide concentrations depend on the levels of cells in these foods. The shoots of plants are good nutritional choices. Growing plants are good, too; they contain more cells because they are in the process of adding new cells (along with their attendant nucleotides).

Significant levels of nucleotides are found in protein foods and some high-fiber carbohydrates. One or two servings of fish, other seafood, or poultry is an excellent choice for this longevity nutrient. Vegetarians can choose legumes for this day. Baby corn is a growing plant, and asparagus is a shoot, so these are also good vegetable choices.

Day #2: Saponins

It is too bad we cannot eat starfish, for these small marine animals are loaded with saponins. But until we find a way of cooking starfish—and I am not so sure we would want to anyway—we must content ourselves with eating the standard sources of this valuable longevity nutrient.

Saponins are found predominantly in dry beans or pulses. This is a culinary treat because so many of these foods are found in ethnic dishes. Caribbean and Latin American cuisines are based on dry beans, and eating these cuisines is an excellent way to maximize saponin intake. If preparing or eating ethnic cuisine is not practical for you, add a serving of dry beans to salads, soups, or vegetable dishes. They are low in calories, and if the entree dish is low fat, larger amounts can be eaten. In addition to being one of the most nourishing of foods, dry beans are among the oldest cultivated foods. The ancient Egyptians grew legumes, as did other people of Africa, the Americas, China, and India.

From a nutritional standpoint, all pulses contain similar amounts of protein, carbohydrate, fats, vitamins, and minerals, though they differ in saponin levels. The following are some examples:

- *Pinto beans*: Named from the Spanish word for "painted," because they have a combination of brown and red colors painted on their surface. They are good in chili, refried beans, and other Tex-Mex recipes.
- *Great Northern beans*: Belong to the white bean family. Excellent in soups and stews.
- *Garbanzo beans*: Their history goes back to ancient Rome, where they were a dietary staple. They are also known as chickpeas. Found in Middle Eastern and Caribbean cuisine.
- *Lima beans*: Also known as butter beans. The American Indians used these beans in such dishes as succotash (a combination of corn and lima beans stewed together). They can be included in many vegetable side dishes.
- *Navy beans*: The most widely used of all the beans, especially in such dishes as baked beans and "pork and beans." These also belong to the white bean family.
- *Kidney beans*: So named because their shape resembles the kidney. They have a light red or brown color and are widely used in many different dishes.
- *Black beans*: Used in many ethnic dishes in Latin America, the Caribbean, and the Middle East.
- *Black-eyed peas (cow peas):* So named because of the black dot on their cream-colored skin. They can be cooked without presoaking and are popular in many different ethnic cuisines.
- *Lentils:* Are commonly used in soups and sometimes as sprouts. They are probably eaten in more areas of the world than any other legume.

Saponin levels have only been measured in some beans. However, all members of this family have saponins, and are considered good sources of this longevity nutrient.

Another source of saponins is ginseng, an herb coming from a plant root and used throughout the world as a mild and natural stimulant. Ginseng has many pharmacological effects on the brain and central nervous system, and scientists have discovered that the active principles in it are various types of this longevity nutrient. Although ginseng contains saponins, it is not considered to be a safe source of the longevity nutrient because of the presence of other, untested substances in this plant. Sarsaparilla, used as a flavoring in teas and soft drinks, also contains saponins and produces effects similar to ginseng. Several foods provide unique types of saponins. Tomatoes, for example, contain a saponin called tomatine. Licorice contains the saponin called glycyrrhizin, which can strengthen muscle and prevent infections, actions similar to those of corticosteroid hormones.

Fenugreek, a spice also used as a medicine, is particularly high in saponins. In fact, the active ingredient in many herbal and folk remedies is some type of saponin. For hundreds of years, the Chinese have used an herb called Yunan Bai Yao to promote health. Recently, numerous studies have revealed Yunan Bai Yao to be a rich source of saponins, which selectively target and kill cancer cells, thus preventing the growth of tumors.

You can glean the same effect by eating any of the saponin-rich foods recommended by this program.

Day #3: Phytates

Day number three is devoted to raising the levels of these unique antioxidants. These naturally occurring nutrients have been known by nutritionists for at least 150 years, and new uses for them continue to be discovered. Where can we find phytates? Sources of phytates include seeds of plants, which is why grains in particular are the best sources. High levels of these longevity nutrients are found in seeds often consumed as snacks, such as sunflower seeds and peanuts. Sesame seeds are the highest dietary source of phytates, and eating small amounts of these can significantly raise body levels.

Good breakfast sources of phytates are foods containing bran, including cereals and bread products such as muffins and bagels. You can also eat whole-grain foods, such as wild rice, at lunch and dinner.

The best grain choices for phytate content are whole grains—

those which have not been milled. Milling wheat removes phytates. Most of the phytates in rice are found in the outer layer of this grain, which is removed when rice is milled.

Day #4: Protease Inhibitors

Be careful today because protease inhibitors are affected by food preparation. Prolonged heating of foods inactivates them. Frying food reduces protease inhibitor concentrations and increases the fat content, further suppressing the level of these longevity nutrients. Boiling, baking, and even chopping or slicing foods affect levels as well. Take less time to cook foods rich with protease inhibitors and eat them in their natural state to ensure ample levels of these longevity nutrients in your diet.

While it is true that some protease inhibitors can be synthesized in the body when one follows a low-fat, high-fiber diet, these protease inhibitors are less effective than those gotten directly from food. Meats, poultry, fish, and dairy products don't have protease inhibitors. Cauliflower and spinach, and peaches and plums are the better choices among vegetable and fruit groups. More rich sources include grains, legumes, and tubers. Three stand out: potatoes, sweet potatoes, and corn. About 10 percent of a potato's proteins are made up of protease inhibitors. Use a microwave oven to bake potatoes and sweet potatoes instead of an oven: this method decreases the baking time. Breakfast is not the best time to ingest protease inhibitors, as they are not present in most breakfast cereals due to their processing.

Day #5: Glutamine

Glutamine is a flavor enhancer, which for many years has been used to make monosodium glutamate (MSG). Although MSG has been "generally recognized as safe" (GRAS status by the PDA), the compound has been shown to cause allergic relations in some people and can be avoided without missing out on glutamine. Healthier, more natural sources of glutamine exhibit the same flavorful qualities. For instance, Parmesan cheese goes well with tomato sauce because of the glutamine in both of these foods. The flavor of cheeses in general is due in large part to high glutamine levels. The Japanese use glutamine-rich seaweed as a flavor enhancer.

Glutamine is found in protein foods, such as beef, lamb, chicken breast, turkey, certain fish, and some seafood. Certain grains have glutamine; however, the levels in these foods, like bread and pasta, are lower. The exact amounts in cheeses and cereals are variable. The food chart should be consulted for exact values of glutamine.

Day #6: Exorphins (Carnosine)

This day is devoted to increasing the levels of carnosine with its multitude antiaging effects. In fact, it's safe to say there are probably not any tissues in the body that won't benefit from this amazing longevity nutrient. You can gain the antiaging effects of carnosine by only eating protein-type foods. Although you should eat from the other groups, vegetables, fruit, and grains do not provide carnosine.

Two servings of chicken, turkey, lamb, or beef will significantly boost your body's levels of this longevity nutrient.

Pheasant, partridge, and other wild game as well as fish probably contain carnosine, but measurements of its levels in these foods have not been made.

Day #7: Pyrroloquinoline Quinone (PQQ)

Foods contain extremely small amounts of PQQ. In fact, it can be measured only in nanograms—1 billionth of a gram—the most likely reason its importance went undetected for so long. We may also see its scarcity as an indication that PQQ deficiency is common. Nevertheless, the PQQ levels in a meal are still 5 to 10 times higher than those already present in the body, leading nutritionists to conclude that we must consume PQQ in order to gain its beneficial effects.

This longevity nutrient can be found in vegetables, fruits, and condiments derived from soybeans. Specific vegetable recommendations include spinach and green peppers, while fruit choices include kiwi fruit and papaya. Beverages such as green tea are also good sources.

A salad with green peppers, spinach, and carrots is an excellent

PQQ entree. A serving of cabbage and another vegetable (such as tomatoes), with fruit for dessert, is another combination that will add appreciably to your PQQ intake.

Day #8: Arginine

Arginine is an amino acid that, unlike some amino acids, is found in both foods of animal and vegetable origin. The body can make this amino acid in the liver and kidneys from other chemical substances. A unique problem occurs with arginine in that although it is high in such foods as meats, another amino acid called lysine competes with the assimilation of arginine into the body. So although it is good to eat protein foods such as meat and fish to obtain arginine, cereals, bagels, crackers, muffins, and other foods with wheat are also good sources because, although they don't have as much arginine as meats, they do not have the competing amino acid lysine. Nuts and legumes are also high in arginine and low in lysine.

Day #9: Inulin and Oligofructose

These are present in several foods but only a few contain worthwhile amounts. Food sources are dominated by two vegetables: the Jerusalem and globe artichokes. Eat these when they are in season because they provide maximum inulin and oligofructose levels. A flour made from Jerusalem artichokes is a common ingredient and used in several pasta products.

Chicory, another food considered to be "exotic," also contains high levels of these longevity nutrients and should become a regular dietary staple. The history of chicory use goes back long before the use of Jerusalem artichokes. The ancient Egyptians cooked or roasted chicory and drank it as a beverage. Today, chicory coffee is still popular. Dandelion greens, bitter but pleasing greens to include in salads, are also a principal supplier.

Secondary food sources must be consumed in greater amounts to gain the same effects as primary sources. Garlic contains high levels of both inulin and oligofructose, but since we use it as a condiment, this food becomes a more minor source.

Day#10: Taurine

Taurine may not get as much hype as some of the other longevity nutrients, but nutritionists would agree that it is a very important factor in the functioning of the body's metabolism and age prevention. The amino acid taurine is present in proteins, but its levels vary. Dark meat chicken and turkey contain much greater amounts of taurine than beef, pork, or veal. Although nutritionists often groan at the consumption of dark poultry meat, occasional ingestion for the purposes of obtaining taurine is allowed. However, adequate intakes can be derived from the white meat as well. Shellfish (oysters, clams, mussels, and scallops) contain much higher amounts than shrimp, and the levels in white fish are about four times higher than in tuna.

Day #11: Tannins

Tannins are a complex group of longevity nutrients, and exact measurements of all the different types of tannins in foods have not been made. At the present time, the best tactic is to rank food tannin levels from high to low, with beverages containing the highest levels, followed by fruits and vegetables.

This would be a good day to switch from coffee or other beverage consumption to tea. Many studies indicate tea is a more healthful beverage than coffee or soda. Tea is harvested from the leaf of the tea plant, and three general types of teas exist: green, oolong, and black tea. Green tea is made by steaming the leaves and drying them in the sun: this type contains high amounts of tannins called catechins, which may constitute more than 30 percent of the dry weight of the leaves. If the tea leaves are allowed to stand for less than an hour in the sun, the product is oolong tea, a popular beverage in Taiwan. A further change in the type of tannins occurs if the tea leaves are allowed to stand for up to 6 hours, resulting in the formation of black tea.

Different countries favor different types of teas. In North Africa, green tea is the most popular variety, while in Asia, either green or oolong tea is consumed. In Canada, Ireland, and the United Kingdom, black tea is the favorite beverage. The United States, by the way, is the only country to drink iced tea as a customary beverage.

Red wine is a unique beverage not only because of its alcohol content, but much more because of its tannins. Tannins come from the grapes used to make wine, which are converted to this substance during the wine's aging.

Tannins are also present in fruits such as currants, blueberries, and raspberries.

Day #12: Monoterpenes

Tangy citrus fruits are great food choices for this longevity nutrient. More specifically, the oils derived from the citrus peel—made into lemon, lime, and orange beverages—are the best sources. Another significant source is marmalade, which contains the fruit peels. Cherries, too, are monoterpene-rich in both their skins and their sweet flesh. Monoterpenes may be the most fun of the longevity nutrients. You can enjoy the benefits of monoterpenes in cool fruit smoothies or colorful fruit salads you can pack to eat on the go. Surprisingly, even mint and spearmint, widely used as condiments and in jams and jellies, contain this longevity nutrient.

At the present time, we can only estimate the levels of monoterpenes in foods. We should not be dissuaded from using them, though, since we have such a good idea which foods contain them and where in food they are located. Small amounts of dietary monoterpenes have been shown to significantly raise body levels of this longevity nutrient, so eating foods with this longevity nutrient will add appreciably to your ability to benefit from them. Remember, look for products containing the peel (beverages, marmalades, jams, jellies) of the citrus fruits.

Day #13: Conjugated Linoleic acid

This is a day for dairy products! Because they come from grain-eating animals, dairy foods provide potent amounts of the longevity nutrient called conjugated linoleic acid (CLA). Natural cheeses that have not been ripened for more than several months generally contain higher amounts of CLA than those ripened longer. Good choices include Colby, ricotta, brick, and Muenster. Milk is an excellent source of CLA, as are sour cream and lamb.

Day #14: Organosulfur Compounds (OC)

Foods containing organosulfur compounds (OC) have been a staple of the human diet for centuries. They can be distinguished by their distinct smell and taste, due to the presence of sulfur compounds in them. I am sure you could recognize any one of these foods even if you were blindfolded—onions, garlic, shallots, scallions, chives, leeks.

Although the foods in this family each contain different types of sulfur compounds, all contain about the same levels. Because studies have shown that eating any of these foods readily raises OC blood levels, 2 servings a day are more than adequate.

Day #15: Lignans

The best sources of lignans are grains, such as barley and whole wheat. Processing is an important determinant when choosing grain foods because modern milling techniques remove most lignans. Therefore, whole grains are the best sources. Of these, flaxseed and its products contain the highest lignan levels. Foods with flaxseed may be difficult to find, but if you check the ingredients of breads, muffins, and cereals at your supermarket, you may be able to find ones that contain flaxseed flour. You can also buy flaxseed flour and breads, pancakes, or pizza dough yourself.

As with other longevity nutrients, not all foods in a particular group have been checked for lignans. The chart, however, includes the most accurate determinations of known lignan values. Among legumes, many beans, cowpeas, and peanuts are particularly good sources of this longevity nutrient. Sunflower and pumpkin seeds are also excellent choices. Various foods with wheat such as cereals, breads, rolls, and pasta contain unknown levels of this longevity nutrient.

Day #16: Quercetin

Quercetin is a flavonoid, which—like other members of this group—is found in the outer parts of plants; only trace amounts are found beneath the soil's surface. Onions are an exception to this rule, as they contain high amounts of this longevity nutrient. Sources vary around the world. In Japan, tea is the principal dietary quercetin source, while in Italy, it is red wine. In the United States, it is onions.

At the present time, not all foods have been analyzed for their flavonoid levels. Fresh or cooked onions are recommended. A salad with red peppers, lettuce, and other vegetables is another way to ingest quercetin. Apples eaten whole, as a snack, or in applesauce also provide significant levels, as does apple juice. Red wine and black tea are also sources. Milk added to tea prevents your body from absorbing quercetin, so have your tea without it.

Day #17: Phytoestrogens

(Genistein and Daidzein)

Despite their group name, both men and women benefit from these longevity nutrients, though women benefit more from the estrogenic/hormonal effects of coumestans.

Genistein and Daidzein

It's easy to figure out food choices for this longevity nutrient because the principal sources are legumes. There are many different members of this food family and phytoestrogen levels vary from zero in some legumes to very high in legumes such as soybeans. People in Asia have eaten soybeans for more than a thousand years, but only quite recently has the western world begun to use this amazing legume. Soy foods, which include entrees, desserts, beverages, and snacks, can be divided into two categories: fermented and nonfermented. Traditional fermented soy foods include soy milk products, tofu, tempeh and miso.

The most popular soy foods in the United States are tofu, soy milk, soy sauce, miso, and tempeh. Also look for veggie burgers, soy yogurt, and soy-based cheeses. Tofu comes in various consistencies and is the base for desserts such as soy "ice cream."

Day #18: Isothiocyanates

Isothiocyanates belong to the cruciferous family of plants, which are chemically identified by the mineral sulfur and visually identified by the cross-like arrangement of their flowers ("Cruciferae" comes from the Latin for cross). The isothiocyanates in these foods are responsible for the pungent flavor and odor of these vegetables and the condiments made from them, such as mustard and horseradish.

Vegetables, while varying in their isothiocyanate levels, are the primary source of this longevity nutrient. Brussels sprouts and collards hold twice the amount of other foods, and only one serving of these provides the highest intake of this nutrient. A serving of broccoli, cauliflower, and cabbage at dinner or lunch—while not as concentrated in isothiocyanates—will add appreciably to your daily intake.

Condiments do not add as much to the diet because we eat them in such small quantities.

Day #19: Carnitine

Carnitine is represented in several food groups, but has a wide range of levels in various foods. For example, ice cream has about eight times more of this longevity nutrient compared to butter. Beef has much more carnitine than chicken. In general, fruits and vegetables have significantly lower values of carnitine than protein foods such as meats, chicken, and fish. Fish is a less important source of this longevity nutrient compared to beef.

Day #20: Phytosterols

Phytosterols, unlike their distant cousin, cholesterol, are found in plants. Although three different types exist, nutritionists don't distinguish among them when making recommendations.

Phytosterols are widely distributed among vegetables, spices, and nuts.

This longevity nutrient is widely distributed in vegetables. High amounts are found in brussels sprouts, cauliflower, and okra. Unlike other longevity nutrients, phytosterol values have been determined in several spices, which means you can spice up your longevity nutrient intake. Peanuts, pecans, pine nuts, and pistachios are especially rich in phytosterols. Cereals can also be added to the list, but at the present time phytosterols levels are not known. Because of the tremendous variety of foods with phytosterols, I have never met anyone who has had trouble designing a diet for this day.

Day #21: Glutathione

Here we are! You made it to the final day of *The New Longevity Diet*, and I hope you have enjoyed trying new foods and revisiting familiar ones during the last 3 weeks. I especially hope that you have come to appreciate the antiaging properties of the choices offered each day. Today, you will concentrate on the powerful antioxidant glutathione. Even though the body can produce this substance by itself, the body's stores must be fortified. Dietary glutathione reaches and aids all the body's vital tissues—especially the liver where it detoxifies and serves as an antioxidant.

This longevity nutrient is found mainly in fruits and vegetables. Among the best fruit choices are peaches and melons. Among vegetables, squash, broccoli, and spinach provide excellent glutathione levels. Two servings of any of these foods—alone or in combination—will give your body all the glutathione it needs for protection.

The New Longevity Diet Antiaging Maintenance Program

Now that you have completed the 21-day program, you are probably wondering what to do next. There are two ways to approach this point: you can start over and continue to use the 21-day program as you did before, or you could choose a daily longevity nutrient from the list on your own. If you think you have gained enough familiarity with the longevity nutrients, and you want to try something new, you can also follow *The New Longevity Diet* antiaging maintenance program.

It is not enough to use the 21-day program and go back to your old eating habits. You must continue to eat these substances because the body constantly calls on them to prevent aging and disease. As far as we know, the majority of these are not stored in the body, and none is always available to be called upon when needed. Therefore, it is important to maintain regular intake.

At the same time, like all good things, it is hard to get enough of the longevity nutrients. As they are present in so many different foods, it would not be feasible to eat all of them in adequate amounts every day. Meal planning and restaurant dining would be a real headache!

The maintenance program is simple and provides flexibility and choice, but it helps you keep your longevity nutrient levels up with ease. Choose two longevity nutrients each day to concentrate on. At the end of a week, you will have gone through 14, and, in the process, greatly improved your nutrition. Continuing to choose two different longevity nutrients per day will provide you with optimum intakes of the longevity nutrients in your diet. Experience with patients and program participants has shown this maintenance program to be effective and easy to follow.

LONGEVITY NUTRIENT VALUES (in mg per serving*)

Food	Serving Size	NUC	SAP	PHY	PI	GLU	EXO	PQQ	ARG	IO	TAU	TAN	MON	CLA	GLU	OC	LIG	QUE	PHE	ISO	CAR	PHS
aduki beans	1/2 cup		X		XX																	
alfalfa sprouts	1/2 cup		422														XX		0.067			
allspice	1 tsp																					1
almonds	1/4 cup chopped			422		1228			586													47
apple	1 average			87				0.00084				46			2.00			7	0.017			22
apple juice	4 oz. glass											19						0.37	X			
apple sauce	1/2 cup												X					XX	X			X
apricot	1 average											3										23
artichoke, globe	1 average			35						5760												28
asparagus	1/2 cup chopped	89	1350			374				3060					20						0.22	28
avocado	1 average			2											15		0.21					
bacon bits	1 Tbsp			196																		
bagel, cinnamon-raisin	1 average					1847			215													
bagel, egg	1 average					2022			225													
banana	1 average							0.0015		1190		X			4.00		0.012					14
barley	1/4 cup			100	X				350			95					0.016					
basil	1 tsp																					106
beef, brisket	3 slices, 5"x1/4" each (2 3/4 oz.)	68				2648	250		1114		29			29	9						71	
beef, chuck	five 1" cubes (3 oz.)	77				4217	283		1774		32			30	11						81	
beef, ground	1 medium pattie (3 oz.)	77				3650	283		1535		32			22	11						80	
beef, rib	2 medium ribs	122				5560	539		2339		52			21	17						130	
beef, round	3"x2"x3/4" slice (3 oz.)	106				3494	283		1470		32			22	11						81	
beef, steak	8 oz.	134				10579	356		4451		41			55	13							
beef, tenderloin	3 1/4"x3 1/4"x3/4" (4 1/4 oz.)	148				4272	393		1796		45			45	15						112	
beef, top sirloin	4 1/2"x3"x3/4" (5 1/2 oz.)	188				7112	500		2990		57			24	19						143	
Beerwurst salami, beef	1 average	X				XX	XX		349		XX			X	X						X	
Beerwurst salami, pork	1 average					XX	XX		405		XX			X							X	
beet	1 medium		X	2													0.8					20
beet greens	1/2 cup																					15
biscuit	1 medium					693			86													
black beans	1/2 cup		X		XX										1				X			

Key
*In cases where the exact value is unknown, the following approximations apply:

X—has low levels of the longevity nutrient

XX—has adequate level of the longevity nutrient

Abbreviations
NUC—Nucleotides
SAP—Saponins
PHY—Phytates
PI—Protease Inhibitors
GLU—Glutamine
EXO—Exorphins
PQQ—PQQ
ARG—Arginine
IO—Inulin and Oligofructose
TAU—Taurine
TAN—Tannins
MON—Monoterpenes
CLA—CLA
GLU—Glutathione
OC—OCs
LIG—Lignans
QUE—Quercetin
PHE—Phytoestrogens
ISO—Isothiocyanates
CAR—Carnitine
PHS—Phytosterols

LONGEVITY NUTRIENT VALUES (in mg per serving*)

Food	Serving Size	NUC	SAP	PHY	PI	GLU	EXO	PQQ	ARG	IO	TAU	TAN	MON	CLA	GLU	OC	LIG	QUE	PHE	ISO	CAR	PHS
black-eyed peas (cowpeas)	1/2 cup		X	815	XX							X			1		0.18		0.081			
black tea	6 oz.											14						3				
black tea, Ceylon	6 oz.											90										
Blood sausage	1 average					X	XX		351		XX			XX			X				X	
blueberry	1/2 cup			3								3										
bologna, beef	1/8" slice (1 oz.)					X	XX		210		9			X	X						X	
bologna, pork	1/8" slice (1 oz.)					X	XX		281		34			X	X						X	
bologna, turkey	1/8" slice (1 oz.)					X	XX		251		34			X								
Brazil nuts	1/2 cup			1259		2206			1673			X										
bread, banana	3"x2 1/2"x1/2" slice			X		668			119			X					X					X
bread, corn	2x2x7/8" slice			489	X	524			86													X
bread, cracked-wheat	1 regular slice			XX	X	831			104								X					
bread, French	4 3/4"x4"x1/2" slice			6		747			80													
bread, Irish soda	4 3/4"x4"x1/2" slice			X		1095			174								X					
bread, Italian	4 3/4"x4"x1/2" slice			X		598			63								X					
bread, mixed grain	4 3/4"x4"x1/2" slice			XX		775			115								X					
bread, oat bran	4 3/4"x4"x1/2" slice		XX	XX		949			134								XX					X
bread, oatmeal	4 3/4"x4"x1/2" slice		XX	XX		652			107								X					X
bread, pita	1 average			43		1820			197								X					
bread, pumpernickel	4 3/4"x4"x1/2" slice			34		707			93								X					14
bread, raisin	1 slice			14		612			94								X					
bread, rye	1 regular slice			39	X	833			104								X					16
bread, wheat	1 slice			65	X	727			95													
bread, white	1 regular slice			21		753			89													
bread, whole wheat	1 regular slice			120	X	828			126								XX					10
broad (fava) bean	1/2 cup		3145	22	XX	885		0.0018				629					0.08	2	0.02			124
broccoli	1/2 cup			8		137			144						4		0.35		0.014	86		12
brownie	1 piece			31		X			X								X					X
brown rice	1/2 cup			761	X																	
brussels sprouts	1/2 cup														2					176		19
buckwheat	1 cup																X					
buffalo meat	4 1/2"x3"x3/4" slice (4 oz.)	X					572															

Key

*In cases where the exact value is unknown, the following approximations apply:

X—has low levels of the longevity nutrient

XX—has adequate level of the longevity nutrient

Abbreviations

NUC—Nucleotides
SAP—Saponins
PHY—Phytates
PI—Protease Inhibitors
GLU—Glutamine
EXO—Exorphins
PQQ—PQQ
ARG—Arginine
IO—Inulin and Oligofructose
TAU—Taurine
TAN—Tannins
MON—Monoterpenes
CLA—CLA
GLU—Glutathione
OC—OCs
LIG—Lignans
QUE—Quercetin
PHE—Phytoestrogens
ISO—Isothiocyanates
CAR—Carnitine
PHS—Phytosterols

LONGEVITY NUTRIENT VALUES (in mg per serving*)

Food	Serving Size	NUC	SAP	PHY	PI	GLU	EXO	PQQ	ARG	IO	TAU	TAN	MON	CLA	GLU	OC	LIG	QUE	PHE	ISO	CAR	PHS
bun	1 hamburger type			43		744																
burrito, bean	1 regular		X		X	XX			596								X		X			X
burrito, beef	1 regular	X	X		X	XX	XX		1310		XX			X			X				X	
butter	1 Tbsp					25			4					54							0.5	
cabbage	1/2 cup							0.0006							0.73		0.024	X		41		8
cabbage, Chinese	1/2 cup							0.0006							X		XX	0.0091		XX		
cabbage, green	1/2 cup							0.0006							X		XX	X		XX		
cabbage, oxheart	1/2 cup							0.0006							X		XX	X		XX		
cabbage, red	1/2 cup							0.0006							X		XX	X		XX		
cabbage, savoy	1/2 cup							0.0006							X		XX	X		XX		
cabbage, white	1/2 cup							0.0006							X		XX	0.0014		XX		
cake, angel food	1/12 of 9 3/4" diam.					291			86													
cake, Boston cream pie	1/8 of 9" diam.					502			104													
cake, cheesecake	1/8 of 8" diam.					818			201					XX								
cake, chocolate w/frosting	1/12 of 9" diam.			18		511			133													X
cake, coffeecake	2 5/8"x2 3/4"x 1 1/4" slice			X		1195			195													
cake, pound	3 1/2"x3"x1/2" slice			X		348			74													
cake, white	1/6 of 9" diam.			X		1016			174													
cake, yellow w/ icing	1/10 of 9" diam.			X		500			118				X									
calabrese	1/2 cup																			24		
Canadian bacon	2 slices						XX		736		XX										23	
candy, chocolate	1 oz.			36																		XX
candy, chocolate mint	1 box			XX									XX									XX
candy, Dots	1 box												XX									
candy, fruit jellies	1 box												XX									
candy, LifeSavers	1 piece												XX									
candy, peppermint	1 piece												XX									
candy, wintergreen	1 piece												XX									
cantaloupe	1/2 cup chopped														8		0.15					
caraway seeds	1 tsp			30									X				0.005					2
cardamom	1 tsp																					1
carrot	1 medium			8				0.0013							5		0.16					9
cashews	1/4 cup			650		1241			596			X					0.091					55

Key
*In cases where the exact value is unknown, the following approximations apply:

X—has low levels of the longevity nutrient

XX—has adequate level of the longevity nutrient

Abbreviations
NUC—Nucleotides
SAP—Saponins
PHY—Phytates
PI—Protease Inhibitors
GLU—Glutamine
EXO—Exorphins
PQQ—PQQ
ARG—Arginine
IO—Inulin and Oligofructose
TAU—Taurine
TAN—Tannins
MON—Monoterpenes
CLA—CLA
GLU—Glutathione
OC—OCs
LIG—Lignans
QUE—Quercetin
PHE—Phytoestrogens
ISO—Isothiocyanates
CAR—Carnitine
PHS—Phytosterols

LONGEVITY NUTRIENT VALUES (in mg per serving*)

Food	Serving Size	NUC	SAP	PHY	PI	GLU	EXO	PQQ	ARG	IO	TAU	TAN	MON	CLA	GLU	OC	LIG	QUE	PHE	ISO	CAR	PHS
cauliflower	1/2 cup	30			X										6		0.066			42		21
celery	1/2 cup chopped							0.00038									0.069					5
cereal, Apple Jacks	1 oz.			50		217			X				X				X					
cereal, Bran Chex	1 oz.			375		480			XX						X		XX					X
cereal, Cheerios	1 1/4 cup		X	XX		180			XX								XX					X
cereal, Cheerios, apple	1 1/4 cup		X	XX		160			XX								XX					X
cereal, Cocoa Krispies	1 oz.			38		120			X								X					X
cereal, Cocoa Pebbles	1 oz.			53		192			296								X					X
cereal, corn bran	1 oz.			65		320			XX								XX					X
cereal, cornflakes	1 cup			20		323			X													50
cereal, Cream of Rice	1 4-oz. pkg.			X		342			176								X					X
cereal, Cream of Wheat	1 4-oz. pkg.			5		1413			166								1420					X
cereal, 40% bran flakes	2/3 cup			305		322			XX								XX					X
cereal, Froot Loops	1 oz.			45		336			X				X				X					X
cereal, Fruity Pebbles	1 oz.			41		260			193				X				X					X
cereal, granola	1/2 cup			175		275			155													X
cereal, Grape-Nuts	1 oz.			151		320			173													X
cereal, Honey Smacks	1 oz.			51		162			X								X					X
cereal, instant oatmeal	1 4-oz. pkg.	40	160	133		1327			426								0.017					X
cereal, Life	2/3 cup			XX		240			XX													X
cereal, oatmeal apple	1 4-oz. pkg.	40	XX	XX		296			XX			X					0.017					46
cereal, 100% bran	1/3 cup			887		342			XX								XX					X
cereal, Product 19	3/4 cup			X		140			XX													
cereal, puffed rice	1 cup			58		142			73								X					X
cereal, puffed wheat	1 cup			X		597			85								X					X
cereal, Raisin Bran	1 oz.			184		190			130								XX					X
cereal, Rice Krispies	1 cup			58		240			X								X					X
cereal, Shredded Wheat	6 biscuits			415		320			X													X
cereal, Special K	1 1/4 cup			186		308			X								X					X
cereal, Total	1 cup			X		276			X													X

Key
*In cases where the exact value is unknown, the following approximations apply:

X—has low levels of the longevity nutrient

XX—has adequate level of the longevity nutrient

Abbreviations
NUC—Nucleotides
SAP—Saponins
PHY—Phytates
PI—Protease Inhibitors
GLU—Glutamine
EXO—Exorphins
PQQ—PQQ
ARG—Arginine
IO—Inulin and Oligofructose
TAU—Taurine
TAN—Tannins
MON—Monoterpenes
CLA—CLA
GLU—Glutathione
OC—OCs
LIG—Lignans
QUE—Quercetin
PHE—Phytoestrogens
ISO—Isothiocyanates
CAR—Carnitine
PHS—Phytosterols

LONGEVITY NUTRIENT VALUES (in mg per serving*)

Food	Serving Size	NUC	SAP	PHY	PI	GLU	EXO	PQQ	ARG	IO	TAU	TAN	MON	CLA	GLU	OC	LIG	QUE	PHE	ISO	CAR	PHS
cereal, Trix	1/2 cup			X		208			X				X				X					X
cereal, wheat bran	1/2 cup			843		386			XX								XX					43
cereal, wheat germ	1/4 cup			XX		356			167													X
cereal, Wheaties	1 cup			411		440			X													X
chapatis (flat bread)	1 average			1920		146			X													X
cheese, American	1 oz.	0.56				1287			260					35							4	
cheese, blue	1 oz.	X				1468			202					47							X	
cheese, brick	1 oz.	X				1564			248					60							X	
cheese, Brie	1 oz.	X				1224			208					XX							X	
cheese, Camembert	1-1/3 oz.	X				1583			265					XX							X	
cheese, caraway	1 oz.	X				1746			270					XX							X	
cheese, cheddar	1 oz.	7				1711			264					39							X	
cheese, Cheshire	1 oz.	X				1621			250					96							X	
cheese, Colby	1 oz.	X				1648			255					56							X	
cheese, cottage	1/2 cup	10				3033			639					21							X	
cheese, cream	1 oz.	X				461			76					21							X	
cheese, feta	1 oz.	X				686			133					48							X	
cheese, Gouda	1 oz.	X				1740			273					72							X	
cheese, Gruyere	1 oz.	X				1696			276					60							X	
cheese, mozzarella	1 oz.	X				1609			295					30							X	
cheese, Muenster	1 oz.	X				1575			250					56							X	
cheese, Parmesan	1 Tbsp	X				477			77					5							X	
cheese, provolone	1 oz.	X				1768			290					XX							X	
cheese, ricotta	1/2 cup	X				3068			792					90							X	
cheese, Romano	1 Tbsp	X				2070			332					4							X	
cheese, Roquefort	1 oz.	X				1040			202					96							X	
cheese, Swiss, reduced-fat	1 oz.	X				1602			260					26							X	
cheese, Velveeta	1 slice	X				XX								XX							X	
Cheez Whiz	1 oz.	X				985			155					92								
cherries	1/2 cup											11	XX									9
chestnut	1 average			12		62			34			X										2
chewing gum, peppermint	1 piece												X									
chewing gum, wintergreen	1 piece												X									
chicken, dark meat	1/2 cup (2 1/2 oz.)	92				2438	87		982		139			6	5						X	

Key
*In cases where the exact value is unknown, the following approximations apply:

X—has low levels of the longevity nutrient

XX—has adequate level of the longevity nutrient

Abbreviations
NUC—Nucleotides
SAP—Saponins
PHY—Phytates
PI—Protease Inhibitors
GLU—Glutamine
EXO—Exorphins
PQQ—PQQ
ARG—Arginine
IO—Inulin and Oligofructose
TAU—Taurine
TAN—Tannins
MON—Monoterpenes
CLA—CLA
GLU—Glutathione
OC—OCs
LIG—Lignans
QUE—Quercetin
PHE—Phytoestrogens
ISO—Isothiocyanates
CAR—Carnitine
PHS—Phytosterols

LONGEVITY NUTRIENT VALUES (in mg per serving*)

Food	Serving Size	NUC	SAP	PHY	PI	GLU	EXO	PQQ	ARG	IO	TAU	TAN	MON	CLA	GLU	OC	LIG	QUE	PHE	ISO	CAR	PHS
chicken breast	1/2 breast (3 oz.)	113				3995	344		1609		13			3	7						4	
chicken gizzard	2 pieces	24				1569	22		690		36			1	1						X	
chicken leg	1 leg (3 1/2 oz.)	125				3845	118		1548		139			7	7						X	
chicken wing	1 piece (1 oz.)	28				958	26		349		36			2	2						X	
chick pea, dry	1/2 cup		1302	129	XX												0.0035		0.084			15
chicory	1/2 cup									9625												
chili con carne	1 cup			X		3928	XX		1403		X			X							X	
chili powder	1 tsp																					
chives	1 Tbsp															0.092	0.038			X		
cider	8 oz.											386						XX	X			
cinnamon	1 tsp																					1
citrus- or mint-flavored ice cream	2/3 cup												XX	X								
clove	1 tsp ground																					6
cocoa	1 cup			117					154			X										X
coconut, shredded	1/4 cup			65					133													
coconut milk	1/4 cup					315			226													
coffee	1 cup																0.0079					
coleslaw	1/2 cup					267			85						X		XX	0.0014		41		
collards	1/2 cup			5													X			147		
cookie, chocolate chip	1 cookie			89		192			X													X
cookie, coconut	1 cookie			29		132			73													
cookies, Fig Newton, apple, strawberry, or raspberry	2 cookies			10		292			38				X									
cookies, ginger snap	1 cookie			X		X			X													
cookies, lemon creme	1 cookie			X		X			X				X									
cookies, mint chocolate	1 cookie			X		X			X				X									
cookies, oatmeal	1 cookie		X	X		405			91													X
cookies, oatmeal and raisin	2 cookies		X	50		X			57													X
cookies, Oreo	1 cookie			X		X			X													
cookies, peanut butter	1 cookie		X	4		X			128													X
cookies, shortbread	1 cookie			X		X			X													
cookies, vanilla wafers	2 cookies			7		X			X													

Key

*In cases where the exact value is unknown, the following approximations apply:

X—has low levels of the longevity nutrient

XX—has adequate level of the longevity nutrient

Abbreviations

NUC—Nucleotides
SAP—Saponins
PHY—Phytates
PI—Protease Inhibitors
GLU—Glutamine
EXO—Exorphins
PQQ—PQQ
ARG—Arginine
IO—Inulin and Oligofructose
TAU—Taurine
TAN—Tannins
MON—Monoterpenes
CLA—CLA
GLU—Glutathione
OC—OCs
LIG—Lignans
QUE—Quercetin
PHE—Phytoestrogens
ISO—Isothiocyanates
CAR—Carnitine
PHS—Phytosterols

LONGEVITY NUTRIENT VALUES (in mg per serving*)

Food	Serving Size	NUC	SAP	PHY	PI	GLU	EXO	PQQ	ARG	IO	TAU	TAN	MON	CLA	GLU	OC	LIG	QUE	PHE	ISO	CAR	PHS
coriander	1 tsp																					3
corn	1/2 cup			26	X	524			180						1							142
corn bran	1/2 cup			65	X	680			600								XX					X
corn bread	2"x2"x7/8" piece			544	X	480			320													X
corn cheese chips	1 oz.			20	X	500			320													X
corn chips, Comquistos, Snack Master	1 oz.			65	X	XX																X
corn chips, Doritos	1 oz.			178	X	300			290													X
corn chips, Fritos	1 oz.			142	X	260			160													X
corn chips, Nacho Doritos	1 oz.			142	X	320			130													X
corn germ	1 Tbsp			6400	X	XX			X													X
Cornish game hen	1 bird					X	XX		3248													
cornmeal	1 Tbsp	XX		107	X	460			340													X
crackers, animal	4 pieces			8		228			28													
crackers, graham	4 pieces			50		322			41													
crackers, Ritz	4 pieces			11		360			X													
crackers, saltine	4 pieces			19		368			44													
crackers, Wheat Thins	2 pieces			95		166			X													
cranberries	1/2 cup											XX					1					
cranberry juice	4 oz.											XX										
cranberry sauce	1/2 cup											XX					XX					
cream	1 Tbsp													XX								
croissant	1 medium					1150			170													
croutons	1 cup					1351			160													
cucumber	1 average				X										6		0.043					11
cultured buttermilk	8 oz.													XX								
cumin	1 tsp																					
custard-style yogurt	1 cup													X								
dandelion greens	1/2 cup									8692												
Danish pastry	4 1/4" diam. x 1"					1314			210													
dates	1 average											XX										
dill	1 tsp																					3
dinner rolls	1 medium					430			240													
doughnuts, frosted	3 1/4" diam. x 1"					514			115													

Key

*In cases where the exact value is unknown, the following approximations apply:

X—has low levels of the longevity nutrient

XX—has adequate level of the longevity nutrient

Abbreviations

NUC—Nucleotides
SAP—Saponins
PHY—Phytates
PI—Protease Inhibitors
GLU—Glutamine
EXO—Exorphins
PQQ—PQQ
ARG—Arginine
IO—Inulin and Oligofructose
TAU—Taurine
TAN—Tannins
MON—Monoterpenes
CLA—CLA
GLU—Glutathione
OC—OCs
LIG—Lignans
QUE—Quercetin
PHE—Phytoestrogens
ISO—Isothiocyanates
CAR—Carnitine
PHS—Phytosterols

LONGEVITY NUTRIENT VALUES (in mg per serving*)

Food	Serving Size	NUC	SAP	PHY	PI	GLU	EXO	PQQ	ARG	IO	TAU	TAN	MON	CLA	GLU	OC	LIG	QUE	PHE	ISO	CAR	PHS
doughnuts, sugared	3 1/4" diam. x 1"					626			107													
duck	1/2 breast					XX			XX													
egg	1 medium								140					4							0.016	
eggnog	4 oz.								183												X	
eggplant	1/2 cup				X							X					0.103					1
Enchirito (Taco Bell)	1 regular		X			3827			1,047		X										X	
endive	1/2 cup																	0.025				
English muffins	1 muffin			48		726			X													
fennel	1 tsp																					1
fenugreek	1 tsp																0.00032		0.00074			5
fig	1 average			5																		4
fig bars	1 1/2"x1 3/4"x1/2" (1/2 oz.)			X									X									X
fish, anchovy	4 pieces	33				486			195		28				1						X	
fish, bass	1 fillet	X				2224			891		XX				X						X	
fish, caviar	1 Tbsp	33				581			254		28				1							
fish, cod	1 medium	81				2897			1,161		112				4						4	
fish, flounder	1 fillet	65				1575			632		96				4						X	
fish, haddock	1 medium	99				3076			1,233		136				6						X	
fish, halibut	1 medium fillet	156				3386			1,357		215				10						X	
fish, herring	3 1/2"x2"x3/4" piece (2 3/4 oz.)	155				2922			1,171		129				6						X	
fish, ocean perch	1 medium piece	81				1807			781		112				4						X	
fish, salmon	3 oz.	106				2518			1,009		146				7						X	
fish, sardine	1 medium	25				441			177		21				1						X	
fish, smelt	4 pieces	100				2868			1,149		138				6						X	
fish, sticks	3 sticks	99				2671			711		144				7						X	
fish, trout	1 small	143				3534			1,417		196				9						X	
fish, tuna, albacore	1/2 cup	106				3794			1,522		36				7						X	
fish, whitefish	3 oz.	99				2970			1,191		146				7						X	
fish sandwich	1 regular					3070			793		X				X						X	
flaxseed flour	1 cup				X										X		53					
Frankfurter, beef	1 average					XX	X		331		XX			X	X						X	
Frankfurter, beef and pork	1 average	X				XX	X		382		XX			X	X						X	
Frankfurter, chicken	1 average	X				X	X		401		XX			X	X						X	

Key
*In cases where the exact value is unknown, the following approximations apply:

X—has low levels of the longevity nutrient

XX—has adequate level of the longevity nutrient

Abbreviations
NUC—Nucleotides
SAP—Saponins
PHY—Phytates
PI—Protease Inhibitors
GLU—Glutamine
EXO—Exorphins
PQQ—PQQ
ARG—Arginine
IO—Inulin and Oligofructose
TAU—Taurine
TAN—Tannins
MON—Monoterpenes
CLA—CLA
GLU—Glutathione
OC—OCs
LIG—Lignans
QUE—Quercetin
PHE—Phytoestrogens
ISO—Isothiocyanates
CAR—Carnitine
PHS—Phytosterols

LONGEVITY NUTRIENT VALUES (in mg per serving*)

Food	Serving Size	NUC	SAP	PHY	PI	GLU	EXO	PQQ	ARG	IO	TAU	TAN	MON	CLA	GLU	OC	LIG	QUE	PHE	ISO	CAR	PHS
Frankfurter, turkey	1 average	X				X	X		419		XX			X	X							
Fresca	1 can												X									
frog leg	1 medium						53															
frozen yogurt	1 cup													XX								
fruit, canned	1/2 cup												X									
fruit bar	1 bar												XX									
fruit juice, frozen from concentrate, bottled, or boxed - cherry, grape, raspberry, orange, white grape, lime, or lemon	1 cup											X	X									
Fruit Roll-Up, Sunkist	1 roll												XX									
garlic	1 average clove					24				525						12	0.01					X
Gatorade, tropical, lemon lime, or orange	1 cup												X									
ginger	1/2 oz.																					
goose	3x2 1/8x3/4" slice (2 3/4 oz.)	XX					X		1,331													
grape, red Magala	1/2 cup					236						64			X							3
grape juice	4 oz.					317						3									0.12	
grapefruit	1/2 average					11						X	X		7							17
grapefruit juice	4 oz.					23						X	XX									X
Great Northern beans	1/2 cup																0.1		0.053			
green beans	1/2 cup		34	56	X												0.092		0.05			X
green peas	1/2 cup	41	1599	24	XX	445			506						4		0.0064					115
green pepper	1 medium							0.0046							6		0.2					14
green tea, Chinese	6 oz.											96										
green tea, Japanese	6 oz.							0.0053				0.159					X		0.09			
grits, corn	1/2 cup			344		1285			341													X
guinea hen	1/2 bird (9 1/2 oz.)					X	X		5,092													
ham	2 4 1/2"x 2 1/4" x1/4" slices (1 oz.)	41				XX	XX		XX		14				4						XX	
ham and cheese loaf	1 slice (1 oz.)	X				X	X		313		X				X						X	
hazelnut	1/4 cup					1289			768								0.042					

Key

*In cases where the exact value is unknown, the following approximations apply:

X—has low levels of the longevity nutrient

XX—has adequate level of the longevity nutrient

Abbreviations

NUC—Nucleotides
SAP—Saponins
PHY—Phytates
PI—Protease Inhibitors
GLU—Glutamine
EXO—Exorphins
PQQ—PQQ
ARG—Arginine
IO—Inulin and Oligofructose
TAU—Taurine
TAN—Tannins
MON—Monoterpenes
CLA—CLA
GLU—Glutathione
OC—OCs
LIG—Lignans
QUE—Quercetin
PHE—Phytoestrogens
ISO—Isothiocyanates
CAR—Carnitine
PHS—Phytosterols

LONGEVITY NUTRIENT VALUES (in mg per serving*)

Food	Serving Size	NUC	SAP	PHY	PI	GLU	EXO	PQQ	ARG	IO	TAU	TAN	MON	CLA	GLU	OC	LIG	QUE	PHE	ISO	CAR	PHS
Hi-C	1 cup												XX									
homogenized milk	1 cup								281					49							3	
homogenized milk, strawberry	1 cup								XX					49							XX	
honeydew melon	1/2 cup														4							
horseradish	1 Tbsp																					
hot chocolate, instant	6 oz. cup			2					X			X										X
ice cream	2/3 cup													39.00							4	
ice milk, soft serve	2/3 cup					956			156					X								
ices, peppermint	1/2 cup												XX									
Italian sausage	1 medium						X		185		X			X							X	
jam, apricot	1 Tbsp												X									X
jam, blackberry	1 Tbsp			X								0.103	X				X					
jam, blueberry	1 Tbsp			X								X	X				X					
jam, grape	1 Tbsp											X	X									X
jam, lemon	1 Tbsp												XX									X
jam, marmalade	1 Tbsp												XX									
jam, orange	1 Tbsp												XX									X
jam, pineapple	1 Tbsp				X								X									X
jam, raspberry	1 Tbsp											0.107	X				X					
jam, red currant	1 Tbsp											X	X									
jam, strawberry	1 Tbsp			X								0.032	X									X
Jell-O, watermelon, apple, berry, black cherry, strawberry, orange, lemon, or lime	1/2 cup											X	X									
Jerusalem artichoke	1 medium			35						37800												28
kale	1/2 cup			6														6		79		
ketchup, tomato	1 Tbsp			1																		
kidney bean, red	1/2 cup	42	1152	282	XX	476			300								0.065		0.014			118
kielbasa	5 3/8" long x 1" diam. (2 3/4 oz.)					X	X		716		XX										X	
kiwifruit	1 average							0.0027				X										
kohlrabi	1/2 cup																			33		
Kool-Aid (lemon, lemon tea, pink lemonade)	4 oz. glass												X									

Key
*In cases where the exact value is unknown, the following approximations apply:

X—has low levels of the longevity nutrient

XX—has adequate level of the longevity nutrient

Abbreviations
NUC—Nucleotides
SAP—Saponins
PHY—Phytates
PI—Protease Inhibitors
GLU—Glutamine
EXO—Exorphins
PQQ—PQQ
ARG—Arginine
IO—Inulin and Oligofructose
TAU—Taurine
TAN—Tannins
MON—Monoterpenes
CLA—CLA
GLU—Glutathione
OC—OCs
LIG—Lignans
QUE—Quercetin
PHE—Phytoestrogens
ISO—Isothiocyanates
CAR—Carnitine
PHS—Phytosterols

LONGEVITY NUTRIENT VALUES (in mg per serving*)

Food	Serving Size	NUC	SAP	PHY	PI	GLU	EXO	PQQ	ARG	IO	TAU	TAN	MON	CLA	GLU	OC	LIG	QUE	PHE	ISO	CAR	PHS
lamb, foreshank	2 servings/ shank (3 1/2 oz.)	116				4463	129		1,827					48	24							
lamb, loin	1 medium (2 oz.)	63				2187	85		895					21	13							
lamb, rib	1 medium	55				1731	61		709					25	11							
lamb chop	1 medium (2 oz.)	63				3000	70		952					21	13							
lamb leg, whole	2 slices 4 1/8"x2 1/4"x1/4" (3 oz.)	109				3490	161		1,429					33	22							
laurel	1 tsp																					151
leek	1/2 cup									2457						0.5	0.2	35				
lemonade, pink or white	1 cup												XX									X
lemon juice	1 Tbsp												XX				0.0092					X
lemon sorbet	1/2 cup												XX									X
lemon tea	1 cup											XX	X				X					
lentils	1/2 cup	162	400	495	XX	1235						678					0.011		0.04			
lettuce, green leaf	1/2 cup														0.3			0.52	11		0.0011	5
lettuce, romaine	1/2 cup														0.3							X
lima beans	1/2 cup	48	95	800	XX	837													0.023			X
liverwurst	1/2 cup	XX							568						2							
low-fat yogurt	1 cup								X					15.00								
luncheon meat, beef	1 slice	X				X	X		531		X			X							X	
macadamia nuts	1/4 cup			X		748			462			X										X
mace	1 tsp																					1
Mandarin tea	1 cup											XX	X									
mango	1/2 average														4							
margarita mix	1 package												XX									
marjoram	1 Tbsp																					1
mayonnaise	1 tsp																					
melba toast	1 package of 2					331			35													
millet, dry	1/4 cup			124	X																	
miso (bean paste)	1 Tbsp		X	X				0.0028											25			
miso soup	1 cup		X	X				X											8			
molasses cookies	1 cookie					X																
Motts Fruit Punch	1 cup												XX									X
Mountain Dew	1 cup												X									
muffin, blueberry	1 average			X		1084			173													X

Key

*In cases where the exact value is unknown, the following approximations apply:

X—has low levels of the longevity nutrient

XX—has adequate level of the longevity nutrient

Abbreviations

NUC—Nucleotides
SAP—Saponins
PHY—Phytates
PI—Protease Inhibitors
GLU—Glutamine
EXO—Exorphins
PQQ—PQQ
ARG—Arginine
IO—Inulin and Oligofructose
TAU—Taurine
TAN—Tannins
MON—Monoterpenes
CLA—CLA
GLU—Glutathione
OC—OCs
LIG—Lignans
QUE—Quercetin
PHE—Phytoestrogens
ISO—Isothiocyanates
CAR—Carnitine
PHS—Phytosterols

LONGEVITY NUTRIENT VALUES (in mg per serving*)

Food	Serving Size	NUC	SAP	PHY	PI	GLU	EXO	PQQ	ARG	IO	TAU	TAN	MON	CLA	GLU	OC	LIG	QUE	PHE	ISO	CAR	PHS
muffin, corn	1 average			X		756			182													X
muffin, wheat bran	1 average			199		517			109								XX					X
mung bean	1/2 cup		291	XX	XX												0.24		0.045			X
mushroom	1/2 cup	63				243			1,266													
mustard	1 tsp																					
mustard greens	1/2 cup																					4
Mystic fruit drink, assorted flavors	1 cup												X									
Nantucket Nectars fruit drink, cranberry, apple, or watermelon	1 cup											X	X									
natto (fermented soybeans)	1/2 cup		X		X			0.0061											55			4
navy bean	1/2 cup	45	1185	564	XX												0.082		0.4			X
nectarine	1 medium														8							
nonfat frozen dairy dessert	1/2 cup													X	X							
noodles, chow mein	1 oz.			114																		
nutmeg	1 tsp																					1
okra	1/2 cup			4											9							19
olive, black	1 medium			0.5																		
olive, green	1 medium			0.5																		
onion, red	1 medium															3	0.091	XX				
onion, white	1 medium					303				9030						2	0.091	35				13
onion, yellow	1 medium															6	X	XX				
onion powder	1 tsp															0.019	X	X				2
oolong tea	6 oz.							0.005		X		39					X					X
orange	1 medium							0.0084							10		0.1					31
orange juice	4 oz.							XX					XX		3.00							
orange peel	1 medium												XX									X
orange seltzer	1 cup												X									
orange tea	1 cup												X				X					
Orangina drink	1 cup												XX									
oregano	1 tsp																					2
pancakes	4" diam.			X		504			84													X
pancakes, buckwheat	4" diam.			XX		796			172								X					
pancakes, whole wheat	4" diam.			244		866			190								X					X

Key

*In cases where the exact value is unknown, the following approximations apply:

X—has low levels of the longevity nutrient

XX—has adequate level of the longevity nutrient

Abbreviations

NUC—Nucleotides
SAP—Saponins
PHY—Phytates
PI—Protease Inhibitors
GLU—Glutamine
EXO—Exorphins
PQQ—PQQ
ARG—Arginine
IO—Inulin and Oligofructose
TAU—Taurine
TAN—Tannins
MON—Monoterpenes
CLA—CLA
GLU—Glutathione
OC—OCs
LIG—Lignans
QUE—Quercetin
PHE—Phytoestrogens
ISO—Isothiocyanates
CAR—Carnitine
PHS—Phytosterols

LONGEVITY NUTRIENT VALUES (in mg per serving*)

Food	Serving Size	NUC	SAP	PHY	PI	GLU	EXO	PQQ	ARG	IO	TAU	TAN	MON	CLA	GLU	OC	LIG	QUE	PHE	ISO	CAR	PHS
papaya	1 average							0.003							7		0.037					
paprika	1 tsp																					4
parsley	1 tsp							0.001							0.0036							2
parsnip	1 cup			21																		
partridge	1/2 breast	135																				
pasta	1/2 cup			112		490			330						X						0.13	
pastrami	3 1/4"x1/8" piece (1 oz.)	XX				XX	XX		361		XX			X							XX	
peach	1 medium											2.00			6							10
peach juice	4 oz.					39						2										
peach pie	1 slice			4																		X
peanut	1/4 cup		1440	684	XX				1,201			X					0.12		0.048			49
peanut butter	1 Tbsp		XX	200	X							X					XX		X			15
pear	1 medium											10			6							13
pear juice	4 oz.											5										
pecans	1/4 cup			397	X	647			371			XX										32
pepper, black	1 tsp																					2
pepper, white	1 tsp																					1
pepperoni	1 slice	X				X	X		377		X			X							X	
persimmons	1 average											XX										5
pheasant	1/2 breast (6.5 oz. raw)						X		2,699													
pickle, dill	1 medium																0.043					
pie, apple	1/7 of 9" diam.			X		1218			149			XX						XX	X			X
pie, blueberry	1/7 of 9" diam.			X		725			90			XX										
pigeon pea	1/2 cup		X														0.04		0.6			X
pineapple	1 slice				X	1071			153													7
pine nut	1/4 cup			X		1389			1,587													25
pinto bean	1/2 cup	144	1047	122	XX	371						X			0.29		0.046		0.31			
pistachio	1/4 cup			X		1280			680			X										33
pizza, cheese	1 slice					1826			287					X								
pizza, pepperoni	1 slice					3705	X		629		X			X							X	
plain yogurt	1 cup								X					X								
plantain	1/2 cup			16								X										
plum	1 medium				X	9						15					0.0014					2
pomegranate	1 medium								703			X										47
popcorn, popped	1 cup			37																		

Key

*In cases where the exact value is unknown, the following approximations apply:

X—has low levels of the longevity nutrient

XX—has adequate level of the longevity nutrient

Abbreviations

NUC—Nucleotides
SAP—Saponins
PHY—Phytates
PI—Protease Inhibitors
GLU—Glutamine
EXO—Exorphins
PQQ—PQQ
ARG—Arginine
IO—Inulin and Oligofructose
TAU—Taurine
TAN—Tannins
MON—Monoterpenes
CLA—CLA
GLU—Glutathione
OC—OCs
LIG—Lignans
QUE—Quercetin
PHE—Phytoestrogens
ISO—Isothiocyanates
CAR—Carnitine
PHS—Phytosterols

LONGEVITY NUTRIENT VALUES (in mg per serving*)

Food	Serving Size	NUC	SAP	PHY	PI	GLU	EXO	PQQ	ARG	IO	TAU	TAN	MON	CLA	GLU	OC	LIG	QUE	PHE	ISO	CAR	PHS
poppy seed	1 tsp			58	X												0.000754					2
Popsicle	1 pop												X									
Pop-Tart, cherry or berry	1 piece												X									
pork, barbecue	1/2 cup (2 1/2 oz.)	84				3246	260		1,288		40			2.00	13						19	
pork, leg (ham)	3 1/4"x2 7/8"x1/2" slice (3 oz.)	73				3913	235		1,554		48			X	16						24	
pork loin, chop	2 medium (3 oz.)	101				3787	391		1,504		39			8.00	43						28	
pork loin, ribs	4" rib (1/2 oz.)	19				645	75		256		48			3.00	3						4	
pork loin, roast	3 slices (3 oz.)	102				4023	396		1,598		51			7.00	20						24	
potato chips	1 oz.			55		159			X						6		X				0.02	11
potatoes, french fried	1/2 cup			50		159		X	X						6		X				0.02	11
potatoes, mashed	1/2 cup			50	X	159		0.0026	X						6		X				0.02	11
potato salad	1/2 cup			63	X	209		0.0026	X						17		X				0.02	11
potato w/skin, baked	1 average			X	X	159		0.0026	X						17		0.025				0.02	11
pretzels	2 pieces			63					X													
prunes	1 average					2																
pumpkin	1/2 cup				X																	15
quail	1 breast					X			716													
rabbit	3 oz.								X												18	
radish	1 medium			3	X												0.0016			6		6
radish greens	1/2 cup																			X		20
raisin, seedless	1/4 cup																					
raspberry	1/2 cup											16					0.086					
red pepper	1 medium														9			0.0018				21
red wine	3 1/2 oz. glass											27			0.73		1	0.013				
rhubarb	1/2 cup											XX										
rice, white	1/2 cup	6		32					2,678						0.82		0.014				0.015	
roasted soybeans	1/2 cup		XX	XX													0.14		7			
rolls, cinnamon	1 roll																					
rosemary	1 tsp																					1
rose wine	3 1/2 oz. glass											2						X				
rutabaga	1/2 cup																XX			118		
sage	1 tsp																					2

Key

*In cases where the exact value is unknown, the following approximations apply:

X—has low levels of the longevity nutrient

XX—has adequate level of the longevity nutrient

X**Abbreviations**

NUC—Nucleotides
SAP—Saponins
PHY—Phytates
PI—Protease Inhibitors
GLU—Glutamine
EXO—Exorphins
PQQ—PQQ
ARG—Arginine
IO—Inulin and Oligofructose
TAU—Taurine
TAN—Tannins
MON—Monoterpenes
CLA—CLA
GLU—Glutathione
OC—OCs
LIG—Lignans
QUE—Quercetin
PHE—Phytoestrogens
ISO—Isothiocyanates
CAR—Carnitine
PHS—Phytosterols

LONGEVITY NUTRIENT VALUES (in mg per serving*)

Food	Serving Size	NUC	SAP	PHY	PI	GLU	EXO	PQQ	ARG	IO	TAU	TAN	MON	CLA	GLU	OC	LIG	QUE	PHE	ISO	CAR	PHS
salad dressing, ranch, Caesar, Italian, Russian, or citrus variety	2 Tbsp												X									
salad dressing, vinaigrette, Blue Cheese, French, or Thousand Island	2 Tbsp																					
salami	2 thin slices (1 oz.)					X	X		260		16			451							X	
savory	1 tsp																					
scallion	1 medium															0.27						
seafood, clam	1 medium	23				591			317		88			X								
seafood, crab	1/2 cup	XX				2805			1,437		XX			X								
seafood, lobster tail	1 medium	XX				2972			1,522		XX			X								
seafood, mussels	1 medium	18				550			295		111			X								
seafood, oyster	1 average	18				134			72		59			X								
seafood, scallops	1 medium	18				343			184		198			X								
seafood, shrimp	1/2 cup	XX				785			1,552		21			X	X							
seeds, sesame	1 tsp		6	1272		119			79													171
seeds, pumpkin	1/4 cup			529		1489			1,392								8					
seeds, safflower	1/4 cup			X		2098			992													
seeds, sunflower	1/4 cup		X	722		2009			865								0.23					203
7-Up, diet	12 oz. can												X									
7-Up, diet cherry	12 oz. can												X									
shallots	3 medium					2545										2						3
sherbet, orange, lemon, or lime	1/2 cup												XX									
sherry wine	3 1/2 oz glass											5										
Slice soda	12 oz. can												X									
snow peas	1/2 cup		10		XX														X			
soda, black cherry	12 oz. can												X									
soda, lemon	12 oz. can												X									
soda, lime	12 oz. can												X									
soda, orange	12 oz. can												X									
soda, strawberry	12 oz. can												X									
sorbet, peach, raspberry, mixed berry, or lemon	2/3 cup												X									

Key
*In cases where the exact value is unknown, the following approximations apply:

X—has low levels of the longevity nutrient

XX—has adequate level of the longevity nutrient

Abbreviations
NUC—Nucleotides
SAP—Saponins
PHY—Phytates
PI—Protease Inhibitors
GLU—Glutamine
EXO—Exorphins
PQQ—PQQ
ARG—Arginine
IO—Inulin and Oligofructose
TAU—Taurine
TAN—Tannins
MON—Monoterpenes
CLA—CLA
GLU—Glutathione
OC—OCs
LIG—Lignans
QUE—Quercetin
PHE—Phytoestrogens
ISO—Isothiocyanates
CAR—Carnitine
PHS—Phytosterols

LONGEVITY NUTRIENT VALUES (in mg per serving*)

Food	Serving Size	NUC	SAP	PHY	PI	GLU	EXO	PQQ	ARG	IO	TAU	TAN	MON	CLA	GLU	OC	LIG	QUE	PHE	ISO	CAR	PHS
sorbet, chocolate or coconut	2/3 cup																					X
soup, vegetable	1 cup																					X
sour cream	2 Tbsp													28			X					X
soy bacon	2 slices		XX	248				X									X		4			X
soybean chips	1/2 cup		XX	X				X									X		54			X
soy breakfast sausage	2 links		XX	X	X			X									X		3			X
soy Cheddar cheese	1 oz.		XX	X	XX			X									X		1			X
soy cream cheese	2 Tbsp		XX	X	XX			X									X		1			X
soy flour	1 cup		XX	X	XX			X									X		300			X
soy hot dog	1 medium		XX	X	X			X									X		10			X
soy ice cream	1/2 cup		X	X	XX			X									X		7			
soy milk	1 cup		X	X	XX			X											10			
soy mozzarella cheese	1 oz.		XX	X	XX			X									X		1			X
soy noodles	1 cup		XX	X	XX			X									X		9			X
soy nuts	2 Tbsp		XX	X	XX			XX									XX		42			X
soy Parmesan cheese	1 tsp		XX	X	XX			X									X		0.2			X
soybeans	1/2 cup		5440	1260	XX	2190		0.0083									0.14		73			45
soy sauce	1 Tbsp		X		X			X									0.0049		X			
soy yogurt	1 cup		X	X	XX			X									X		34			X
spinach	1/2 cup	32	4230		X			0.002				XX			3			2				9
split peas	1/2 cup		X		XX												0.01		0.025			X
Sprite	12 oz. can												X									
squash	1/2 cup				X										11							
squash, acorn	1/2 cup				X										14							
squash, zucchini	1/2 cup				X										9							
squid	1/2 cup										356											
star anise	1 tsp																					2
strawberry	1/2 cup					33						20			8		1	0.7				9
Sunkist	12 oz. can												X									
Sunny Delight	12 oz. can												X									
Surge	12 oz. can												X									
sweet potato	1 medium				X			0.0019							3							19
swordfish	1 fillet	XX							1,196		XX										X	
taco, beef	1 regular	X		110		1978	XX		513		XX			X							XX	

Key

*In cases where the exact value is unknown, the following approximations apply:

X—has low levels of the longevity nutrient

XX—has adequate level of the longevity nutrient

Abbreviations

NUC—Nucleotides
SAP—Saponins
PHY—Phytates
PI—Protease Inhibitors
GLU—Glutamine
EXO—Exorphins
PQQ—PQQ
ARG—Arginine
IO—Inulin and Oligofructose
TAU—Taurine
TAN—Tannins
MON—Monoterpenes
CLA—CLA
GLU—Glutathione
OC—OCs
LIG—Lignans
QUE—Quercetin
PHE—Phytoestrogens
ISO—Isothiocyanates
CAR—Carnitine
PHS—Phytosterols

LONGEVITY NUTRIENT VALUES (in mg per serving*)

Food	Serving Size	NUC	SAP	PHY	PI	GLU	EXO	PQQ	ARG	IO	TAU	TAN	MON	CLA	GLU	OC	LIG	QUE	PHE	ISO	CAR	PHS
taco salad	1 regular					3189			882													
tangerine	1/2 cup																740					
taro	1 average											X										11
tarragon	1 tsp																					1
tea, cinnamon apple, ginger peach, peppermint, lemon, raspberry, wild berry, or orange	1 cup											XX	X									
tea, chamomile or chai	1 cup											XX										
tea, Earl Grey	1 cup												XX				X					1
tea, instant, Nestea	6 oz.			2								XX	X									
tea, Lipton, Constant Comment, Luzianne, or Tetley	1 cup											XX	X									
tempeh	1/2 cup		XX		XX			X											55			X
tempeh burger	1 medium		XX		X			X									X		25			X
thyme	1 tsp																X					2
tofu (bean curd)	1/2 cup		XX		XX			0.0031											28			X
tofu yogurt	1 cup		XX		XX			X									X		68			X
tomato	1 medium					172		0.0011							9		0.071					9
tomato, canned	1/2 cup			8		X									X		XX					X
tomato juice	4 oz.			X		320									2		X				0.006	
tomato soup	1/2 cup			8		X									X		X					X
tostada, beans and cheese	1 regular		X		X	1844											X		X			X
tostada, beef and cheese	1 regular	X			X	3923	XX	1			X			X			X				X	
Triscuit	7 pieces			X																		
Triticale	1/2 cup			1195													X					
turkey, back meat	1 piece (7 oz.)	252				8300	449		3,755		298			27								
turkey, wing	1 piece (2 oz.)	79				2445	140		1,111		93			6								9
turkey breast	3"x2 1/8"x 3/4" piece (3 oz.)	482				3908	1372		1,717		103			2								
turkey leg	1 leg (8 oz.)	343				10206	573		4,450		750			21								
turmeric	1 tsp																					2

Key
*In cases where the exact value is unknown, the following approximations apply:

X—has low levels of the longevity nutrient

XX—has adequate level of the longevity nutrient

Abbreviations
NUC—Nucleotides
SAP—Saponins
PHY—Phytates
PI—Protease Inhibitors
GLU—Glutamine
EXO—Exorphins
PQQ—PQQ
ARG—Arginine
IO—Inulin and Oligofructose
TAU—Taurine
TAN—Tannins
MON—Monoterpenes
CLA—CLA
GLU—Glutathione
OC—OCs
LIG—Lignans
QUE—Quercetin
PHE—Phytoestrogens
ISO—Isothiocyanates
CAR—Carnitine
PHS—Phytosterols

LONGEVITY NUTRIENT VALUES (in mg per serving*)

Food	Serving Size	NUC	SAP	PHY	PI	GLU	EXO	PQQ	ARG	IO	TAU	TAN	MON	CLA	GLU	OC	LIG	QUE	PHE	ISO	CAR	PHS
turnip	1 medium			4											1					90		9
veal	4 1/8"x2 1/2"x1/2" piece (3 oz.)	122				4742	XX		1,836		40			25.00	22						XX	
vegetable soy burger	1 burger		XX	X	X												X		26			X
Vienna sausages	2 links	X					XX		184		XX			17.00							X	
walnuts	1/4 cup			613	XX	1629			1,144			2			0.7		0.05					33
watermelon	1/2 cup									16					21							2
wheat crackers	16 pieces			X		X																X
wheat flour	1 cup			386		X																X
wheat germ	1/2 cup			X		X			X													X
white wine	4 1/2 oz. glass											7			2							
wild rice	1/2 cup			1936																		
wine vinegar	2 Tbsp.											3						X				
winged beans	1/2 cup		X	1958															X			
yam	1/2 cup			94								X										10
yeast	1/4 oz.			35																	X	
yellow peas	1/2 cup		80		X														X			X
yogurt, cherry, berry, banana, or peach	1/2 cup											X		X								
yogurt, lemon, lime, or orange	1/2 cup												X	X								
Yoo-Hoo chocolate drink	1 cup													X								

Key

*In cases where the exact value is unknown, the following approximations apply:

X—has low levels of the longevity nutrient

XX—has adequate level of the longevity nutrient

Abbreviations

NUC—Nucleotides
SAP—Saponins
PHY—Phytates
PI—Protease Inhibitors
GLU—Glutamine
EXO—Exorphins
PQQ—PQQ
ARG—Arginine
IO—Inulin and Oligofructose
TAU—Taurine
TAN—Tannins
MON—Monoterpenes
CLA—CLA
GLU—Glutathione
OC—OCs
LIG—Lignans
QUE—Quercetin
PHE—Phytoestrogens
ISO—Isothiocyanates
CAR—Carnitine
PHS—Phytosterols

Recommended Longevity Allowance Chart

The following values represent an optimal intake *on a day when you are concentrating on that nutrient.* For practical purposes, this level of longevity nutrient intake is difficult to maintain. However, frequent daily consumption is the ideal. Look to these values as your goals. At the very least, you should consume the indicated amounts of each nutrient once a week.

Longevity Nutrient	Recommended Dietary Longevity Nutrient Allowance (mg/day)
Nucleotides	150–190
Saponins	2,000–2,500
Phytates	460–870
Protease Inhibitors	Too small to calculate
Glutamine	2,350–4,000
Exorphins	400–550
PQQ	0.004–0.005
Arginine	890–1,740
Inulin and Oligofructose	10,250–12,530
Taurine	150–185
Tannins	125–250
Monoterpenes	Too small to calculate
CLA	60–75
Glutathione	14–17
OCs	5–7
Lignans	.05–.07
Quercetin	3–7
Phytoestrogens	25–30
Isothiocyanates	125–155
Carnitine	40–65
Phytosterols	30–60

8

THE 21-DAY *NEW LONGEVITY DIET* FOR "MENU-STYLE" EATERS

The following section should make all of you who are "menu plan" eaters very happy. For each day of the *New Longevity Diet*, I've included a menu and recipes for any dish that's not obvious. These recipes have been thoroughly researched and tested to provide optimum levels of longevity nutrients.

Obviously, it would be ideal if you made every dish, but that's not practical for everybody. So aim to get at least two of those recipes (or a similar prepared food) into your diet each day.

At the end of the 21 days of this plan, you will have substantially increased your longevity nutrient content and had some delicious food to boot!

At that point you can either start all over again or begin to expand your repertoire using the advice and tables in the previous chapter. As you integrate these foods into your diet, you'll be surprised by how natural longevity eating is. Before long, you won't be relying on these menus—you'll be getting your share of longevity nutrients without a second thought.

Don't be put off by the rigidity of this program. It's designed that way so that you can change your eating style without much thought. It's been my experience with clients that after you've been through the cycle once, your thinking about food will have changed. You won't need to pay so much attention because the longevity nutrients will be part of your life.

Another thing to remember: I've created this menu plan as an ideal—just as I did with the designer-style plan. If you don't follow it to the letter—especially after the first three weeks—it's no problem. Adding any of these foods into your diet on a regular basis will have an enormous impact on your health.

The following are sample menus for each day. Recipes are located at the end of the book in the appendix and each features a longevity nutrient. If you change the recipes, be sure not to touch the key ingredients—remember each recipe has been chosen for a particular longevity nutrient.

Once you have gained familiarity with using these recipes, you will see how easy it is to choose your own recipes for the menu style plan. An asterisk indicates an item containing the longevity nutrient of the day. The recipe number is located in parentheses next to the food item.

DAY #1: NUCLEOTIDES

✦ **BREAKFAST**

Omelette with Smoked Ham (1)*
Cantaloupe
Skim milk

✦ **LUNCH**

Grilled Tuna with Papaya Salsa (24)*
Warm Spring Salad with Baby Vegetables (25)*
Coffee

✦ **SNACK**

Baby carrots*

✦ **DINNER**

Shrimp and Fresh Herbs (73)*
Mediterranean Couscous Salad (74)*
Lentil Soup (75)*

Chocolate Flan (76)
Lemonade

DAY #2: SAPONINS

✦ **BREAKFAST**

Scrambled egg substitute or egg whites with low-fat Cheddar cheese and peas*
1 slice whole wheat toast
Peach
Coffee or tea

✦ **SNACK**

Peanuts*

✦ **LUNCH**

Frijoles con Arroz Picante (26)*
Sparkling mineral water

✦ **DINNER**

Lemon Chicken (77)*
Pea and Mushroom Risotto (78)*
Asparagus with Parmesan (optional) (79)
Crunchy Berries (80)*
Tea

DAY #3: PHYTATES

✦ **BREAKFAST**

Wheat Cereal with sliced banana and skim milk*
Orange juice
Coffee

✦ **LUNCH**

Sunflower Seed Sandwich (27)*
Tomato juice

✦ **SNACK**

Orange

✦ **DINNER**

Grilled Sesame Chicken Breasts* (81)
Barley, Tomato, and Spinach Pie (optional) (82)*
Asian Eggplant, Green Beans, and Tomatoes with Peanuts (83)*
Cantaloupe Sorbet (84)
Mineral water

DAY #4: PROTEASE INHIBITORS

✦ **BREAKFAST**

Low-fat cottage cheese with sliced peach*
One-half toasted bagel with margarine
Coffee or tea

✦ **LUNCH**

Roasted Green Pepper Soup (28)
Croutons
Soy milk

✦ **SNACK**

Cucumber

✦ **DINNER**

Zucchini and Smoked Salmon with Linguine in Lemon Cream Sauce (85)*
Roasted Cauliflower with Spices (86)*
Peaches with non-dairy light whipped topping*
Wine

DAY #5: GLUTAMINE

✦ **BREAKFAST**

Golden Honey Milk Shake (2)*
Grapefruit*
Coffee or tea

✦ **SNACK**

Dried prunes*

✦ **LUNCH**

Spicy Potato Quesadillas with Guacamole (29)*
Tomato juice*

✦ **DINNER**

Baked Ziti with Eggplant (87)*
Spicy Lobster Salad (88)
Angel Food Cake (89)*
Coffee

DAY #6: EXORPHINS (CARNOSINE)

✦ **BREAKFAST**

Turkey bacon*
Bagel
Coffee or tea

✦ **SNACK**

Slices of turkey breast*

✦ **LUNCH**

Chicken Cashew Stir-Fry (30)*
Steamed rice
Jasmine Tea

✦ **DINNER**

Southwest Spicy Pork Skewers (90)*
Green Rice (91)
Pineapple Parfait (92)
Espresso coffee

DAY #7: PYRROLOQUINOLINE QUINONE (PQQ)

✦ **BREAKFAST**

PQQ Fruit Compote* (3)
Low-fat cottage cheese
Green or oolong tea*

✦ **LUNCH**

Savory Stuffed Green Peppers (31)*
Carrot and celery sticks*
Grape juice

✦ **SNACK**

Papaya*

✦ **DINNER**

Indonesian and Chinese Fusion Stir-Fry (93)*
Steamed rice
Wilted Spinach Salad (94)*
Kiwi Cocktail (95)*

DAY #8: ARGININE

✦ **BREAKFAST**

Banana Almond Muffins (4)*
Orange
Coffee or tea

✦ **LUNCH**

Turkey Roll-Ups with Provolone Cheese (32)*
Sparkling mineral water

✦ **SNACK**

Nuts*

✦ **DINNER**

Thai Chicken and Rice Noodles (96)*
Steamed brown rice
New England Baked Apples with Maple Glaze (97)*
Thai Iced Coffee (98)

DAY #9: INULIN AND OLIGOFRUCTOSE

✦ **BREAKFAST**

Whole wheat toast
Sliced banana* with low-fat yogurt
Grapefruit juice

✦ **LUNCH**

Artichoke Soup (33)*
Mineral water

✦ **SNACK**

Low-fat yogurt with wheat germ*

✦ **DINNER**

Barbecued Tuna with Marinated Arugula Salad (99)
Spring Salad with Dandelion Greens (100)*
Chicory with Scallion Oil (optional) (101)
Coffee or tea
Nutty Bananas (102)

DAY #10: TAURINE

✦ **BREAKFAST**

Turkey bacon*
English muffin
Orange
Coffee or tea

✦ **LUNCH**

Seafood Casserole (34)*
Mineral water

✦ **SNACK**

Grapes

✦ **DINNER**

Angel Hair Pasta with Asparagus and Speck (103)*
Collard Soup (104)*
Scallops with Sizzling Herbs (optional) (105)*
Seltzer water
Honeydew Sherbet (106)

DAY #11: QUERCETIN

✦ **BREAKFAST**

Low-fat yogurt with strawberries*
Bagel
Apple juice*

✦ **SNACK**

Apple*

✦ **LUNCH**

Chicken Salad with Peanut Dressing and Apples (35)
Soy Curried Chickpeas with Sunflower Seeds (optional) (36)*
Romaine and Black Olive Salad (37)*
Apple juice

✦ **DINNER**

Salmon with Wilted Arugula (107)
Baked Endives with Apples and Cloves (optional) (108)
Spinach, Apple, and Potato Salad (109)*
Apple Harvest Pudding (110)*
Black tea*

DAY #12: PHYTOESTROGENS

✦ **BREAKFAST**

Miso Omelette (5)*
Soy bacon*
Orange juice

✦ **SNACK**

Tofu yogurt*

✦ **LUNCH**

Vegetable and Soybean Hot Pot (38)*
Carrot sticks
Tea

✦ **DINNER**

Spaghetti with Tempeh Tomato Sauce (111)*
Steamed green beans*
Whole wheat roll
Very-Berry Tofu Smoothie (112)*

DAY #13: LIGNANS

✦ **BREAKFAST**

Whole or bran cereal* with skim milk

Strawberries*
Coffee or tea

✦ **SNACK**
Sunflower seeds*

✦ **LUNCH**
Vegetarian Lunch (39)*
Raspberry Smoothie (40)

✦ **DINNER**
Barbecued Halibut with Bean Salad (113)
Stuffed Summer Squash (114)*
Pear Delight (115)*
Iced tea

DAY #14: CONJUGATED LINOLEIC ACID (CLA)

✦ **BREAKFAST**
Low-fat yogurt*
Egg substitute or egg whites scrambled with Colby or Cheddar cheese*
Orange juice

✦ **SNACK**
Cottage cheese*

✦ **LUNCH**
Stilton Sandwich (41)*
Cool Cucumber Soup (42)*
Skim milk*

✦ **DINNER**
Herbed Lamb Chops (116)*
Baked Cheese Polenta with Escarole (117)*
Mineral water
Melon with low-fat frozen yogurt*

DAY #15: ISOTHIOCYANATES

✦ **BREAKFAST**
Low-fat cottage cheese
Peach
English muffin
Coffee or tea

✦ **LUNCH**
Broccoli Tart with Pine Nuts (43)
Seltzer

✦ **SNACK**

Radishes

✦ **DINNER**

Flounder with Lemon Champagne Beurre Blanc (118)
Broccoli with Squash and Corn (optional) (119)
Baked Red Cabbage (120)*
Honeydew Granite (121)
Iced tea

DAY #16: CARNITINE

✦ **BREAKFAST**

Whole wheat bagel with melted American cheese
Mango
Whole milk*

✦ **LUNCH**

Favorite Fajitas (44)*
Mineral water

✦ **SNACK**

Whole wheat toast

✦ **DINNER**

Herbed Chicken with Wine (122)*
Steamed rice
Tennessee Banana Pudding (123)
Iced tea

DAY #17: PHYTOSTEROLS

✦ **BREAKFAST**

Rice bran cereal with skim milk*
Figs*
Orange juice
Coffee or tea

✦ **LUNCH**

Chicken and Melon Salad with Pine Nuts (45)*
Whole wheat roll
Diet soda

✦ **SNACK**

Peanuts*

✦ **DINNER**

Beef and Basil (124)*

Steamed rice
Sweet Glazed Carrots with Sesame Seeds (optional) (125)*
Asparagus with Lemon and Sage (126)*
Honeyed Figs (127)
Apple juice

DAY #18: TANNINS

✦ **BREAKFAST**

Tropical Rhubarb (6)*
Whole wheat toast
Green or Black tea*

✦ **LUNCH**

Open-Faced Ham Sandwich (46)
Strawberry Rhubarb Soup (optional) (47)
Cider*

✦ **SNACK**

Hot cocoa* with low-fat whipped topping

✦ **DINNER**

Scallops with Limes (128)
Cranberries and Rice (129)*
Green Tea Ice Cream (130)*
Red wine

DAY #19: MONOTERPENES

✦ **BREAKFAST**

Lemon Almond Pancakes with English Lemon Curd (7)*
Grapefruit*
Skim milk

✦ **SNACK**

Cherries*

✦ **LUNCH**

Fish Salad with Mint (48)*
Iced tea

✦ **DINNER**

Orange Grilled Chicken with Spicy Salsa (131)*
Corn with Chipotle Lime Vinaigrette (132)*
Tangerine Ice (133)*
Lemonade*

DAY #20: ORGANOSULFUR COMPOUNDS

✦ **BREAKFAST**

Puffy Chive Omelette (8)*
½ Grapefruit
Coffee or tea

✦ **LUNCH**

Potato Leek Soup (49)*
Tomato juice

✦ **SNACK**

Carrot sticks

✦ **DINNER**

Savory Shrimp Stir-fry (134)*
Steamed rice
Snow Peas (135)*
Fresh pineapple slices
Jasmine tea

DAY #21: GLUTATHIONE

✦ **BREAKFAST**

Breakfast Ambrosia (9)*
1 slice whole wheat toast
Orange juice

✦ **LUNCH**

Orange Rice Salad (50)*
½ Pita bread
Mineral water

✦ **SNACK**

½ Grapefruit*

✦ **DINNER**

Marinated London Broil (136)
Squash Baked with Leeks (137)*
Seasoned Baked Potatoes (138)*
Peach Crisp (139)*
Tea

9

THE NEW LONGEVITY DIET WEIGHT-LOSS PROGRAM

If you plan to live to a ripe old age, you're limiting your chances of doing so if you're overweight. That's because excess fat interferes with the function of practically *every* organ in the body. In fact, you'd be very hard-pressed to find a system that isn't affected directly or indirectly by obesity. Fat can accumulate inside the cells of an organ, strangling various cell functions. Or the excess fat may change the way your hormones operate. It's tempting to say that obesity is a direct cause of aging—but that can't be said for sure right now. It is safe to say that obesity accelerates it, however, and it is a factor that *must* be dealt with so that the longevity nutrients can perform their antiaging functions effectively.

Excess fat generates free radicals. Try this: take some butter from the refrigerator, and leave it out in a warm room for a couple of days. Take a sniff. That's free radicals in action! This same biochemical process occurs in the body. Free radicals are generated from fat, and an overweight person produces many more of these harmful substances than are already being produced in the body. By losing weight, you immediately start to take an important step in reaching your maximum life span because you are already attacking the overproduction of free radicals—or ROS—a proven cause of aging.

Another problem with fat is that it is a repository for all kinds of harmful chemicals. These upset homeostasis and can cause disease. In addition to being an energy reserve for the body, fat *sequesters* harmful chemicals and foreign agents that enter the body every day. Ordinarily, the liver is the main site of the detoxification of these chemicals. For poorly understood reasons, however, a lot of these substances end up full strength in the fat stores on the hips, thighs, and abdomen. While it is better for toxic chemicals to be in the fat cells than to be, for example, in the skin, when that fat gets rotated out, the toxic chemicals get released. This increased toxicity to the body has the potential to be harmful, and is another reason to make sure you get enough of the longevity nutrients.

Excess fat is also a significant factor in a number of diseases that significantly impair the body's capacity to reach its maximum life span. We can get a better idea of the effect fat has on the body and its potential for shortening your life span by looking at different body systems. Excess fat affects hormone levels in the body. For example, it is associated with insulin resistance, considerably destructive to several organs such as the liver, pancreas, and muscle.

Physicians have known for years that excess fat contributes to diseases of the cardiovascular system. When this system is impaired and an adequate blood supply is compromised, the brain can't get nutrients, the kidneys can't remove toxic products, and the liver can't carry out its detoxification program. Muscles and joints can't get the nutrients they need, and the skin can't get its longevity nutrients to counteract the effects of aging. The effects of fat on the cardiovascular system are far-reaching indeed.

Excess weight is thought to be one of the major risk factors of atherosclerosis, or hardening of the arteries. The longevity nutrients are powerful antiaging substances, but they must be able to get to where they can function—an impossible task if arteries are clogged with cholesterol and don't function properly.

Excess fat affects every organ. Obesity can result in excessive fat buildup in the liver, seriously impairing its important functions. Too much weight causes excess strain on the joints, which may affect the progression of certain diseases such as osteoarthritis.

The immune system helps protect us against the invasions of foreign substances and agents. In overweight people, the cells of the immune system do not have the same ability to guard the body against bacteria and viruses as they do for a person of normal weight. Obesity and the aging process each suppress the immune system in certain ways. But if you are overweight as you age, the effect is a double whammy.

There's no doubt that being overweight is a life-threatening condition. It is estimated that obesity is second only to tobacco use as a significant cause of illness and death in the United States. The more excess weight you carry around, the greater your risk of high blood pressure, diabetes, arthritis, cancer, and even infertility. Among Americans, excess weight is probably responsible for *90 percent* of the cases of non-insulin-dependent diabetes, 20 percent of all cases of hypertension, and 37 percent of all reported incidents of coronary heart disease. With cancer, the link is thought to be very strong between excess weight and cancer of the breast, endometrium, gallbladder, and prostate.

How Big Is the Obesity Problem?

The extent of the problem of obesity in this country is staggering. Currently, one-third of Americans are overweight! Severe obesity afflicts 22 percent of all Americans. This compares with 14 percent in Britain and just 7 percent in France—a country associated with rich sauces and wonderful meals.

Signs of health consciousness are everywhere—except at people's waistlines. Low-fat foods, health clubs, and athletic gear have become multi-billion-dollar industries. Statistics suggest that this health awareness is paying off. Since the early 1960s, blood pressure and blood cholesterol levels have been dropping, while rates of coronary heart disease mortality have declined by more than half of what they were. Given these trends, we might expect to see a trim, well-toned population, but we don't.

According to the most recent federal statistics, the number of overweight Americans has almost doubled over the past 25 years. Currently, 22.5 percent of the U.S. population is considered to be clinically obese, compared to only 14.5 percent in 1980. The end to this increase does not appear to be in sight.

Although many researchers blame increased food availability and lack of exercise for this increase, officials at the Centers for Disease Control and Prevention (CDC) have been quoted as saying, "We have not clearly identified the major changes in eating behavior or activity sufficient to account for the recent rapid increase in obesity."

Although other countries do not have as accurate long-term data as the United States has, obesity is increasing at an alarming rate in other countries, too. In Brazil, for example, it has increased from 3.1 percent to 5.9 percent in men and from 8.2 percent to 13.3 percent in women between 1976 and 1989. In Australia, obesity has increased from 9.3 percent to 11.5 percent in men and from 8.0 percent to 13.2 percent in women between 1980 and 1989. Some places like Western Samoa have even higher increases where rates of obesity have gone from 38.8 percent to 58.4 percent in men and from 59.1 percent in 76.8 percent in women between 1978 and 1991.

Perhaps even more disturbing is the finding that obesity is on the rise in all segments of the population. Teenagers—especially girls—middle-aged and elderly people are all overweight. Even children ages 6 to 11 are gaining weight at an alarming rate. Teenage girls probably have one of the biggest problems with obesity, which can lead to bulimia, which involves binging and purging, anorexia nervosa, an eating disorder that involves self-starvation and weight loss and can be fatal in some cases.

Why Do People Get Fat?

After spending millions of dollars on research, scientists have not been able to come up with a good reason why some people weigh more than they should. Is it as simple as social obligations that involve a lot of eating? Or is excess weight related to an overindulged sweet tooth?

Over the years, a number of theories have been proposed and then discarded. One of these theories was that people gained weight because of low metabolism. But several studies showed that bodies are more efficient at burning up excess calories than had been previously thought. In other words, energy intake is pretty well balanced by energy expenditure. However, if this system is out of balance and slightly favors the intake of calories over expenditure, it is easy to see why, over a 30-year span (from age 22 to 55, when most people gain weight), it is possible to put on a significant amount of weight. Just a one-percent-per-year weight gain in a normal weight man or woman over 30 years adds up to an extra 22 pounds!

Up until a few years ago, nutritionists had little understanding of how fat cells functioned in the body. In fact, fat cells—or adipocytes, as nutritionists call them—seemed very uninteresting because they were thought to simply store and then "liberate" calories (energy) from foods. Today, however, there has been an explosion of knowledge about how the brain, the nervous system, the gastrointestinal system, and the endocrine system interact with fat cells and control how they function. We now know that it is this complex, interconnected system that regulates fat cells in the body and, along with it, determines whether we are overweight, underweight, or just right.

The number of fat cells and their composition is largely determined by the amount and type of food eaten. The amount of food eaten is influenced to a large degree by appetite. We often hear, "He has a big appetite," or "I have no appetite today," but it is really a very complex system that makes people want to start or to stop eating. This system is regulated by a vast array of hormones, such as insulin and glucagon, along with many substances secreted from the gastrointestinal system at the direction of the brain. The part of the brain that helps regulate energy and controls appetite, called the hypothalamus, is still poorly understood and much more complex than originally thought. So, today we still have no clear understanding of why we are sometimes not hungry at all and, at other times, feel positively ravenous.

Regarding appetite, there are other areas, such as the biochemical and physiological ones, in which much remains to be learned. Psychologists who study the factors that control appetite have come up with different ideas about what affects one's eating behavior. One of these is the *palatability* of food. Most people tend to eat more when the food is more palatable and/or readily available. In addition, there are many social influences that affect eating behavior. Seeing others eat may induce one to eat and even overeat in such situations even though one is not hungry. This is an example of a psychological force that directs eating.

Another factor has to do with cognitive considerations. These are the powerful forces that dictate eating behavior, *especially* in dieters. Dieters, usually, are advised to consume a select amount of calories at a meal, for the week, and so forth. This pattern is *not* helpful because it puts guidelines on eating instead of requiring the dieter to listen to his body's inner signaling of true hunger and satiety. Consequently, the dieter tries to lose weight by overriding these physiological signals. This approach often fails because it does not instruct the dieter to deal with these signals—a problem which may have led to the dieter's weight problem in the first place.

Recently, biochemists were excited by a new substance thought to be involved in regulating body fat. Called leptin, this molecule is synthesized by the body's fat cells and then secreted into the bloodstream. There, it interacts with the nervous system to help control the desire for food, depending on how much energy is being expended at any particular time for any particular activity. Although leptin has worked predictably in animal testing, it does not hold great promise as the missing link in the obesity question for humans because studies have found no difference in the amount of leptin in overweight people compared with people of normal weight. Like many other substances involved in the way fat cells function, leptin has been shown to be only one part of the puzzle, and more research needs to be done.

Blame It on Genetics?

The human body seems to be endowed with genes that favor calorie storage. Hundreds of thousands of years ago, when food was scarce, those who survived probably did so because they had the capacity to store fat. Many biologists think that these "survival of the fattest" genes have been inherited by us all. This means that the body's natural inclination is to store calories rather than to burn them. Such a genetic trait may have been essential for our ancestors but it works against us because we live in a country where we have too much food to eat and, due to our hectic schedules, too little time to exercise to burn it off.

It is true that the tendency toward being overweight may be inherited. For example, our body shape, which is determined largely by the distribution of fat, is inherited by as much as 40 percent from our parents and grandparents. Other factors that contribute to obesity also appear to be inherited. For example, one's resting metabolic rate, the level of physical activity enjoyed, changes in energy expenditure in response to eating, the amount of certain fat-controlling hormones in the body, and even food preferences seem to be passed on from generation to generation. However, in spite of many studies of the human genetic code, no one has come up with an "obesity gene" to explain why some are overweight and others are not. Rather, scientists believe there are many genes that may be involved in being overweight, and these are expressed *only* when there is an interaction with the environment. For example, one individual may have a gene that causes an increased secretion of a hormone that promotes fat accumulation in the fat cells. In this individual, the gene presents a problem only if he or she overeats. Conversely, a person without this gene may not gain weight despite overeating. This explains why some people seem to be able to eat anything, and everything, without gaining a pound.

There are also genes that control behavior, especially behavior related to eating and exercise. If one has a genetic trait to like fatty foods, for example, he or she is more likely to indulge in those foods. The same is true in relation to exercise. There may be a gene that makes some folks tend to dislike exercise—the "couch potato" syndrome—and others to feel a need to be moving constantly. These genes may make it harder for some people to maintain a desirable weight, but—with effort—these traits can be overruled.

Periodically, the United States government conducts what is called the National Health and Nutrition Examination Survey (NHANES). The last two surveys (1988–91 and 1976–80) showed a significant increase in the problem of obesity. During this time, people became fatter but not taller. If obesity were a genetic disease, then we would expect people to get taller to compensate. This is further proof that genetics is not the *prime* factor in the cause of obesity, because if this were so, people would also have become taller.

Not All Fat Is Alike

Although all experts agree that most everyone should slim down to some degree, some insist that the *location* of fat on the body is more important that total body weight.

The term used to explain fat breakdown is lipolysis. Lipolysis is under the control of certain hormones that direct fat to be broken down. These hormones have more effect in liberating fat from the stomach area than from fat that's just under the skin. If you're overweight, more free fatty acids are released from the stomach into the blood system, especially the blood vessels that go to the liver. A high concentration of these free fatty acids is bad for the liver, inhibiting the breakdown of the hormone insulin, which can lead to diabetes and other health problems.

Muscle is also affected by this increased level of free fatty acids from the abdomen. The effect is to inhibit or prevent muscle from taking up glucose from the blood, resulting in increased blood sugar levels. The combination of the effects on the liver, which raise insulin and cause an increase in blood glucose, is certainly counterproductive to good health and a long life.

Excess fat in the stomach may also be a problem because of a certain stress hormone called cortisone. Studies have shown that people who have high levels of cortisone in their blood because of chronic stress carry more abdominal fat. The connection here may be that fat cells in the stomach have receptors to which cortisone attaches and, by doing so, stimulates absorption. When planning to lose weight, especially from the stomach—getting rid of that spare tire—it is important to reduce stress, as high levels prove to be counterproductive.

Diagnosing Your Weight Problem

An important tool in diagnosing weight problems is the body-mass index (BMI) equation. Without it, it is hard to determine how much weight you have to lose. The BMI is based on a simple equation: weight divided by the square root of height in inches. An easy way to do this is to weigh yourself, then measure your height, and plot the numbers using the chart on page 159. Where these values intersect is your BMI. From this chart, you can see if you are overweight. Most experts agree that a BMI above 26 carries a higher than normal risk of stroke, cardiovascular heart disease and diabetes, along with other weight-related problems. If you are in this range, you should reduce your weight. Studies done by George L. Blackburn and his colleagues at the New England Deaconess Hospital (now the Beth Israel Deaconess Medical

Center) in Boston showed that a 10 percent loss of body weight in a group of people 50 to 100 percent overweight produced significant drops in blood pressure, triglycerides, and blood sugar in addition to increasing high-density lipoprotein. Since then, studies in medical centers around the world have confirmed these results.

Another way to gauge your weight problem is to examine where in your body you store your excess fat. The health risks associated with being overweight often depend on how body fat is distributed. Excess fat on the stomach or abdomen (more common in men than women) increases the risk of diabetes and heart disease. Nutritionists think this is because fat cells in this part of the body are released into the bloodstream more easily and upset the actions of the hormone insulin. Because of this, it is important not to carry around a spare tire in addition to love handles.

Another measurement, the waist-to-hip ratio (WHR) is used to determine whether you have a problem with your midsection. See page 164.

The BMI and WHR are means to determine your health risks and degree of obesity based on scientific standards. Your values based on these measurements may indicate that you don't have health risks for obesity. However, you may still be concerned about your appearance. Even though your BMI value doesn't indicate a health risk, you still can and should use the program to lose the weight that you want to lose. Of course, you should always talk to your doctor before starting a weight-loss program.

Essential Components of a Weight-Loss Program

Too often, people are convinced that a weight-loss program involves only dieting and calorie restriction. This type of program *never* works because the other key ingredients to weight loss are missing. In fact, there are three important components to a successful weight loss program: eating the right foods, exercise, and a positive outlook on life—the right mental attitude, which involves changing eating behavior.

Losing weight with the longevity nutrients is different from most other programs because the focus is not on how many calories are consumed or how many fats or carbohydrates are eaten. In fact, the word

BMI CHART

Height \ Weight	100	105	110	115	120	125	130	135	140	145	150	155	160	165	170	175	180	185	190	195	200	205
5′0″	20	21	21	22	23	24	25	26	27	28	29	30	31	32	33	34	35	36	37	38	39	40
5′1″	19	20	21	22	23	24	25	26	26	27	28	29	30	31	32	33	34	35	36	37	38	39
5′2″	18	19	20	21	22	23	24	25	26	27	27	28	29	30	31	32	33	34	35	36	37	37
5′3″	18	19	19	20	21	22	23	24	25	26	27	27	28	29	30	31	32	33	34	35	35	36
5′4″	17	18	19	20	21	21	22	23	24	25	26	27	27	28	29	30	31	32	33	33	34	35
5′5″	17	17	18	19	20	21	22	22	23	24	25	26	27	27	28	29	30	31	32	32	33	34
5′6″	16	17	18	19	19	20	21	22	23	23	24	25	26	27	27	28	29	30	31	31	32	33
5′7″	16	16	17	18	19	20	20	21	22	23	23	24	25	26	27	27	28	29	30	31	31	32
5′8″	15	16	17	17	18	19	20	21	21	22	23	24	24	25	26	27	27	28	29	30	30	31
5′9″	15	16	16	17	18	18	19	20	21	21	22	23	24	24	25	26	27	27	28	29	30	30
5′10″	14	15	16	17	17	18	19	19	20	21	22	22	23	24	24	25	26	27	27	28	29	29
5′11″	14	15	15	16	17	17	18	19	20	20	21	22	22	23	24	24	25	26	26	27	28	29
6′0″	14	14	15	16	16	17	18	18	19	20	20	21	22	23	24	24	25	26	26	26	27	28
6′1″	13	14	15	15	16	16	17	18	18	19	20	20	21	22	22	23	24	24	25	26	26	27
6′2″	13	13	14	15	15	16	17	17	18	19	19	20	21	21	22	22	23	24	24	25	26	26
6′3″	12	13	14	14	15	16	16	17	17	18	19	19	20	21	21	22	22	23	24	24	25	26
6′4″	12	13	13	14	15	15	16	16	17	18	18	19	19	20	21	21	22	23	23	24	24	25

"calorie" isn't even in the vocabulary of *The Longevity Diet*. Rather, the focus is on eating a well-balanced diet that is low in saturated fat and high in the longevity nutrients.

Of course, increasing your physical activity is also important in any weight-loss program—and not just for burning excess fat. Research has shown that exercise may reduce one's desire to eat high-fat foods and may increase one's appetite for carbohydrates. Working out can also lead to better self-image and a more positive feeling about life. Everyone should try to make getting more exercise second nature. Remember the old axiom: Don't sit if you can stand, don't stand if you can walk, don't walk if you can run. Something as simple as using the stairs instead of the elevator whenever possible can make a big difference in the long run.

The third factor in losing weight is mental attitude. Often, people place roadblocks in front of themselves along the path to reaching their ideal weight. Stress, anxiety, depression, or boredom all can play a part in preventing people from reaching their weight-loss goals. It is important to overcome these issues in order to achieve your objective.

Forget about appetite suppressants, fat-blocking drugs, or other weight-loss programs that involve putting foreign substances into your body. Losing weight by following *The Longevity Diet* is the natural way to go. Because the emphasis is on eating in a healthy way—and not on counting calories or grams of fat—long-term success is assured. In other words, this program is different from other diet programs that result in dieters returning to their former eating habits. Once you realize how good you feel when consuming the longevity nutrients, you will work hard to continue to include them in your diet.

What Can the Longevity Nutrients Do for Your Weight Problem?

First of all, we would not be talking about weight loss if all the other programs out there worked. If you are like most people, you have probably tried at least *one* weight reduction program. For at least the last 100 years the public has been bombarded by diets that promise quick and easy weight loss. Sadly, the results have been very poor, although many have captured media and public attention. I think diet book authors are well intentioned, but let's face it, absolutely none of their diets achieve what everyone wants—*a long-term, final solution to their obesity problem.*

Weight reduction programs in diet books usually emphasize one macronutrient over the others. For example, high-protein, high-carbohydrate, and even high-fat diets have all been championed at some point. Another method is emphasizing a certain food or group of foods over the others, for example, the "cabbage soup" or "grapefruit" diet. As varied as these methods are, most of them fail to effect any *long-term* weight loss.

There have also been many scientific approaches to dieting, such as recommending low-calorie food or counting grams of fat or calories. Surprisingly, more often than not, the weirdest diet, such as the "ice cream" diet, works just as well as a scientifically devised diet.

One of the main problems here is use of the term "diet," meaning a program to lose weight quickly and, hopefully, without any appetite problems. The problem is diets don't last forever—they are usually an artificial way of eating that most people do not want to follow after they lose weight. I don't think there is anything so fraught with failure as dieting programs and the overwhelming willingness on the part of so many to keep trying to lose weight by trying other programs.

One of the worst ways to go about losing weight is to rely on drugs. Appetite suppressants, mood stimulators, and other diet aids have been used to achieve weight loss for the last 100 years. Appetite suppressants just *don't* work—they may for while, but when you go off them weight gain is inevitable. I remember the admonitions of a famous physician who was prominent in weight reduction many years ago. His advice on appetite suppressants was if you want to use them, go ahead, but use them for the rest of your life because when you stop you'll gain back the weight. Of course, this can be very dangerous.

Too often, well-intentioned individuals start to do something about their weight problem by focusing only on diet, and although eating too many calories may be at the heart of one's weight problem, there are other factors that are just as important. These include previously mentioned lifestyle factors such as emotional and social problems that must be solved to be successful in losing weight. If you are having marital troubles, financial difficulties, or problems at work or elsewhere, then you are not going to be successful in losing weight with any program. Such stressful situations must be dealt with to be successful in a weight reduction program. You have to get your mental house in order before you can deal with your weight.

The Longevity Nutrients and Weight Loss

Aging and obesity are closely related, therefore maintaining your ideal weight will put you on the road to living your maximum life span. This diet is designed to help you lose weight while at the same time gaining the antiaging effects of the longevity nutrients.

Lignans raise the blood levels of the sex hormone binding globulin (SHBG) and, by so doing, keep the levels of certain hormones in check. One of these is insulin, an anabolic hormone, which too much of, as we learned before, can lead to insulin resistance and the depositing of fat in the body. In cases of insulin resistance, the insulin becomes less able to do its work, so blood sugar levels build up and cause aging effects on protein molecules. Moderating insulin levels is one of the main effects of lignans.

Arginine can help with the changes during the somatopause when growth hormone levels decrease. Decline in growth hormone correlates with increased obesity, and by using this longevity nutrient, its levels are increased, which helps in weight loss.

Many women gain weight during and after menopause, especially in the stomach area. There are many factors—loss of estrogen being one of them—as it may protect women from excess weight gain before menopause. The phytoestrogens, genistein and daidzein, that are longevity nutrients with estrogenic properties, have been shown to help prevent weight gain after menopause.

Conjugated linoleic acid (CLA) is an important substance with numerous antiaging effects. This helps reproportion the composition of the body as weight is being lost. Although definitive studies have not been carried out, preliminary studies indicate a significant role in attaining ideal body composition.

Excess fat disappears after it is burned by the mitochondria. The longevity nutrient carnitine has an important role here in facilitating the delivery of fats into the mitochondria for their disposal. At the same time, this cell part benefits from carnitine's antiaging effects.

Phytosterols help to regulate cholesterol absorption and work with the liver in its function to metabolize and break down fat. Also, these foods have been historically eaten by those people who have very little obesity and are generally lean and healthy.

Inulin and oligofructose, by virtue of their fibrous structure, are excellent to ingest because they reduce appetite and they have a much lower carbohydrate value than other carbohydrates that are normally eaten. They also help modulate blood sugar levels, preventing the development of hypoglycemia and its attendant effects on energy levels and appetite.

PQQ (pyrroloquinoline quinone) is essential for muscle metabolism. Muscles burn fat and glucose, which is crucial to losing weight. The combination of exercise and longevity nutrients can make muscles a serious player in reaching your ideal weight. All of the longevity nutrients have chemical functions that boost various body systems involved in weight reduction.

By now, you know that losing weight is more than just cutting back on calories. Scientists believe that our early ancestors lived where there was an abundance of only natural foods, which contained many of the same substances as the longevity nutrients. Obesity is a phenomenon of modern man who has turned his eating habits away from natural foods and has paid a steep price along the way in terms of health and the problem of obesity.

So, let's get started losing weight with *The New Longevity Diet*.

Step #1

It's important to know whether or not you truly have a weight problem. In order to find this out, refer to the chart of BMIs. Using your height and weight, plot these on the chart. If you are between 26 and 28, or above, then you probably have excess weight.

Another way to assess one's weight problem is to examine where one's excess fat is stored in the body. The health risks associated with being overweight often depend on how body fat is distributed. Excess fat on the stomach or abdomen increases the risk of diabetes and heart disease. Nutritionists think that this is because fat cells in this part of the body are released into the bloodstream more easily and upset the actions of the hormone insulin. Because of this, it is important not to carry around a spare tire.

The waste-to-hip ratio, or WHR, is used to determine whether a problem exists in the midsection. To figure out your WHR, measure the narrowest part of your waist and then measure the widest part of your hips. Men are considered at risk for the complications of obesity if their WHR is greater than 0.9 and women if their WHR is greater than 0.8. The WHR along with the BMI will help you to determine the extent of your weight problem.

Has adulthood brought with it an extra 10 or 20 pounds? You're not alone. Most people add a few pounds every decade of adulthood. Is this unhealthy? It depends. Did your excess weight settle around your middle, giving you an apple shape? Or did it sink to your buttocks, hips, and thighs, leaving you with a pear shape?

If you have an apple shape—a pot belly or spare tire—you carry fat in and around your abdominal organs. Fat around your middle alters the way your body uses fat, which can lead to diabetes, coronary artery disease, and cancer. Even very thin "apples" run the same health risks as obese "apples," because fat in your abdomen is more likely to break down and enter your blood where it can clog your arteries.

If you have a pear shape—large buttocks, hips, and thighs—you may not have much greater health risks than someone who's not overweight. Pear shapes are generally inherited. If your mom has "thunder thighs," you may have them too. Although apple shapes can also be inherited, the health risks of overeating, drinking alcohol regularly, and not getting enough exercise are worse for "apples" than for "pears."

How your waist-to-hip ratio is calculated:

1. Measure your waist at your navel.
   ___ inches or centimeters
2. Measure your hips at their widest point (over your buttocks)
   ___ inches or centimeters
3. Divide your waist measurement by your hip measurement.

For example, if you have a 27-inch waist and 38-inch hips, divide 27 by 38 to get a waist-to-hip ratio of 0.71.

For most women, the waist-to-hip ratio should fall below 0.80. For most men, the waist-to-hip ratio should be no greater than 1.0.

Step #2

None of the longevity nutrients contain significant calories that could lead to weight gain. Just the opposite, as already pointed out, these amazing substances aid the weight reduction process because of their diversified effects on the body's physiology. The amount and speed of weight loss varies from person to person and is also highly related to one's level of exercise.

Follow the 14-day menu plan. This plan allows three meals each day. At no times are foods eaten after dinner, and it is essential to follow the instructions on cooking tips and portion sizes. Numbers of recipes (located in the appendix) are given in parentheses.

At the end of the 14 days, reevaluate your BMI and WHR to see what progress you've made. You can continue on for another 14-day cycle, mix and match these recipes into your own menu plan, or design your own diet. If you can choose the last option, you should try to include as many foods as possible with high concentrations of the following longevity nutrients:

- lignans
- arginine
- phytoestrogens
- CLA
- carnitine
- phytosterols
- inulin and oligofructose
- PQQ

Step #3

Exercise. As with any weight-loss program, exercise is a vital component of *The New Longevity Diet*. Refer to chapter 10 for information on exercise and how it relates to this program.

The 14-Day New Longevity Weight-Loss Program

DAY #1

✦ **BREAKFAST**

Kiwi and Banana Granola Yogurt (10)*
Orange juice

✦ **LUNCH**

Salad Niçoise (51)*
Mineral water

✦ **DINNER**

Spice-Rubbed Filets Mignons (140)*
French Country Potatoes (141)*
Green Beans with Almonds (142)*
Berry Yogurt Parfaits (143)*
Diet soda

DAY #2

✦ **BREAKFAST**

Banana Cinnamon Toast (11)*
Coffee

✦ **LUNCH**

Tarragon Hamburgers with Pickled Red Onions (53)
Lemonade

✦ **DINNER**

Salt-Crusted Breast of Chicken with Artichokes (144)*
Rice Topped with Tomato Sauce (145)*
Lime Blackberry Pudding (146)
Sparkling mineral water

DAY #3

✦ **BREAKFAST**

Carrot-Apple Whole Wheat Muffins (12)*
Grapefruit juice

✦ **LUNCH**

Cream Cheese and Pineapple Sandwiches (54)*
Skim milk

✦ **DINNER**

Orange-Flavored Poached Salmon (147)*
Country Asparagus Soup (148)*
Kiwi-Mango Sherbet (149)*
Coffee

DAY #4

✦ **BREAKFAST**

Scrambled Tofu with Mushrooms and Tomatoes (13)*
Coffee

✦ **LUNCH**

Barley and Smoked Turkey Salad (55)
Skim milk

✦ **DINNER**

Flounder Fillets Coated with Pine Nuts (150)*
Carrot Salad with Cilantro Dressing (151)*
Cinnamon Baked Bananas (152)*
Sparkling mineral water with lime

DAY #5

✦ **BREAKFAST**

Peach and Blueberry Breakfast Parfait (14)*
Cider

✦ **LUNCH**

Grilled Tempeh Sandwiches (56)*
Iced tea

✦ **DINNER**

Roast Pork with Spice Crust (153)*
Rice with Lemon and Cilantro (154)*
Papaya Ice (155)
Mineral water

DAY #6

✦ **BREAKFAST**

All-Wheat Pancakes (15)*
½ Grapefruit
Tea

✦ **LUNCH**

Japanese Crabmeat salad (57)*
Mediterranean Artichokes (58)
Diet drink

✦ **DINNER**

Dandelion Green Salad (156)*
Salmon with Mediterranean Sauce (157)*

Broiled Apples with Maple Syrup (158)
Lemon flavored carbonated water

DAY #7

✦ **BREAKFAST**

Raspberry and Almond Muesli (16)*
Cranberry juice

✦ **LUNCH**

Marissa's Favorite Turkey Burgers (59)
Sparkling mineral water

✦ **DINNER**

Lemon Shrimp and Asparagus Fettuccine (159)*
Papaya Salad with Lime Vinaigrette (160)*
Apple, Pear, and Cranberry Gratin (161)*
Jasmine Iced Tea (162)

DAY #8

✦ **BREAKFAST**

Baked Cheese Toast (17)*
Orange juice

✦ **LUNCH**

Chicken Salad with Exotic Mushroom Vinaigrette (60)*
Grapefruit Lime Cooler (61)

✦ **DINNER**

Steamed Dover Sole in Olive and Pine Nut Sauce (163)*
Artichokes with Roman Vinaigrette (164)*
Honey Apple Sorbet (165)*
Tea

DAY #9

✦ **BREAKFAST**

Pear Cashew Muffins (18)*
Skim milk

✦ **LUNCH**

Tofu Salad and Sprout Sandwiche (62)*
Mineral water

✦ **DINNER**

Sun Salad (166)
Sesame and Ginger Asparagus (167)*

Roast Chicken with Mushroom and Pecan Stuffing (168)*
Orange Almond Iced Tea (169)*

DAY #10

✦ **BREAKFAST**

Smoked Ham and Cheese Omelette (19)
Coffee

✦ **LUNCH**

Vegetable Noodle Soup with Cheddar (63)
Tuna Sandwiches with Basil and Tomato (64)*
Mineral water

✦ **DINNER**

New Potatoes with Chicory (170)*
Herbed Grilled Lamb Chops (171)*
Swiss Vegetable Soup (172)*
Sliced watermelon
Wine

DAY #11

✦ **BREAKFAST**

Breakfast Fruit Compote (20)*
Skim milk

✦ **LUNCH**

Roasted Garlic and Avocado Crab Sandwich (65)*
Grapefruit Cooler (66)

✦ **DINNER**

Cannelloni and Cauliflower Sauté (173)*
Curly Chicory and Red-Leaf Lettuce Salad (174)*
Chocolate Almond Mousse with Raspberries (175)
Iced Tea

DAY #12

✦ **BREAKFAST**

Hearty Omelette (21)*
Orange juice

✦ **LUNCH**

French Fruit and Cheese Sandwich (67)*
Ginger Lime Tea (68)

✦ **DINNER**

Green Beans with Pine Nuts (176)*
Honey Glazed Carrots (177)
Oyster and Romano Soufflé (178)
Pineapple Grape Sorbet (179)
Mineral water

DAY #13

✦ **BREAKFAST**

Triple Berry Breakfast Shake (22)*
Coffee

✦ **LUNCH**

Turkey and Avocado Tortilla Rolls with Black Bean-Corn Salsa (69)*
Tomato Juice (70)

✦ **DINNER**

Roasted Red Snapper with Potatoes and Red Wine (180)
Stirred Rice with Spinach (181)
Warm Goat Cheese Salad with Dried Cherries and Pancetta Vinaigrette (182)*
Chocolate Walnut Angel Cookies (183)*
Mineral water

DAY #14

✦ **BREAKFAST**

Flaxseed Pancakes (23)*
Orange juice

✦ **LUNCH**

Marinated Green Pepper Hamburgers on Whole Wheat Rolls (71)*
Honey Darjeeling Iced Tea (72)

✦ **DINNER**

Black and White Salad (184)*
Glaze-Grilled Swordfish (185)*
Berries in Meringue Baskets (186)
Mineral water

How to Use *The New Longevity Diet*

How-to-Diet Cooking Tips

- When you eat beef or veal, always choose lean cuts and trim away all visible fat. That means you'll have to forget about those richly marbled porterhouse steaks, but I think you'll find a flank steak, strip steak, or sirloin just as enjoyable. Also, be especially careful about the ground beef you buy. I allow hamburgers on *The New Longevity Diet,* but only if you make them with the leanest ground beef you can find. Go for ground sirloin or ground round, not chuck. And ask your butcher to trim off as much fat as possible before he grinds it.
- Be sure to broil, grill, or roast both beef and veal. Don't fry.
- When you eat lamb, keep the same rules of the game in mind. Buy the leanest cuts; trim off all the fat; broil, grill, or roast.
- When you eat pork, make an extra effort to avoid fatty cuts. You'll have to avoid pork roasts, unless it's a trimmed pork tenderloin. Pork chops need their fat trimmed as well, and avoid the richly marbled ones. While I don't advise eating fatty cured pork products such as bacon, you can enjoy some ham and Canadian bacon on occasion.
- Chicken is a wonderful food for dieters. Remember to stick to the white meat, because that is leaner than the dark meat. Always trim off fat and skin before cooking. Broil, grill, or roast your chicken—never fry it.
- Fish is also a wonderful food for dieters, and you'll see that I recommend a lot of it on *The New Longevity Diet*. It's hard to trim the skin off fish before cooking it, but be sure not to eat it. Also, never fry your fish; enjoy it broiled, grilled, or oven-baked.
- Eat only fresh or frozen fish. Avoid the canned or smoked varieties unless they're preserved in water or mustard. Avoid the kinds packed in oil.
- *The New Longevity Diet* allows you to eat cheese, but let me add a special word of caution here. Cheese often contains lots of fat, calories, and salt—three things you generally want to avoid on a diet. When you have cheese, stick to the low-fat variety. Many cheeses are made with skim milk and low sodium, while others like feta

cheese, are naturally lower in calories. Also, when you have cottage cheese or cream cheese, be sure to stick to the low-fat brands.

- Substitute plain yogurt for any sour cream. And be sure to use low-fat yogurt. When you're having yogurt alone, instead of as a condiment, try buying the plain kind and adding your own fresh fruits.
- When you use even small quantities of fat in cooking, try to use a reduced-calorie margarine. Even better, use a nonstick cooking spray, which contains virtually no fat or calories.
- If you're uncomfortable using reduced-calorie products, but enjoy sautéing, try doing so with only a teaspoon of oil in a nonstick pan along with a couple of tablespoons of defatted chicken or beef broth. Some of my patients even add Worcestershire sauce or wine (the calories in alcohol burn off during cooking).
- Add flavor to your food by cooking with herbs and spices. That will help you avoid excess fat and salt in your diet.
- You can even have a little pizza on this diet. But be careful to avoid the kind with meat toppings. There are lots of delicious vegetable toppings now—broccoli, spinach, and eggplant as well as the more traditional mushrooms, peppers, and onions.
- When you eat cereal on *The New Longevity Diet,* I must ask you to be careful about your choices. When it comes to fat and calories, not all cereals are created equal.

  Avoid the granola types and the packaged brands that have lots of added sugar. There are even some reduced-calorie cereals that use sugar substitutes that you may want to try. If you don't like sugar or sugar substitutes, I encourage you to stick to the non-processed cereal varieties, such as good old oatmeal.
- When you have a potato, I recommend baking, boiling, and steaming as the best cooking methods. Whatever you do, don't fry. And don't lather on the sour cream and butter. Stick to reduced-calorie margarine and reduced-calorie sour cream, or better yet, just plain yogurt. Mix in some chives or hot sauce for a change.
- When you have corn, feel free to enjoy it on the cob or in kernels. But remember to avoid butter and salt.
- When you have vegetables, be sure to boil or steam them. No frying, and don't smother vegetables in butter or oil at the table. I recommend a little lemon juice; it enhances the flavor of almost every vegetable.

- You'll see that *The New Longevity Diet* is filled with fruits and vegetables. Sometimes the menu plans may call for varieties that are out of season or otherwise unavailable in your area. If that happens, just consult the appropriate Longevity Food List, and you'll find a suitable substitute.
- Eat fresh fruit whenever possible. If you must have canned varieties, be sure they are packed in fruit juice with no added sugar.
- Let me add a word of caution about raisins, currants, dates, and other dried fruits. They have more calories than fresh fruits, so use them sparingly and only where specifically called for in the menus. Even though they are technically fruits, they are not good snack foods.
- Enjoy fruit juices as much as possible on the diet. Look for low-calorie cranberry juice and other-reduced calorie varieties. Or, if you prefer regular kinds, I suggest having about an ounce of juice with a glass of carbonated water. I call these juice spritzers and they are a great friend to dieters. This trick will allow you to drink more fluids throughout the day. I don't recommend that you drink glass after glass of pure fruit juice. It has more calories than you might think. As you'll see later in the book, I often treat fruit juices as side dishes or appetizers, rather than as simple beverages. Juice spritzers, on the other hand, you may drink as often as you like.
- Every now and then, on *The New Longevity Diet,* I recommend hot chocolate. Please keep in mind that I mean only the reduced-calorie cocoa drinks available at your supermarket. And be sure you make them with skim milk or water, not whole milk.
- I also suggest that you occasionally enjoy frozen yogurt while you're on the diet. This can be a delightful alternatives to ice cream. Please keep in mind that I mean only the low-fat varieties.
- Enjoy the soups I recommend, but make sure that none is cream-based. Creamed soups are too high in fat and calories. Also, be sure to defat soups and broths before eating them or using them in cooking.
- *The New Longevity Diet* does not strictly forbid alcoholic beverages, but I certainly do not advise drinking them regularly. Alcohol has a lot of calories, and it is the kind of disinhibitor that can trip you up on the best of diets. If you feel you must have alcohol, I rec-

ommend you stick to only one or two drinks a week. Be sure to have only the reduced-calorie beers or reduced-calorie wine spritzers. And remember, even those drinks have a significant amount of calories, at least as much as a glass of juice or skim milk.

- One helpful hint to many a dieter is herbal tea. It's caffeine free, so even if you're sensitive to that chemical, you can drink it.

How to Diet—Portion Tips

There's a marvelously useful word that can be a big help when you're dieting, and that's the word *one*, as in:

One slice of bread
One muffin
One egg
One container of low-fat yogurt
One waffle
One sandwich
One scoop of ice cream
One potato
One slice of bacon

You get the idea!

If *one* is the word that can make a big difference when you're dieting, "Don't overeat" is the short sentence you should also commit to memory.

You won't be hungry if you follow *The New Longevity Diet,* and there's no reason to keep eating when you're not hungry. Eat enough so that you feel satisfied, but not so much that you feel stuffed, full, or uncomfortable from too much food.

There may be times when you know you have had enough, even though you haven't eaten every morsel of food listed on the menu or food plan for the day. *This is the moment to stop eating!* Even if, according to the plan, you may have a dessert or snack, don't eat if you're not hungry.

In addition to that important word *one*, and the essential rule to never overeat, the following will explain the quantities and serving sizes you may have of the food on *The New Longevity Diet.*

- **A SERVING OF MEAT OR POULTRY** means you may have one lamb chop, one lean pork chop, a lean hamburger, two thin slices of roast beef, or half a chicken breast. The meat (without bone) should weigh between four and six ounces. I don't recommend that you have red meat more than three times a week. As a dieter, you should emphasize poultry and fish.
- **A SERVING OF FISH** means a filet, steak, whole fish, or portion of a large fish. The fish flesh should weigh between four and six ounces.
- **A SERVING OF SHRIMP** means about a cup of shrimp, which is usually three large ones, or six to eight medium ones, or a cup of small ones. Be careful with shrimp salad you don't make at home; it can be made with high-fat ingredients. Half a cup is usually ample.
- **A SERVING OF SCALLOPS** means about four to six ounces.
- **A SERVING OF OYSTERS OR CLAMS** means anywhere from six to twenty plain oysters or clams. Oysters and clams themselves are low in calories, but most people like only a half a dozen at a time. Also, be careful of recipes like oysters Rockefeller and clams casino that include lots of high-fat, high-calorie ingredients. Keep in mind, too, that these foods are high in cholesterol and you'll want to limit your intake, if that is a concern of yours.
- **A SERVING OF PASTA** as a main dish means a moderate, filling amount, which is about two ounces of dry pasta. As most pasta comes in sixteen-ounce boxes, it's easy enough to figure out when you've taken approximately two ounces or one eighth from the box. When you're having pasta as a side dish, I think you should have only one half to one ounce. That should be enough to accompany any main dish.
- **A SERVING OF PIZZA** means one quarter of a ten-inch-diameter pie.
- **A SERVING OF SOUP** means about a bowl, or twelve to sixteen ounces of soup, which is enough for a filling meal.
- **A SERVING OF BEAN SOUP** means about a cup, or eight to ten ounces.
- **A SERVING OF MEAT, FISH, OR CHEESE FOR A SANDWICH** means approximately two ounces. If it's turkey or chicken, you may have up to three ounces. Avoid those overstuffed deli sandwiches.
- **A SERVING OF VEGETABLES** means . . . well, I've never met anyone who got fat from eating broccoli, brussels sprouts, green beans, cabbage, asparagus, or similar vegetables. Just be sure you eat those vegetables without butter, margarine, oil, or sauce. You may

have as much as you want of the vegetables listed in the Longevity Nutrient Value List.

- **A SERVING OF POTATO** means one potato. Potatoes of all varieties (new potatoes, sweet potatoes, red bliss potatoes, Idahos) are special vegetables. You can't indulge in potatoes the way you can in other, less starchy vegetables. So, one serving of potato means only one. You may have it baked, steamed, or boiled. If you're having red bliss or new potatoes, you may have three small ones, the approximate equivalent of one baking potato.
- **A SERVING OF CORN** means one ear of corn on the cob or one-half cup of kernels.
- **A SERVING OF BEANS** means about one-half cup of beans. Like potatoes, beans are higher in calories than most other carbohydrates.
- **A SERVING OF RICE** means one-half cup of cooked rice.
- **A SERVING OF COLESLAW** means one-half cup.
- **A SERVING OF SALAD** means you may have as much as you like of salad ingredients such as lettuce, celery, onions, and radishes. As with other vegetables, I haven't seen anyone get fat on salad, as long as you remember that eggs, cheese, and meat are not salad ingredients. Also, stick to moderate amounts of low-fat, low-calorie dressing.
- **A SERVING OF BREAD** means one slice, even if you're having a sandwich. If the bread is not presliced, a serving means one half-inch slice. If you're using reduced-calorie bread, you can have two slices as a single serving.
- **A SERVING OF A ROLL** means one roll.
- **A SERVING OF A MUFFIN** means one muffin. If it's the baked variety, it should weigh two and a half to three ounces. Avoid the super big muffins that weigh as much as five or six ounces.
- **A SERVING OF BAGEL** means one bagel.
- **A SERVING OF CEREAL** means you may have one to one and one-half ounces of cereal.
- **A SERVING OF PANCAKES OR FRENCH TOAST** means two pancakes (4"x 4"x½") or one piece of French toast.
- **A SERVING OF SKIM MILK ON YOUR CEREAL** means you shouldn't use so much that you turn your cereal soggy. Use one-third to one-quarter cup on your cereal.
- **A SERVING OF CREAM CHEESE** means you may have one ounce of a reduced-calorie kind.

- **A SERVING OF YOGURT** means eight ounces of plain, low-fat yogurt. Try adding a couple ounces of fresh fruit if you want to flavor it.
- **A SERVING OF COTTAGE CHEESE** means about four ounces of a low-fat brand.
- **A SERVING OF SOUR CREAM** means one tablespoon of a reduced-calorie brand.
- **A SERVING OF JELLY** means you may have one or two tablespoons of reduced-calorie jelly.
- **A SERVING OF SYRUP** means you may have one or two tablespoons of reduced-calorie syrup.
- **A SERVING OF MAYONNAISE** means you may use no more than one-half tablespoon of reduced-calorie mayonnaise.
- **A SERVING OF MARGARINE** means one pat (about a teaspoon) of a reduced-calorie kind.
- **A SERVING OF KETCHUP** means you may have up to two or three tablespoons.
- **A SERVING OF MUSTARD** means you may have as much mustard as you wish. This is a nice alternative for those of you who don't like using low-calorie products on sandwiches, salads, and the like.
- **A SERVING OF HORSERADISH** means you may have as much as you wish. This is another underappreciated, low-fat, low-calorie condiment that's wonderful on sandwiches. Have half a teaspoon with turkey or cold beef and see what I mean.
- **A SERVING OF APPLESAUCE** means you may have one-half cup of unsweetened applesauce. Don't have the presweetened kind.
- **A SERVING OF SALAD DRESSING** means you may use two tablespoons of bottled reduced-calorie dressing. It's not free, so don't pour it on.
- **A SERVING OF SAUCES** means that when you're putting sauce on spaghetti, use a light hand. I recommend one-third to one-half cup of meat sauce and one-half to three-quarters cup of vegetable or seafood sauce.
- **A SERVING OF CHEESE AS A CONDIMENT** means that you're sprinkling Parmesan and Romano on spaghetti; don't overdo. One or two tablespoons should be enough.
- **A SERVING OF CHEESE AS A SNACK** means a slice of cheese that is low in fat and salt. It should weigh about an ounce.

- **A SERVING OF POPCORN** means you may have one to two cups of unbuttered and unsalted popcorn.
- **A SERVING OF CRACKERS** means you may have two or three, not the whole box.
- **A SERVING OF RICE CAKES** means you can have one.
- **A SERVING OF DRIED FRUIT** means no more than one-eighth cup.
- **A SERVING OF ICE CREAM, ICE MILK, FROZEN YOGURT, TOFUTTI, OR SHERBET** means one two-ounce scoop. Most scoopers serve up just that amount.
- **A SERVING OF PIE OR CAKE** means only one slice. And one slice does not mean one-quarter of the pie. You know what one slice means. A nine-inch pie divides nicely into eight pieces.
- **A SERVING OF FRUIT** means in general one piece of fruit. But this, like vegetables, is the place to overindulge. If you're feeling hungry, a second piece of fruit is not going to ruin the diet. If you're having berries, three-quarters to one cup is fine. But be more careful with cherries and grapes. Stick to one-half to three-quarter cup of these more calorie-laden fruits. Mangoes and papayas are exceptions. They're pretty rich in calories, so you should limit yourself to one per serving.
- **A SERVING OF MELON** means half a cantaloupe, one-quarter to one-eighth of a honeydew, and a 4" x 8" inch wedge of watermelon.
- **A SERVING OF ANY FRUIT OR VEGETABLE JUICE** means a four- to six-ounce serving, the size of an average juice glass.
- **A SERVING OF JUICE SPRITZER** means you may have as much as you want. They only contain about an ounce of fruit juice, so they're a great way to quench your thirst throughout the day.
- **A SERVING OF SKIM MILK** means an eight-ounce serving.
- **A SERVING OF WINE** means a three-and-one-half-ounce glass or a twelve-ounce wine spritzer.
- **A SERVING OF BEER** means one bottle, twelve ounces, of low-calorie beer.
- **A SERVING OF SKIM MILK IN YOUR COFFEE OR TEA** means you shouldn't turn these beverages white; after all, you want to retain that delicious coffee or tea flavor. Approximately one to two tablespoons of skim milk should do it.
- **A SERVING OF COFFEE OR TEA** means that, while there is no strict limit on the amount you can drink (since these beverages contain

no fat or calories that contribute to weight gain), I do recommend that you don't have more than two to three cups a day.

- **SODAS.** Stay away from regular sodas. They're loaded with sugar and calories. Diet sodas aren't fattening, and if they're caffeine free, there's no strict limit to how many you can drink a day. However, the long-term effects of sugar substitutes are still being debated, so I recommend no more than one or two diet sodas a day.
- **MINERAL OR CARBONATED WATER.** Enjoy! There are no health or weight-gain risks here, and the lightly flavored carbonated waters can be truly delicious. (Be careful of those brands high in sodium.)

10

EXERCISE, DISUSE, AND THE LONGEVITY NUTRIENTS

The bad news first: lack of exercise or physical inactivity hastens the general breakdown of the body. In other words: if you don't use it, you will lose it.

But there is good news: exercise not only staves off the loss of bone and muscle mass associated with aging, it also facilitates metabolization of our longevity nutrients, enhancing their disease-preventing and anti-aging effects.

Why Exercise?

Nowhere are the effects of physical inactivity as obvious as in our muscles, whose usefulness is determined by the energy-producing fibers that make them up. Without exercise, muscles atrophy—the muscle mass and total number of fibers decrease measurably. Leg muscles of people in their 80s average 140,000 fewer fibers than those of 30- to 40-year-olds. The remaining fibers simply cannot produce adequate energy for muscle function.

Along with the reduction of fibers, a general change in the muscle composition occurs as we age. The size of muscle decreases, due in large part to an infiltration of fat and connective tissue in a process that begins as early as age 18 in women and the early 30s in men. So now we're looking at a muscle that has fewer energy-producing fibers, is composed in increasing proportions of non-muscle tissue, and there are still more disheartening changes to come!

In the muscle, nerves called motor neurons stimulate the fibers into action. The number of motor neurons also decreases as a result of disuse and aging, and each time nerves are lost to poor diet or inactivity, the fibers to which they are attached atrophy. The consequences of all of these changes in our muscles can be measured in performance: endurance, peak force production, and explosive power all decrease when muscles atrophy. Consider the fact that 40 percent of women between the ages of 55 and 64 cannot lift a 4.5-kg weight (about 10 lbs.).

Now consider the silver lining to all of this: more exercise, along with increased intake of our longevity nutrients, restores motor neurons and results in a regeneration of muscle fibers.

Physical Fitness Method and Styles

The notion that exercise is a factor in health and longevity isn't a new one. In the fourth century B.C., Hippocrates stressed the concept of physical exercise in the practice of medicine. In the 1100s, the physician and philosopher Maimonides wrote extensively about the importance of exercise.

Modern science has verified Maimonides' ideas that exercise arms the body to fight disease and helps it perform better in general. He also believed that exercise and proper diet went hand in hand in health maintenance. But although the ancient scholars suspected the value of exercise, they simply didn't know enough about the workings of the body to determine the best type of exercise. Now we know. From tracking the health and fitness of individuals in long-term studies, we have learned that there is no one type of exercise that will confer total physical fitness. The best programs entail both major types of exercise, aerobic and anaerobic.

Let's Get Physical

Aerobic exercise came in vogue in the United States in the 1970s and 1980s when many people learned that it promoted weight loss and that the risks for heart disease associated with high cholesterol could be mitigated by exercise that taxed the cardiovascular system. But aerobic exercise should be combined with anaerobic exercises, which promote strength and flexibility in the major muscle groups in our bodies. Aside from building muscle power, anaerobic exercise also benefits our body's overall health.

Most exercise regimens are devised to work around the "training effect," which is the theory that an overloaded system will respond by adapting to a level of function higher than its starting level. The training effect works in stages, beginning with the systemic overload. Your heart or any other muscle group is given a task of sufficient intensity and duration to be stimulated to the point of fatigue. When the exercise is over, the stimulus is withdrawn; and the system enters the recovery period. In order for the training effect to take place, the recovery period must be long enough to permit an adaptation for the system.

Finally, exercises must be repeated, or the adaptation gained from the last workout will be lost between sessions—a phenomenon familiar to any frequent exerciser who has ever skipped a couple of sessions.

Aerobic Exercise

This category includes exercises such as walking, running, and playing tennis or volleyball. The common denominator for all of these is cardiovascular and respiratory stimulation—your heart beats faster and you breathe harder. In order to obtain what is called an aerobic effect (systemic overload and greater endurance), a certain number of calories must be expended. The amount of calories used for a given exercise is an index to the level of intensity. For example, all of the exercises named above, when engaged in for 5 to 10 minutes, are considered to be of moderate intensity. When you choose an exercise, you should consider the intensity in relation to your own level of fitness and your health status.

There are a few ways to determine whether your chosen exercise has an aerobic effect. The most commonly used method is measuring heart rate, because heart rate is easily measured and corresponds reliably to the much more difficult to measure quantity of oxygen consumed during exercise. Monitor carefully, though: as your heart adapts to increasing demands, your heart rate response decreases, so subsequent workouts must be made more difficult to reach the same heart rate. A heart rate target zone of up to 90 percent of maximum heart rate has been found to be efficacious in eliciting an aerobic training effect. Once you've determined your heart rate target zone, you can achieve a training effect by planning your exercise so that your heart rate is within the target zone for between 15 and 60 minutes two to five times a week.

Strength Training

In addition to an aerobic program to promote cardiovascular fitness, all exercise programs should contain a strength and endurance training component. This is critical to build muscle and bone mass, two things that will dramatically improve the quality of your later years.

The fundamental principle behind muscular strength programs is very simple: if resistance is applied to a muscle as it contracts, the muscle will adapt by becoming stronger. In the muscle itself, this increase in strength is visible as enlargement of muscle fibers. Progressive increases in resistant force result in progressively greater adaptations. Therefore, all muscular strength programs apply more resistant force than the muscle is normally exposed to. But that is where the similarity between such programs usually ends, and there are widely varying views on how best to apply this resistance.

Before I go into detail about the three types of resistance exercises, I want to remind you that they all have the same goal: *to build muscle strength and endurance*. Whether you choose isotonic, isokinetic, or isometric exercise, you will be able to measure results for yourself and determine which is the most satisfying. Even though scientists don't agree on the best means to develop your muscles, they all agree with the basic ideas proposed so many years ago by Maimonides and Hippocrates: exercise is a critical part of staying healthy longer.

Isotonic Exercise

Muscle contraction is the term for the way a muscle develops tension to overcome resistance. The principle behind isotonic exercise has to do with the two ways in which muscles contract. The best way to understand this is to do a simple exercise.

Hold a weight, like a hardcover book or an apple, in your hand with your arm parallel to your spine and your wrist forward. Using your free hand, hold the muscle in your upper arm as you raise the weight from abdomen to chest height. Feel the muscle hunching up under your skin? The muscle is hunching up because it is shortening. When a muscle is said to contract concentrically, it shortens as it contracts, just as you can feel here.

Now, while still feeling the muscle, lower the weight from your chest to below your waist, and you should feel the muscle stretching out. Although the muscle is lengthening, it's still resisting force, so it's still contracting. This type of contraction, where a muscle lengthens as it contracts, is known as eccentric contraction.

Generally speaking, eccentric contraction generates more tension in the muscle than the concentric kind. Because of this, it's important to limit eccentric contraction exercises early on to reduce the chance of muscle strains.

Isokinetic Exercise

Whether it involves concentric or eccentric muscle contractions, isokinetic exercise involves carefully controlling muscle lengthening or shortening throughout exercise periods. This control is achieved through the use of equipment of variable resistance.

Isometric Exercise

In isometric exercise, muscular force is exerted against an immovable object. Even though the notion of pushing as hard as you can against a wall might first strike you as silly, give it a try. You'll see that even though nothing happens externally, a great deal of tension contracts the muscles.

Muscular strength increases as a result of sustaining the contraction against the resistance long enough for peak tension to develop within the muscle. Since there's no joint movement in this type of exercise, strength develops only at the position in which the exercise is performed. Even a resistance of only 60 to 80 percent of the muscle's capacity will lead to appreciable increases in strength.

All resistance exercise, irrespective of type, improves functional ability of the muscles. Muscular strength increases—as a result of the enlargement of existing muscle fibers along with recruitment of new fibers—as long as the muscle contraction is stressed by increasing levels of tension. Endurance also increases with sustained strength training. If enough muscles are recruited during prolonged mild resistance exercise, total body endurance can be increased as well.

Finally, resistance exercises increase muscular performance, also known as power. Two factors determine power. The first is the rate at which a muscle contracts and develops force throughout the range of motion. The second is the relationship between speed and force. Power can be increased by moving either a high load for a low number of repetitions or a low load for a high number of repetitions to the point of muscular fatigue.

When we talk about power, we often distinguish between aerobic and anaerobic power. This is because within the same muscles, there are two types of muscle fiber. Aerobic power, which is built by low-intensity exercise sustained over a long period of time, involves Type I, or *slow twitch* muscle fibers. These generate low levels of muscle tension but can sustain contraction for longer intervals than Type II fibers. Because they fatigue very slowly, these are more suited to aerobic activity. The Type II or *fast twitch* muscle fibers that determine anaerobic power, however, are capable of generating a great amount of tension very quickly and are therefore involved in high-intensity bursts of energy such as sprinting or heavy weight lifting. Because they gather energy so quickly, they also fatigue quickly and do not contribute much to muscular endurance.

Interactions of Exercise and the Longevity Nutrients

The more we know about the health benefits of exercise, the more we appreciate the need for good nutrition in conjunction with this process. It's a fairly recent development that has doctors advising their patients on how to balance their intake of carbohydrates, fats, vitamins, and minerals to gain maximal benefits of exercise. As counterintuitive as it seems to us in retrospect, for many years nutrition was a completely separate discipline.

The longevity nutrients augment the health benefits of exercise, and use of the longevity nutrients in conjunction with an exercise program gives you an edge in preventing aging and disease.

The Longevity Nutrients and Aerobic Exercise

Using an aerobic program has several advantages for your health. The best known of these is the prevention of coronary heart disease (CHD) as well as its corollaries atherosclerosis and blood clots in the blood vessels. Physicians agree that exercise lowers the risk of CHD, based on dozens of studies conducted worldwide, which consistently demonstrate that individuals in higher fitness categories have fewer incidents of cardiovascular disease. There are several mechanisms by which exercise reduces risk of CHD. For one thing, exercise reinforces the heart against fatal arrhythmias. Then, aerobic training bolsters the blood vessels' ability to transport oxygen, making the heart more capable of ensuring an adequate supply for itself. Exercise also prevents the formation of deadly clots that block supply of blood to the heart and lower blood pressure overall. Finally, exercise changes your blood cholesterol profile, boosting HDL levels and keeping LDLs from building up on the blood vessel walls.

Having said that, let me introduce another weapon in your arsenal against CHDs. Saponins and phytosterols work to inhibit accretion of deadly LDLs while exercise promotes synthesis and retention of HDLs. Certain flavonoids, such as quercetin, also fight the effects of LDLs, by functioning as an antioxidant specific to the LDL molecule.

One of the main goals of aerobic exercise is cardiovascular fitness, which in turn results in improved heart function and deterrence of CHD. The longevity nutrient taurine works to regulate the level of calcium in the heart. This is critical because in order for the heart to pump blood, calcium moves across the membranes of the heart's cells to produce a contraction. Exercise improves the ability of the heart to pump, but without taurine, this function can be compromised. Taurine works in concert with exercise for maximal cardiovascular fitness.

If you're at risk for CHD, pay special attention to your intake of saponins, phytosterols, quercetin, and taurine—especially in conjunction with an anaerobic exercise program.

The Longevity Nutrients and Anaerobic Exercise

One of the most visible results of resistance training is an increase in muscle mass. The increase can even be measured by taking a cross-sectional measurement of the muscle before and after exercising. At a microscopic level, there is an increase in the size of individual muscle fibers in resistance-trained muscles. Muscle fibers that have grown, especially those that function aerobically, have a greater need for antioxidants, such as the longevity nutrient carnosine.

Increasing muscle mass also requires nutrients to support mitochondrial function. In muscles, mitochondria have a pivotal role in energy production. The longevity nutrient carnitine is used in our bodies to transport fat molecules into the mitochondria. The heart and muscles are particularly vulnerable to lower levels of carnitine, and serious problems can develop if supplies are not adequate.

Yet another aspect of resistance training concerns the increase of blood supply to the fibers of the muscle. This is seen as an increase in density of small blood vessels that carry nutrients to the muscle fibers. Without a corresponding increase in blood supply, the new fibers would atrophy. The longevity nutrient arginine is an important modulator of the ability of blood vessels to meet supply, and flavonoids such as quercetin protect new blood vessels in resistance-trained muscles.

Resistance training's most obvious results may be in muscle, but the most important ones, for many people, concern bones. Osteoporosis, a condition in which bone loss results from a hormonal, nutritional, or mechanical deficiency, causes the bone to become more porous and therefore less able to withstand stress.

Like muscle, bone responds to changes in mechanical strain, albeit nowhere near as quickly. But don't be fooled—even though response isn't as obvious on the surface, consider this: an individual who spends a week in bed may suffer up to one percent loss in spinal density, and restoration to the earlier level could take four months, provided the individual attends to his diet and exercise. The exercises most likely to increase bone mass are those that involve resistance training. In fact, people who have high levels of resistance training have denser bones than those who only engage in aerobic exercises.

Again, resistance exercises work best to improve bone health when nutrition and hormones are also monitored. It has been conventional wisdom for some time that estrogen, calcium, and vitamin D are key components of any plan to reinforce bones. But we can now add one more name to this list: the longevity nutrient genistein has been shown to produce changes similar to the hormone estrogen in bone, and it is therefore another critical component of any plan to fight osteoporosis.

The Immune System

The effects of exercise on the immune system are wide-ranging, and they have been documented extensively in humans and animals. In regular exercisers, the number of immune cells in the blood increase significantly; moreover, they work better. Many of these studies demonstrate heightened immune defenses against cancer and other chronic diseases in the exercising subjects. As we have seen, many of the longevity nutrients stimulate the immune system. Arginine, phytates, and glutamine are three of these.

There is an undeniably important relationship between exercise and diet. Inactivity results in reduced muscle mass, which in turn slows down metabolism, hindering the efficacy of nutrients and digestion. Regular exercise, on the other hand, promotes muscle metabolism and the efficient handling of nutrients. And whether through direct action on muscles or indirect action on supporting tissues, exercise keeps us healthy longer.

The Least You Can Do: *The New Longevity Diet* Exercise Program

The number of Americans who do not participate in regular exercise has been called an epidemic. This may, in part, be caused by the widespread belief that all exercise involves very strenuous activity at a health club, when really the opposite is true: one can follow a program that is neither strenuous nor time-consuming.

Before starting any exercise program, it is important to have a physical exam conducted by a physician. The purpose of this is to identify any diseases or conditions that put you at risk when you start to exercise. Your physician may, for example, do a stress test to determine your cardiovascular status or measure your bone density to find out if your bones are particularly vulnerable to fracture. Only after you have identified all potentially risky activities should you start an exercise program, and it should be constructed so as to avoid all such activities, of course.

Frankly, exercise isn't mandatory to gain the antiaging effects of *The New Longevity Diet*, but it is my fervent hope, as well as that of most health experts in the world, that you'll make it a part of *your* antiaging program. Furthermore, exercise has a synergistic effect on functions maximizing your body's need for and benefit from these molecules. Because a diet that is rich in the longevity nutrients energizes people, you may find yourself eager to exercise.

There are a lot of levels of commitment and investment with exercise, and while many people get greater knowledge and incentive from joining a health club or hiring a personal trainer, there are just as many who derive equal enjoyment and benefits from a cheap set of weights they picked up at the nearest sporting goods store and a good pair of running shoes. These are really all you need to design your own cardiovascular and resistance training program.

Bearing in mind that most of us experience about a 1 percent decline in aerobic capacity per year as we age, you'll want to include some exercises that require high repetitions of muscle contractions with less resistance. Aerobic activity will stem the decline of your systems, and it will also moderate your blood sugar levels and increase your glucose tolerance—thereby lowering your risk of adult-onset diabetes.

I recommend a program of 3 to 5 exercise sessions per week. Begin at 20 minutes per session and gradually increase to 45 minutes. Your program should include both aerobic and anaerobic activity. Consult a trainer, exercise physiologist, health club, or book to find advice on tailoring a program that's right for you.

By combining the antiaging, weight loss, and overall health-wise *New Longevity Diet* with exercise, you will not only afford yourself the opportunity to live the full human life span, but do it as an emotionally and physically healthy, fit, and active person.

11

THE NEW LONGEVITY DIET RECIPES

Ingredients marked with an asterisk contain the longevity nutrient for the day. At the end of each recipe, all of the longevity nutrients found in the recipe are listed.

BREAKFASTS

1 · Omelet with Smoked Ham

nonstick cooking spray
2 *thin slices smoked ham (1½ ounces),* cut into strips*
4 *eggs*
2 *tablespoons nonfat milk*
pinch of salt
pinch of black pepper

1. Spray a nonstick skillet with cooking spray. Add the ham and cook while stirring with a fork until the fat runs, 1 or 2 minutes. Set aside.

2. Whisk the eggs in a small bowl with the milk, salt, and pepper. Spray a 9-inch omelette pan with cooking spray, add eggs, and turn heat to moderate high. Stir eggs with a spatula; when eggs are runny on top and set on bottom, place ham on one side. Raise pan to an angle and roll omelette with the spatula. Remove from skillet by turning omelette onto a warmed plate.

MAKES 2 SERVINGS.
nucleotides

2 · Golden Honey Milk Shake

*1 cup puffed wheat**
½ cup skim milk
½ cup crushed ice
1 tablespoon half-and-half
1 tablespoon honey
1 teaspoon vanilla

1. In a blender combine all of the ingredients.
2. Blend until smooth and creamy.

MAKES 1 SERVING.
glutamine, arginine, CLA

3 · PQQ Fruit Compote

3 tablespoons lime juice
3 tablespoons superfine sugar
2 tablespoons chopped crystallized ginger
2 star fruits, peeled and thinly sliced
1 mango, peeled, seeded, and chopped
1 papaya, peeled, seeded and chopped*
*1 orange**
3 kiwis, peeled and sliced
2 bananas, peeled and thinly sliced*
6 strawberries

1. In a large bowl, whisk together the lime juice, sugar, and ginger. Set aside 6 slices of the star fruit. Stir in the remaining star fruit, the mangoes, papayas, oranges, kiwis, and bananas.

2. Assemble 6 serving bowls and spoon equal amounts of the fruit mixture into each one. Garnish each with a starfruit slice and a strawberry. Chill before serving.

MAKES 6 SERVINGS.
PQQ

4 · Banana Almond Muffins

nonstick cooking spray
⅔ *cup (about 2 small) mashed ripe bananas**
⅔ *cup orange juice*
⅓ *cup maple syrup or honey*
⅓ *cup vegetable oil*
2 *teaspoons grated lemon zest*
2 *tablespoons crushed almonds**
2 *cups whole wheat pastry flour**
1 *cup toasted wheat germ*
1 *teaspoon baking soda*
1 *teaspoon baking powder*
½ *teaspoon salt*

1. Preheat oven to 375°F. Spray 12 muffin cups with nonstick spray. In the bowl of a food processor, puree the banana, orange juice, maple syrup or honey, oil, and lemon zest. Add the crushed almonds.

2. In a bowl mix the dry ingredients, reserving ¼ cup of the wheat germ. Make a well in the center and fold in the liquid. Spoon the batter into the muffin cups and sprinkle equal amounts of the remaining wheat germ over every muffin.

3. Bake the muffins for 20 to 25 minutes. Cool the muffins in the pan on a rack for 5 to 10 minutes, and serve.

MAKES 12 MUFFINS.
arginine, glutamine, PQQ

5 · Miso Omelette

*6 eggs**
2 tablespoons water
nonstick cooking spray
2 tablespoons miso mixed with 2 teaspoons water*
1 medium tomato, diced
*4 tablespoons alfalfa sprouts**

1. Place eggs and 2 tablespoons water in a bowl and whisk.
2. Spray a skillet with nonstick spray. Add the eggs and stir until partially set. Place the miso, tomatoes, and alfalfa sprouts in the middle and spread into a long strip. Fold the omelette into thirds. Lift the omelette onto a plate and cut into quarters and serve immediately.

MAKES 3–4 SERVINGS.
phytoestrogens, nucleotides, arginine

6 · Tropical Rhubarb

*2 pounds fresh rhubarb (properly aged)**
⅛ cup grapefruit juice
⅛ cup pineapple juice
½ cup sugar
½ cup water

1. Trim the ends of the rhubarb and discard the leaves. Peel off the outer covering by pulling or scraping.
2. Cut the stalks into 1½-inch lengths and place in a saucepan with the pineapple, grapefruit juice, and sugar.
3. Boil until tender (about 5 minutes).
4. Let cool; then chill in refrigerator overnight.

MAKES 6 SERVINGS.
tannins, glutamine, monoterpenes

7 · Lemon Almond Pancakes with English Lemon Curd

1 cup all-purpose flour
⅓ cup sugar

1¼ teaspoons baking powder
pinch of salt
*grated zest of 1 lemon**
1 cup low-fat milk
1 large egg
2 tablespoons reduced-calorie margarine, melted
1 teaspoon pure almond extract
*½ teaspoon pure lemon extract**
nonstick cooking spray
English Lemon Curd (recipe follows)
fresh berries for garnish

1. Combine flour, sugar, baking powder, and salt in a medium bowl and whisk together. Add lemon zest. In a separate bowl, thoroughly blend milk, eggs, melted margarine, almond and lemon extracts. With a spatula, fold the liquid ingredients into the dry ingredients until just combined.

2. Preheat a nonstick skillet over medium heat. Spray skillet with cooking spray.

3. Using a ladle, spoon ¼ cup of the batter onto the skillet. Flip the pancakes over using a wide spatula when the underside becomes golden. Serve immediately with the English Lemon Curd and fresh berries or keep in a preheated 200°F oven until ready to serve.

MAKES 10 PANCAKES.
monoterpenes

ENGLISH LEMON CURD

¾ cup granulated sugar
2 tablespoons cornstarch
*1 tablespoon grated lemon zest**
*½ cup lemon juice**
2 tablespoons reduced-calorie margarine
½ cup water
2 egg yolks

1. Mix the sugar, cornstarch, and lemon zest in a medium nonstick saucepan. To the mixture, stir in the lemon juice, margarine, and ½ cup water and continue stirring. Over medium heat, bring mixture to a boil, stirring constantly, about 1 minute, until mixture is thick.

2. In a separate small bowl, beat the egg yolks. Add ¼ cup of the lemon mixture into the egg yolks. Then slowly pour the egg yolk mixture into the lemon mixture, stirring constantly. Reduce heat to low and cook for 1 minute. Transfer the lemon curd to a bowl and refrigerate, covered, until chilled.

8 · Puffy Chive Omelette

nonstick cooking spray
3 *large egg whites*
2 *large eggs, separated*
2 *tablespoons low-fat milk*
1 *tablespoon grated Parmesan cheese*
1 *tablespoon dried chives (or 2 teaspoons fresh)**
dash of paprika

1. Spray a 10-inch glass pie plate with nonstick cooking spray; set aside.

2. In medium bowl, with electric mixer on high speed, beat egg whites until stiff but not dry.

3. In another medium bowl, with electric mixer on medium speed, beat egg yolks until thick and lemon-colored. Using rubber spatula, gently fold egg yolks, and remaining ingredients, into egg whites, until completely blended. Pour into prepared pie plate; smooth top to distribute mixture evenly. Microwave on high for 2½ to 3 minutes, or until just set, rotating plate once. Omelette will puff considerably when cooking and will drop as it cools.

4. Gently fold omelette in half and slide onto serving plates.

MAKES 2 SERVINGS.
OC, CLA

9 · Breakfast Ambrosia

1 *cup cantaloupe balls*
1 *cup watermelon balls**
½ *pound seedless green grapes**
3 *kiwi fruit, sliced*
1 *small firm pear,* diced*

2 tablespoons lemon juice
1 tablespoon honey
¼ cup pineapple juice
¼ cup white grape juice

1. Mix cantaloupe balls, watermelon balls, grapes, kiwi fruit and pear together.

2. For the dressing, blend together the lemon juice, honey, pineapple juice, and white grape juice. Toss with the fruit and chill for 2 hours.

MAKES 4 SERVINGS.
glutathione, tannins, glutamine

10 · Kiwi and Banana Granola Yogurt

*1½ ripe bananas**
8 ounces plain low-fat yogurt
½ cup plus 2 tablespoons granola
2 tablespoons low-fat sour cream
1 teaspoon packed dark brown sugar
*1 cup kiwi fruit**

1. Slit the banana lengthwise and slit each side again so that the banana is quartered. Dice the banana into small pieces. In a bowl combine yogurt, granola, sour cream, aand brown sugar. Fold in banana and kiwi.

2. Divide the mixture between 2 bowls. Serve chilled.

MAKES 2 SERVINGS.
PQQ, inulin and oligofructose, tannins, phytosterols, CLA, arginine

11 · Banana Cinnamon Toast

1 ripe medium banana
*¼ cup lite soy milk**
½ teaspoon vanilla extract
2 slices whole wheat bread
nonstick cooking spray
2 teaspoons sugar
⅛ teaspoon ground cinnamon

1. In a blender or food processor, combine banana, soy milk, and vanilla. Blend until smooth.

2. Pour mixture in shallow bowl and dip bread to coat both sides.

3. Place bread in a nonstick skillet sprayed with cooking spray.

4. Drizzle any remaining banana mixture over bread. Cook bread until browned on both sides.

5. In a small bowl, combine sugar and cinnamon and sprinkle over toast.

MAKES 2 SERVINGS.
phytoestrogens, inulin and oligofructose, tannins, phytosterols

12 · Carrot-Apple Whole Wheat Muffins

*1¼ cups whole wheat flour**
*¼ cup all-purpose flour**
2 teaspoons baking powder
1 teaspoon cinnamon
¼ teaspoon salt
2 eggs
1 cup plain, low-fat yogurt
2 tablespoon molasses
1 tablespoon vegetable oil
*¼ cup shredded carrots**
¼ cup grated peeled apples

1. Preheat oven to 375°F. Mix together flours, baking powder, cinnamon, and salt in a small bowl.

2. In a large bowl, blend the eggs with a whisk; add yogurt, molasses, and oil; stir in the carrots and apples. Fold the egg mixture into the flour mixture until well combined. Spoon the batter into paper-lined muffin tins.

3. Bake in the preheated oven for 15 to 20 minutes.

MAKES 12 SERVINGS.
lignans, phytates, glutamine, phytosterols

13 · Scrambled Tofu with Mushrooms and Tomatoes

1 tablespoon olive oil
½ cup finely chopped red bell pepper
½ cup sliced mushrooms
2 medium scallions, chopped
2 cloves garlic
¼ cup chopped onion
*1½ cups mashed, silken, firm tofu (12 oz)**
3 plum tomatoes, cut into ½-inch cubes
2 tablespoons low-sodium soy sauce
1 tablespoon minced fresh, flat-leaf parsley
1 tablespoon minced fresh thyme
1 tablespoon minced fresh oregano
½ teaspoon black pepper

1. Over medium heat, heat the oil in a nonstick skillet. Add the bell peppers, mushrooms, scallions, and garlic. Sauté, stirring occasionally, until the vegetables are tender, about 4 minutes.
2. Turn the heat to low and stir in the tofu, tomatoes, soy sauce, parsley, thyme, and oregano. Cook for 3 minutes and serve with freshly ground black pepper.

MAKES 4 SERVINGS.
phytoestrogens, glutamine, arginine, PQQ, OCs

14 · Peach and Blueberry Breakfast Parfait

*¾ cup nonfat vanilla yogurt**
*½ cup blueberries**
1 teaspoon all-fruit berry syrup
*¼ cup chopped peach**
½ teaspoon granulated sugar
½ teaspoon wheat germ

1. In small mixing bowl, combine yogurt, blueberries, and syrup.
2. In separate small mixing bowl, combine peach and sugar.

3. Into a parfait glass, spoon half of the blueberry mixture; top with peach mixture and remaining blueberry mixture.

4. Sprinkle with wheat germ.

MAKES 1 SERVING.
CLA, tannins, protease inhibitors

15 · All-Wheat Pancakes

¾ *cup whole wheat flour**
¾ *cup all-purpose flour*
2 *cups coarse wheat bran**
½ *teaspoon baking powder*
¼ *teaspoon cinnamon*
¼ *teaspoon ground ginger*
2 *teaspoons salt*
1½ *cups skim milk*
2 *large eggs**
2 *tablespoons firmly packed brown sugar*
1 *tablespoon unsalted butter, melted*
2 *teaspoons pure vanilla extract*
nonstick cooking spray
maple syrup for topping

1. In a medium bowl, whisk together the whole wheat and all-purpose flours, bran, baking powder, cinnamon, ginger, and salt. In another bowl, whisk together the milk, eggs, brown sugar, melted butter, and vanilla to blend thoroughly. Fold the liquid ingredients into the flour mixture thoroughly. Batter will have lumps.

2. Spray a skillet or griddle with nonstick cooking spray and set burner at medium heat or griddle at 350°F.

3. Spoon ¼ cup of batter into the skillet or onto griddle for each pancake. Cook until the underside of the pancake is lightly brown and the tops are speckled with bubbles. Turn and cook on the other side. Top with the syrup and serve immediately.

MAKES 14 PANCAKES.
lignans, phytates, glutamine, arginine

16 · Raspberry and Almond Muesli

*1 cup rolled oats**
*3 tablespoons oat bran**
*3 tablespoons wheat germ**
2 cups low-fat milk plus additional to taste
2 teaspoons honey
¼ teaspoon vanilla
pinch of salt
½ teaspoon cinnamon
⅛ teaspoon nutmeg
*2 cups raspberries**
*1 navel orange, peeled, sectioned, and cut into 2-inch pieces**
*3 tablespoons sliced almonds**
3 tablespoons raisins

1. In a small bowl combine the rolled oats, oat bran, wheat germ, 2 cups of milk, honey, vanilla, salt, cinnamon, and nutmeg. Chill the mixture in the refrigerator, covered, overnight.

2. Divide the mixture between 4 bowls. Place ¼ of the raspberries, orange, and almonds over each serving. Serve the muesli with milk.

MAKES 4 SERVINGS.
lignans, PQQ, nucleotides, saponins, phytates, glutamine, tannins

17 · Baked Cheese Toast

*2 tablespoons part-skim ricotta**
1 egg white
*1 tablespoon low-fat cream cheese**
½ teaspoon granulated sugar
½ teaspoon cornstarch
½ teaspoon vanilla extract
*2 slices whole wheat bread**

1. Preheat oven to 350°F.
2. In small bowl, combine all ingredients except bread.

3. Spread ½ cheese mixture on each slice of bread. Toast in oven until cheese is bubbly, about 5 minutes.

MAKES 2 SERVINGS.
CLA, arginine

18 · Pear Cashew Muffins

- *1½ cups flour*
- *½ cup firmly packed brown sugar*
- *1 teaspoon baking soda*
- *¼ teaspoon salt*
- *1 teaspoon cinnamon*
- *¼ teaspoon nutmeg*
- *1 cup plain low-fat yogurt**
- *½ cup applesauce**
- *3 tablespoons molasses*
- *1 egg, slightly beaten*
- *1 tablespoon vanilla*
- *1 tablespoon lemon zest or grated lemon peel**
- *1½ cups pears, diced**
- *¼ cup chopped cashews**

1. Preheat oven to 400°F. In a large bowl, stir together flour, brown sugar, baking soda, salt, cinnamon, and nutmeg.

2. In another bowl, stir together yogurt, applesauce, molasses, egg, vanilla, and lemon zest until blended.

3. Add yogurt mixture to dry ingredients. Stir in pears and cashews. Spoon batter into muffin tins. Bake 20 to 25 minutes, until browned.

MAKES 12 MUFFINS.
PQQ, CLA, phytates, tannins, quercetin, phytosterols, glutamine, arginine

19 · Smoked Ham and Cheese Omelette

- *1 tablespoon low-fat margarine*
- *1 thin slice raw smoked ham, cut into strips**
- *4 eggs*

salt and pepper
*3 tablespoons grated Gouda cheese**

1. Coat a nonstick skillet with cooking spray. Add the ham and cook gently until the fat runs. Drain and set aside.

2. In a mixing bowl, whisk the eggs with a little salt and pepper until mixed. In a 9-inch omelette pan, melt the margarine over moderately high heat; add the eggs. When the omelette starts to cook on the bottom, pull the cooked egg from the sides to the center of the pan and tilt the pan to allow the uncooked egg to run underneath. When the mixture is set on the bottom but still runny on the top, add the ham and cheese onto omelette. Leave the omelette on the heat until lightly browned on the bottom and almost set on the top.

3. Fold the omelette, tipping the pan away from you, and turning the edge with a spatula. Half roll, half slide onto a warm platter, guiding it to land folding in three. Serve immediately.

MAKES 2 SERVINGS.
arginine, CLA, carnitine

20 · Breakfast Fruit Compote

*½ cup dried cranberries**
*½ cup dried apples**
*½ cup dried pears**
*½ cup dried peaches**
*½ pound dried apricots**
½ cup sugar
1 tablespoon honey
*1 tablespoon freshly grated orange zest**
*1 tablespoon fresh lemon juice**
2 cups water

1. Mix the dried fruits in a bowl and soak in cold water for 2 hours. Drain the fruit.

2. Halve and core the fruits.

3. Combine the fruit in a saucepan with the sugar, honey, zest, lemon juice, and water. Bring the liquid to a boil. Simmer for 10 to 15 minutes.

4. Remove the pan from the heat and let cool. Serve the compote at room temperature.

MAKES 4 SERVINGS.
tannins, monoterpenes, phytosterols, PQQ

21 · Hearty Omelette

2 large eggs
2 large egg whites
1 teaspoon minced, fresh chives
1 tablespoon cold water
salt and pepper to taste
1 teaspoon reduced-fat or margarine
*1 ounce cooked, crumbled turkey sausage**
*2 tablespoons finely chopped fresh mushrooms**
1 teaspoon minced fresh parsley

1. Put the eggs, egg whites, chives, and water into a bowl. Add the salt and pepper. Beat lightly.

2. Heat the omelette pan and when it is quite hot, add the margarine. Sauté sausage and mushrooms until sausage turns slightly brown.

3. Add the beaten eggs, shaking the skillet while holding it flat on the burner. Simultaneously stir the eggs rapidly with the tines of a fork, holding the tines parallel to the bottom of the skillet. Let the omelette cook undisturbed until the edges and bottom are set.

4. With a spatula, fold the omelette in half and place onto plate. Serve garnished with parsley.

MAKES 2 SERVINGS.
arginine, PQQ

22 · Triple Berry Breakfast Shake

*1 cup fresh blueberries, stemmed, rinsed, and drained**
*1 generous cup sliced ripe fresh strawberries**
*1 cup frozen cranberries**
*1½ cups plain yogurt**
1 large ripe banana, peeled and sliced

1 cup fresh orange juice
whole strawberries for garnish

1. Pile the blueberries, strawberries, cranberries, yogurt, banana, and orange juice into a large blender—or do it in batches—and blend at high speed until smooth.

2. Pour into tall glasses, garnish with whole strawberries and serve right away.

MAKES 4 SERVINGS.
lignans, CLA, tannins, glutamine, glutathione, quercetin

23 · Flaxseed Pancakes

1½ cups whole wheat, semolina grind
*½ cup ground flaxseed**
1½ cups flour
¼ teaspoon baking powder
¼ teaspoon baking soda (double if you use flour instead of mix)
1 tablespoon sugar
¼ teaspoon salt
2 egg whites
1 cup low-fat milk

1. Mix ingredients together.

2. Bake on griddle or electric skillet at 375°F, or cook waffles on waffle iron.

MAKES 8 SERVINGS.
phytoestrogens

LUNCHES

24 · Grilled Tuna with Papaya Salsa

2 teaspoons mustard seeds
juice of 4 limes
juice of 1 orange
1½ tablespoons fresh lemon juice

1 teaspoon olive oil
1 firm papaya, peeled, seeded, and cut into ¼-inch pieces
¼ red bell pepper, chopped fine
¼ green bell pepper, chopped fine
1 small red onion, diced
3 tablespoons scallions
2 teaspoons fresh cilantro leaves, chopped
½ fresh poblano chili, seeded and chopped fine (wear rubber gloves)
*4½-pound 1-inch-thick tuna steaks**

1. In a bowl, combine the mustard seeds with lime, orange, and lemon juices. Whisk in the olive oil.

2. In a separate bowl, combine the papaya, red pepper, green pepper, onions, scallions, cilantro, and poblano chilis.

3. Add the contents of the first bowl and mix thoroughly.

4. Prepare a grill or make a charcoal fire. Grill tuna on an oiled rack set 5 inches above the grill or coals. Grill 4 to 5 minutes on each side for medium-rare fish.

5. Divide tuna equally among 4 plates and serve with salsa.

MAKES 4 SERVINGS.
nucleotides, PQQ, OCs, lignans

25 · Warm Spring Salad with Baby Vegetables

1 tablespoon chervil, finely chopped
1 tablespoon chives, thinly sliced
1 tablespoon basil, finely chopped
¼ cup thinly sliced white part of scallion
2 tablespoons extra virgin olive oil
½ pound asparagus, trimmed*
½ pound small dry white beans
*1 cup baby corn**
*2 cups broccolini**
*8 finger (baby) carrots, halved lengthwise**
3 quarts water, as well as other water for soaking beans
¼ pound snap peas, trimmed
8 baby zucchini, quartered and cut into 1-inch lengths
salt and pepper to taste

1. In a large bowl, combine chervil, chives, basil, scallion, and the oil.

2. Discard the bottom part of the asparagus by cutting away a 2-inch piece. Cut the asparagus diagonally into ½-inch pieces.

3. In a saucepan, cover the beans with water, soak for 1 hour, and boil for 1 hour until tender. Let cool and drain the beans in a colander.

4. In a large saucepan, bring 3 quarts of water to a boil. Add the baby corn, broccolini, baby carrots, asparagus tips and pieces. Cook the vegetables for 2 minutes and transfer them to the colander, reserving the boiling water.

6. Drain the vegetables well and place with the herbs and scallions.

7. Using the same boiling water, add the snap peas and zucchini and cook for 1 to 2 minutes. Drain the vegetables in the colander and add to the oil, herbs, and scallions.

8. Toss and add salt and freshly ground pepper to taste.

MAKES 4 TO 6 SERVINGS.
Nucleotides, saponins, protease inhibitors, glutamine, inulin and oligofructose, phytosterols, phytates, tannins, PQQ, glutathione

26 · Frijoles con Arroz Picante

1 pound dried black beans, soaked in cold water overnight, or simmered in water for one hour and drained*
4 ounces Canadian bacon, chopped into small pieces
2 large garlic cloves, minced
1 tablespoon Grey Poupon or other Dijon mustard
1½ teaspoons dried oregano
2 cups coarsely chopped onion
2 green bell peppers, chopped
½ teaspoon paprika
1 tablespoon chili powder
8 cups water
1 28-ounce can whole tomatoes, drained and chopped
⅓ cup finely chopped fresh coriander, or to taste
salt to taste
3 cups steamed rice
chopped radish and red onion as an accompaniment

1. In a large saucepan, combine the beans, Canadian bacon, garlic, mustard, oregano, onion, bell peppers, paprika, chili powder, coriander, and 8 cups of water. Simmer the mixture, covered, stirring occasionally, for 3 hours, or until the beans are tender.

2. Stir in the tomatoes and salt to taste. Simmer the mixture, uncovered, stirring occasionally, for 1 hour, or until the mixture is thickened.

3. Spoon the beans over the rice and garnish with radish and red onion.

MAKES 6 TO 8 SERVINGS.
saponins, arginine, glutamine, OCs, lignans, PQQ, isothiocyanates

27 · Sunflower Seed Sandwich

4 ounces low-fat cream cheese at room temperature
4 ounces low-fat (50%) sharp Cheddar, chopped
2 scallions, thinly sliced including the green part
⅓ cup coarsely chopped bottled pimientos, drained and patted dry
⅓ cup plain nonfat yogurt
¼ cup shelled raw sunflower seeds, toasted lightly*
whole wheat bread

1. Add the cream cheese and the Cheddar to a food processor and process with the metal blade until they are combined. Add the scallions, and blend the mixture.

2. Add the pimiento and the yogurt and blend the mixture until the pimiento is chopped fine.

3. Add the sunflower seeds and blend the mixture until the whole seeds are just incorporated.

4. Spread on slices of whole wheat bread, making sandwiches.

MAKES ABOUT 6 SANDWICHES.
phytates, glutamine, arginine, CLA

28 · Roasted Green Pepper Soup

2 roasted green peppers (recipe follows)
*1½ cups mashed silken firm tofu**

2 cups vegetable stock (below)
*3 tablespoons red wine vinegar**
1 tablespoon extra virgin olive oil
2 teaspoons minced garlic
1 teaspoon sugar
½ teaspoon ground black pepper
¼ teaspoon salt
2 tablespoons minced fresh chives
1 tablespoon minced fresh rosemary
1 tablespoon minced fresh coriander

1. Put the bell peppers, tofu, vegetable stock, vinegar, oil, garlic, sugar, pepper, and salt into a food processor; process until smooth and creamy. Stir in the chives, coriander, and rosemary.

2. Adjust the seasonings to taste. Refrigerate in a covered container for at least three hours before serving chilled.

ROASTED GREEN PEPPERS

2 whole green bell peppers
nonstick cooking spray

1. Preheat the broiler and place rack 3 inches from the broiler.
2. Cut green pepper in half. Remove stem and seeds.
3. On a nonstick pan sprayed with cooking spray, broil for ten minutes until skins are blackened. Cool before using.

VEGETABLE STOCK

*2 large potatoes, quartered**
3 carrots, peeled and coarsely chopped
2 onions, peeled and coarsely chopped
3 celery stalks, coarsely chopped
*2 squash, sliced**
*8 parsley sprigs**
1 teaspoon dried marjoram
1 bay leaf
½ teaspoon salt
10 coarsely cracked peppercorns
3 quarts cold water

1. Combine all ingredients in a large pot.

2. Bring to a boil. Lower heat and simmer partially covered for 1 hour.

3. Strain through a cheesecloth-lined colander. Let cool before refrigerating for 2 or 3 days.

MAKES 6 SERVINGS.
protease inhibitors, phytosterols, PQQ

29 · Spicy Potato Quesadillas with Guacamole

1 tablespoon vegetable oil
1 medium Spanish onion, thinly sliced*
1 large baking potato, peeled and cut into ¼-inch cubes*
1 cup fat-free reduced-sodium chicken broth
salt and pepper to taste
nonstick cooking spray
8 fat-free tortillas (8-inch diameter)
guacamole (recipe follows)
4 ounces reduced-fat Monterey Jack cheese, shredded
½ cup low-fat sour cream
1 tomato, chopped*
½ avocado
2 fresh or pickled jalapeño chili peppers, thinly sliced (wear plastic gloves when handling)

1. Preheat the oven to 400°F.

2. Heat the oil in a medium nonstick skillet over medium heat. Add the onion and cook, stirring often, for 6 minutes, or until golden brown. Stir in the potatoes and cook for 1 minute. Stir in the broth and simmer for 8 minutes, or until the potatoes are very soft and the liquid has been absorbed. Season with salt and pepper.

3. Spray 2 baking sheets with nonstick spray.

4. Arrange 4 of the tortillas on the baking sheets. Divide the potato mixture among the tortillas and spread evenly. Top each with 1 of the remaining tortillas. Coat the tops of the quesadillas with nonstick spray.

5. Bake, turning once, for 10 minutes, or until lightly browned and heated through. Cut each quesadilla into 8 wedges.

6. Serve with guacamole, shredded cheese, sour cream, avocado, and chili pepper.

MAKES 4 SERVINGS (32 WEDGES).
glutamine, inulin and oligofructose, OCs, lignans, protease inhibitors, PQQ, glutathione

GUACAMOLE

- 2 *cloves garlic, peeled*
- 2–3 *tablespoons fresh lemon juice*
- 4 *avocados, peeled, pitted, and cut into slices*
- 1 *teaspoon salt*
- ⅛ *teaspoon chili powder*

1. Using a food processor with a metal blade, process the garlic until finely minced.

2. Add lemon juice and avocados and pulse to combine well. Process until smooth. Season to taste with salt and chili powder.

MAKES 4 CUPS.

30 · Chicken Cashew Stir-Fry

- *nonstick cooking spray*
- 2 *cloves garlic, crushed*
- 1 *teaspoon minced ginger*
- ¾ *pound boneless chicken* breasts, shredded*
- 2 *tablespoons oyster sauce*
- ¼ *pound snow peas, ends trimmed*
- 5–6 *szechuan dried red chili peppers*
- ¼ *cup unsalted cashew nuts*
- 6 *large lettuce leaves*
- 8 *scallions, cut into 1-inch lengths*

1. Coat a wok with nonstick cooking spray and heat at medium; add garlic and ginger and stir-fry until fragrant. Add oyster sauce and chicken and cook for 6 to 8 minutes. Reduce heat.

2. Add the snow peas, scallions, chili peppers, and cashew nuts; mix well. Serve over lettuce on a platter and top with scallions.

MAKES 3–4 SERVINGS.
exorphins, glutamine, arginine, taurine, inulin and oligofructose, OCs, lignans, protease inhibitors

31 · Savory Stuffed Green Peppers

*4 large green bell peppers**
2 teaspoons olive oil
½ cup onions, finely chopped
½ cup red peppers, finely chopped
½ cup sliced mushrooms
*2 cups mashed potatoes**
¼ cup parsley, finely chopped
¼ teaspoon salt
2 large tomatoes, peeled and chopped
*2 cups tomato sauce**

1. Preheat oven to 350°F. Slice tops from peppers, then remove seeds and interior spines. In a saucepan, cook peppers in boiling water for 5 minutes or until slightly tender. Drain upside down and set aside.

2. In a saucepan, heat the oil and cook the onions, red peppers, and mushrooms until soft. Add to mashed potatoes along with parsley, salt, and pepper. Stuff peppers with mashed potatoes and place them in a baking dish. Combine tomatoes with tomato sauce and spread around base of peppers. Bake for about 15 minutes, covered. Uncover and bake 2 minutes longer. Serve warm.

MAKES 4 SERVINGS.
PQQ, glutamine, OCs, lignans, CLA, protease inhibitors, glutathione

32 · Turkey Roll-Ups with Provolone Cheese

*4 pieces Middle East flat bread (6" × 8")**
1 tablespoon low-fat mayonnaise

1 tablespoon red wine vinegar
*½ teaspoon dried oregano**
½ teaspoon paprika
*4 slices provolone cheese, cut into ¼-inch strips**
*1 small red onion, sliced thin and chopped**
4 radishes, trimmed and sliced thin
2 tablespoons chopped tomatoes
*8 ounces turkey breast, preferably fresh baked**
4 leaves of lettuce

1. In a mixing bowl, combine mayonnaise, vinegar, oregano, and paprika. Stir in the cheese, onions, radishes, and tomatoes.

2. Roll out the bread. Place a lettuce leaf on each piece. Then spoon filling over the lettuce. Layer two slices of turkey on top and roll up the bread.

MAKES 4 SERVINGS.
arginine, glutamine, inulin and oligofructose, monoterpenes, OCs, lignans

33 · Artichoke Soup

FOR THE ARTICHOKES:
7 cups water
⅔ cup flour
½ cup lemon juice
1 teaspoon salt
*8 large artichokes**

FOR THE SOUP:
1 tablespoon butter
1 medium onion, chopped
2 celery stalks, chopped
1 garlic clove, minced
3 tablespoons flour
4 cups low-fat chicken stock
1 tablespoon chopped fresh parsley
1 tablespoon chopped fresh tarragon
1 cup half-and-half

salt and pepper to taste
2 *tablespoons lemon juice*
lemon zest, in thin strips

1. In a large saucepan with 7 cups of water, add the flour, whisking slowly. Add the lemon juice and salt. Set over medium heat and bring to a boil, stirring frequently. Turn the heat to low.

2. Pull off the outer leaves of the artichokes. Cut away and discard the remaining inner leaves to expose the choke in the center. Trim the artichoke bottoms, placing each one into the simmering liquid. Cover the pan and cook about 35 to 45 minutes, or until the artichokes are tender when pierced.

3. Remove from burner and let artichokes cool for about an hour in the cooking liquid. Rinse them under cold water. Scrape out and discard the chokes. Refrigerate the bottoms, covered, until you are ready for them.

4. With the meat blade of a food processor, puree the artichoke bottoms in a bowl. Set aside.

5. Melt the butter in a large saucepan. Add the onion, celery, and garlic, and cook gently for about 10 minutes. Add the flour and cook, stirring, for about 2 minutes, then whisk in the stock. Bring just to a boil, stirring frequently, then blend in the artichoke puree, parsley, and tarragon. Add the half-and-half and season with salt and pepper to taste. Stir in the lemon juice. Garnish with the strips of lemon zest. Serve hot.

MAKES 6 SERVINGS.
inulin and oligofructose, OCs, monoterpenes, phytosterols

34 · Seafood Casserole

nonstick cooking spray
12 *ounces boneless and skinless chicken breasts cut into 1-inch pieces*
1 *medium onion, finely chopped*
1 *red or yellow bell pepper, seeded and cut into ¼-inch strips*
2 *cloves garlic, minced*
2 *tomatoes, seeded and cut into ¼-inch pieces*
2 *teaspoons finely chopped oregano*
1 *teaspoon finely chopped fresh thyme*
3 *tablespoons finely chopped fresh parsley*

2 cups short grain rice
⅓ cup dry white wine
4 cups nonfat chicken stock
¼ teaspoon saffron thread, crumbled
12 littleneck clams, scrubbed*
1 pound scallops
1½ pounds shrimp, peeled and deveined*
salt and pepper
½ cup cooked or frozen and thawed peas

1. Preheat the oven to 400°F.

2. Coat nonstick skillet with cooking spray and cook the chicken, stirring often for about 5 minutes or until lightly browned. Transfer the chicken to a plate.

3. In the same skillet, sauté onions, bell peppers, and garlic. Cook until onions and garlic are golden brown. Combine the tomatoes, oregano, thyme, and 2 tablespoons of the parsley and cook for 2 minutes.

4. Add the rice to the skillet and cook for 1 minute, or until the grains are coated. Add the wine and bring to a boil. Add 3½ cups of the stock and the saffron. Return to a boil, reduce the heat to medium and simmer for 10 minutes. Stir in the clams and scallops. Return to a boil, stir in the shrimp.

5. Cover the skillet and transfer to oven. Bake for 20 to 25 minutes. Stir in the peas. The casserole should be moist; if it dries add more stock. Season with salt and pepper and sprinkle with the remaining parsley.

MAKES 6 SERVINGS.
taurine, nucleotides, glutamine, exorphins, arginine, inulin and oligofructose, OCs, lignans, CLA, monoterpenes

35 · Chicken Salad with Peanut Dressing and Apples

2 whole boneless chicken breasts
¼ cup reduced-fat chunky peanut butter
¼ cup honey
½ cup reduced-fat mayonnaise

1 tart apple such as Stayman or Granny Smith, finely chopped*
1 tablespoon lemon juice
½ cup golden raisins
½ cup diced celery
*1 cup chopped red cabbage**
½ teaspoon cayenne
2 tablespoons vinegar
½ cup sliced radishes
salt to taste
*8 leaves Boston or Bibb lettuce**

1. Heat oven to 350°F. Place chicken breasts in a nonstick baking pan. Bake 30–35 minutes. Cube meat.

2. In a medium-size bowl, mix peanut butter, honey, and mayonnaise. Add chicken and mix well. Add apple, lemon juice, raisins, celery, cabbage, cayenne, vinegar, radishes, and salt. Toss until mixed.

3. Spoon chicken mixture on top of lettuce leaves placed on plates.

MAKES 6 SERVINGS.
quercetin, nucleotides, arginine, exorphins, taurine, PQQ, isothiocyanates

36 · Soy Curried Chickpeas

2 tablespoons olive oil
2 onions, thinly sliced*
3 cloves garlic, minced
*2 tablespoons sunflower seeds**
1 tablespoon curry powder
pinch of salt
16 ounces canned chickpeas (garbanzo beans)
3 tablespoons fresh lemon juice
1 teaspoon tamari or light soy sauce
2 tablespoons chopped fresh tarragon
2 cups Jasmine rice, cooked

1. In the olive oil, sauté the onion and garlic until browned, about 15 minutes. Stir in the sunflower seeds and curry powder. Season with salt. Cook uncovered for 5 minutes, stirring occasionally.

2. Drain the chickpeas, reserving ½ cup of the liquid. Add the chickpeas to the pan with the reserved liquid and cook, stirring frequently, until the chickpeas are hot and almost all the liquid has been absorbed.

3. Stir in the lemon juice, tamari, and tarragon. Arrange 4 serving dishes, and serve over rice.

MAKES 4 SERVINGS.
quercetin, phytates, CLA, saponins, monoterpenes

37 · Romaine and Black Olive Salad

*1 medium head Romaine lettuce**
4 tablespoons freshly chopped dill
2 large red radishes, thinly sliced
1 small red onion, thinly sliced
1 green bell pepper, seeded and cut into thin strips
3 large tomatoes, quartered and sliced
12–15 black olives, pitted
½ cup Monterey Jack cheese, grated

VINAIGRETTE:
3 tablespoons olive oil
1½ tablespoons lemon juice
salt and pepper to taste

1. Remove and discard the large outer leaves of the lettuce, shredding the inner part. Rinse, then dry the lettuce in a small towel and place in a large salad bowl. Mix the lettuce with the dill and radishes. Toss in the red onion, green pepper, tomatoes, olives, and cheese.

2. Toss with vinaigrette just before serving.

MAKES 4 SERVINGS.
quercetin, protease inhibitors, lignans, OCs, PQQ, glutamine, monoterpenes

38 · Vegetable and Soybean Hotpot

½ cup soybeans, soaked overnight*
1 tablespoon rice bran or vegetable oil
½ teaspoon chili powder

- 1 *clove garlic, crushed*
- 1 *teaspoon grated ginger root*
- 3 *ounces scallions, diced*
- ¼ *cup green peas*
- ¾ *pound mushrooms, diced*
- ¼ *pound carrots, cut into julienne strips*
- 3 *ounces water chestnuts, thinly sliced*
- 3½ *teaspoons cornstarch*
- 1 *tablespoon sherry*
- 1 *tablespoon tamari*
- *salt and pepper to taste*

1. Drain the soybeans. Place in large saucepan and boil at medium high heat for 1 hour. Reduce the heat and simmer, covered, until they are soft, about 1 more hour. Drain, reserving the stock, and set aside.

2. Heat the oil in a large saucepan and sauté the chili powder, garlic, and ginger root for 2 to 3 minutes. Add the scallions, green peas, mushrooms, carrots, and water chestnuts, and continue cooking, covered, for 10 minutes over gentle heat.

3. In a bowl, whisk together the cornstarch, sherry, and tamari with 1½ cups of the soybean stock. Add mixture to the saucepan together with the cooked soybeans. Stir well, bring to a boil, and simmer, covered, for 10 minutes. Season with salt and pepper. Serve hot.

MAKES 4 SERVINGS.
phytoestrogens, glutamine, OCs, lignans, arginine, PQQ, glutathione

39 · Vegetarian Lunch

- ½ *cup dried kidney beans,* covered with water and soaked overnight*
- 4½ *cups water*
- 1 *cup lentils,* rinsed*
- 2 *teaspoons olive oil*
- 2 *medium onions, chopped**
- 2 *cloves garlic, minced**
- 2 *tablespoons fresh parsley, finely chopped*
- ½ *teaspoon dry mustard*
- ¼ *teaspoon paprika*

½ cup rice
¾ teaspoon salt

1. Boil the beans in their water in a large saucepan. Cover and cook over medium heat until beans turn tender. Add 2½ cups water and the lentils and boil. Cook over medium heat for 30 minutes.

2. In oil, sauté onions, garlic, parsley, mustard, paprika, and salt. Heat for 10 minutes. Add rice and stir-fry for an additional 3 minutes. Combine with the bean and lentil mixture. Add 2 more cups of water and bring to a boil. Cook over medium heat for 20 minutes longer or until the rice is done.

MAKES 8 SERVINGS.
lignans, saponins, glutamine, phytoestrogen, phytates, glutamine

40 · Raspberry Smoothie

*1 cup raspberries, frozen**
*1 cup orange juice**
*2 fresh bananas, frozen and sliced**

1. Pour orange juice in a blender. Add raspberries and bananas. Blend untill smooth.

2. Chill before serving.

MAKES 2 SERVINGS.
tannins, glutamine, PQQ, monoterpenes, inulin and oligofructose, phytosterols

41 · Stilton Sandwich

*2 ounces Stilton cheese**
*2 ounces low-fat cream cheese**
milk for consistency*
1 teaspoon marjoram
2 teaspoons chives, cut into narrow rounds
½ teaspoon horseradish
4 slices bread
½ cucumber, sliced very thin

salt and pepper to taste
handful watercress or garden cress, stems removed

1. Using a food processor, combine the Stilton and cream cheese. Add milk to adjust consistency.

2. Add marjoram, chives, and horseradish. Pulse to combine thoroughly. Stir them into the cheese mixture, and salt to taste.

3. Spread a thick layer of cheese over 2 slices of bread. Place the cucumber slices on top in overlapping layers. Sprinkle with salt and pepper. Finish sandwiches with remaining 2 slices of bread. Garnish with the watercress.

MAKES 2 SERVINGS.
CLA, arginine, glutamine, OCs

42 · Cool Cucumber Soup

6 small pickling cucumbers, peeled and finely diced
salt
3 cloves garlic
*4 cups plain low-fat yogurt**
3 tablespoons chopped, toasted walnuts
fresh chives, finely chopped, for garnish

1. Sprinkle the cucumbers with salt and leave for 1 hour in a colander to drain. Crush the garlic with a little salt.

2. In a bowl, combine yogurt, garlic, cucumbers, walnuts. Cover and refrigerate for 4 to 5 hours. Cucumbers and walnuts can be blended first for a smoother texture.

3. Add ice water to thin to desired consistency.

4. Ladle into individual bowls, and garnish with chives.

MAKES 4 SERVINGS.
CLA, protease inhibitors, arginine, tannins, phytosterols

43 · Broccoli Tart with Pine Nuts

2 tablespoons extra virgin olive oil
2 cloves garlic, finely minced
*1 bunch broccoli, rabe, well rinsed, tough stems removed**
1 tablespoon lemon juice

- ½ *teaspoon salt and black pepper to taste*
- 1 *medium onion, thinly sliced*
- 6 *tablespoons toasted pine nuts*
- ½ *pound frozen puff-pastry dough, thawed*
- 1 *egg, lightly beaten with 1 teaspoon water*
- 1 *tablespoon oregano**

1. Preheat oven to 425°F. In a large saucepan, saute the garlic in 1 tablespoon of the oil until browned. Add the broccoli rabe and cook for about 10 to 12 minutes. Add the salt, pepper, and lemon. Cook for 2 to 3 minutes. Remove from heat, cool, and coarsely chop.

2. In a small nonstick saucepan, cook the onion over medium heat for 10 minutes until golden brown. Set aside and let cool.

3. Roll out the puff-pastry on a lightly floured surface to a thickness of ¼ inch. Cut out a circular section large enough to line an 8-inch circular tart pan. Turn up the edges with a fork to form an edge around the tart.

4. Transfer the onions to a food processor, add two tablespoons pine nuts and oregano. Process with the metal blade of the processor until smooth. Add salt and black pepper to taste.

5. Brush the edges with the beaten egg. Layer the onion and pine nut mixture over the tart. Spread the rabe evenly and sprinkle with remaining pine nuts. Bake for 12 minutes or until lightly brown. Drizzle the remaining olive oil and serve immediately.

MAKES 4 SERVINGS.
isothiocyanates, OCs, arginine, phytosterols

44 · Favorite Fajitas

- 4 *tablespoons cilantro + 1 cup cilantro*
- 4 *cloves garlic, minced*
- ½ *teaspoon dried rosemary*
- ½ *teaspoon cayenne*
- ½ *teaspoon salt*
- 1 *pound beef skirt steak,* or top sirloin steak trimmed of all visible fat*
- ½ *cup lime juice*
- 1 *yellow bell pepper, cut into ½-inch strips*

- 1 *green bell pepper, cut into ½-inch strips*
- 1 *medium red onion, cut into 8 wedges*
- 6 *scallions*
- 8 *fat-free flour tortillas (8-inch diameter)*
- 1 *large tomato, seeded and finely chopped*
- ¼ *cup low-fat sour cream*
- 1 *cup salsa*

1. Combine 4 tablespoons of the cilantro, the garlic, rosemary, cayenne, and salt in a rectangular glass bowl. Rub into the steaks, cover with lime juice, and marinate in the refrigerator for 2 hours.
2. Preheat a charcoal or gas grill or an oven broiler.
3. Grill or broil the steak for 3 to 4 minutes per side for medium-rare to medium, or until cooked to taste. At the same time, grill or broil the bell peppers, onion wedges, and scallions for 6 to 8 minutes, or until they are slightly browned. Thinly slice the steak and arrange on a platter with the grilled vegetables.
4. Warm the tortillas on the grill or under the broiler for 10 seconds per side, or until soft and pliable. Place in a basket. Place the tomatoes, the remaining 1 cup cilantro, sour cream, and salsa in individual serving bowls.
5. Arrange so that diners can make their own fajitas by placing some of the sliced beef and grilled vegetables on a tortilla, spooning tomatoes, red onions, cilantro, sour cream, and salsa on top, and rolling up the tortilla.

MAKES 8 SERVINGS.
carnitine, inulin and oligofructose, glutathione, OCs, PQQ, glutamine

45 · Chicken and Melon Salad with Pine Nuts

- 4 *ounces grilled chicken, thinly sliced*
- 2 *tablespoons dry sherry*
- 2 *tablespoons balsamic vinegar*
- 1 *tablespoon teriyaki sauce*
- 2 *cups shredded lettuce**
- 1 *cup cantaloupe chunks*
- 1 *cup cubanel (Italian) pepper, sliced**
- ½ *cup carrots, shredded**

½ cup celery, finely sliced
¼ cup scallions, diagonally sliced
12 grape tomatoes
1 tablespoon pine nuts
2 ounces seasoned croutons

1. In a bowl, combine chicken, sherry, vinegar, and teriyaki sauce; set aside.

2. Line serving platter with lettuce; decoratively arrange cantaloupe, pepper, carrot, celery, scallions, and tomatoes on lettuce. Arrange chicken on salad. Drizzle sherry mixture over salad and sprinkle with pine nuts and croutons.

MAKES 2 SERVINGS.
phytosterols, nucleotides, glutamine, exorphins, arginine, taurine

46 · Open-Faced Ham Sandwich

1 French baguette
2 slices fresh mozzarella
4 teaspoons Dijon mustard
4 ounces shaved, smoked ham
2 slices tomato
*4 tablespoons finely chopped spinach**
8 large basil leaves

1. Slice French baguettes in half, lengthwise. Place on a nonstick baking sheet. Top each with mozzarella and broil in oven until cheese in melted.

2. Spread mustard over melted cheese.

3. Layer with ham, sliced tomatoes, spinach, and basil leaf.

MAKES 2 SERVINGS.
tannins, glutamine, arginine, PQQ

47 · Strawberry-Rhubarb Soup

1 teaspoon unsalted butter
3 stalks rhubarb, peeled and cut into 1-inch chunks

- 2 *cups hulled and sliced fresh strawberries*
- ½ *cup fresh orange juice*
- ½ *cup sugar*
- 1 *cup nonfat vanilla yogurt*
- 4 *leaves fresh mint*

1. Melt the butter in a medium nonstick pan over medium-high heat. Add the rhubarb and sauté for 1 minute. Reduce the heat to medium. Cover and cook for 7 minutes, or until the rhubarb is tender and has released all of its liquid. Remove from the heat. Uncover and allow to cool slightly.

2. Transfer to a blender or a food processor fitted with the metal blade. Add the strawberries, orange juice, sugar, and ½ cup of the yogurt. Process until smooth. Pour into a medium bowl. Cover and refrigerate for at least 1 hour, or until the soup is well chilled.

3. Pour the chilled soup into 4 small glass bowls. Place 1 tablespoon of the remaining yogurt in the center of each bowl. Place a mint leaf in each bowl.

MAKES 4 SERVINGS.
tannins, glutamine, glutathione, lignans, quercetin, phytosterols

48 · Fish Salad with Mint

- 2 *pounds flounder fillets*
- 1 *tablespoon dill weed, minced*
- 3 *tablespoons chopped fresh mint*
- 2 *tablespoons chopped chives*
- 1 *large green pepper, seeded and chopped into small dice*
- 2 *garlic cloves, minced*
- 1 *tablespoon chopped parsley*
- *juice of 2 large lemons* (more to taste)*
- *zest of one lime**
- *salt and pepper to taste*
- 3 *heads Boston lettuce, halved*

1. Preheat oven to 375°F.

2. Rinse the fillets, place in a nonstick pan, cover with aluminum foil, and bake 10 minutes for each pound or until the fish flakes easily with a fork. Remove from the heat; let cool.

3. In a small bowl, combine the dill weed, mint, chives, green pepper, garlic, parsley, lemon juice, and lime zest. Transfer fish to a large bowl and toss with herbs. Season to taste with salt and pepper, cover, and chill in the refrigerator.

4. Line a bowl or platter with the lettuce leaves. Add the fish and top with the salad.

MAKES 6 SERVINGS.
monoterpenes, glutamine, inulin and oligofructose, OCs, lignans

49 · Potato and Leek Soup

2 *tablespoons reduced-fat margarine*
7 *cups water*
3 *cups leeks,* chopped and thoroughly washed*
1 *bay leaf*
2 *tablespoons fresh parsley, chopped*
2 *tablespoons fresh basil leaves, chopped*
1½ *pounds unpeeled red potatoes, washed and diced*
2 *tablespoons olive oil*
2 *cups peeled tomatoes, seeded and finely chopped*
¼ *cup red wine vinegar*
salt and black pepper to taste
½ *cup garlic-flavored croutons*

1. Melt the margarine in a soup pot with ½ cup of the water and add the leeks, bay leaf, parsley, and basil. Cook over medium low heat until onion is tender and add 2 cups of water and the potatoes. Cover the pot and cook for 6 minutes. Add the remaining water and bring to a boil. Cook for 7 minutes or until the potatoes are tender.

2. Heat the oil in a skillet, add the tomatoes, and cook over medium heat until the tomatoes have thickened slightly. Stir with a spoon to make a smooth sauce. Add sauce to potatoes.

3. Add vinegar and salt and pepper to taste. Serve warm over garlic-flavored croutons.

MAKES 6 SERVINGS.
OCs, protease inhibitors, glutamine, PQQ, glutathione, quercetin, tannins, phytosterols

50 · Orange Rice Salad

FOR THE SALAD
1 cup long-grain rice
*2 cups fresh squeezed orange juice**
1 cup broccoli florets, chopped
¼ pound snow peas, trimmed and sliced
1 small red onion, finely chopped
2 large oranges, peeled and divided into sections*
3 sweet red peppers, drained and cut into strips
6 tablespoons vinaigrette (recipe follows)

1. Combine the rice and orange juice in a saucepan. Bring to a boil. Stir and cover, cooking over low heat until the liquid is absorbed and the rice is tender, about 12 minutes. Remove from stove and let cool.

2. Combine the broccoli and snow peas and steam for 5 minutes, covered.

3. Mix the prepared vegetables into the cooled rice. Fold in the orange sections and red peppers. Place on individual serving dishes and drizzle a tablespoon of the vinaigrette on each.

MAKES 6 SERVINGS.
glutathione, PQQ, monoterpenes, inulin and oligofructose, OCs

VINAIGRETTE
1 teaspoon ground parsley
1 teaspoon cumin
2 tablespoons fresh lemon juice
2 tablespoons balsamic or cider vinegar
salt and pepper to taste
2 tablespoons olive oil
½ teaspoon minced garlic

1. Mix the parsley and cumin with the lemon juice and vinegar. Season with salt and pepper. Stir in the olive oil gradually so that the dressing thickens as you mix it. Stir in the garlic.

2. Let stand up to 30 minutes.

51 · Salad Niçoise

3 ripe plum tomatoes, quartered
6 ounces green beans, steamed until tender
⅓ cup black olives
1 small cucumber, peeled and thinly sliced
1 head Boston lettuce, torn
2 carrots, grated
1 can water packed tuna (6½ ounces), drained
*4 anchovy fillets**
2 hard-cooked eggs, quartered*
1 cup vinaigrette (recipe follows)

1. In a large bowl, combine tomatoes, green beans, olives, cucumbers, lettuce, and carrots.

2. Crumble tuna and add to salad along with anchovies and eggs. Toss in prepared vinaigrette. Chill before serving.

VINAIGRETTE

2 tablespoons fresh lemon juice
3 tablespoons tarragon vinegar
2 cloves garlic, finely minced
1 teaspoon Dijon mustard
1 teaspoon thyme, finely chopped
1 teaspoon chervil, finely chopped
1 teaspoon sage, finely chopped
5 tablespoons low-fat plain yogurt
salt and pepper to taste

1. In a small bowl, combine lemon juice, vinegar, garlic, mustard, and spices.

2. Add yogurt to spices. Salt and pepper to taste.

MAKES 4 SERVINGS.
arginine, taurine, glutamine, PQQ, quercetin

52 · Apricot and Cashew Coleslaw

*2–3 ounces cashew nuts**
2–3 ounces dried apricots
½ pound red or white cabbage, shredded
2 celery ribs, chopped
1 tablespoon red wine vinegar
1 teaspoon horseradish
3 tablespoons low-fat yogurt
3 tablespoons nonfat sour cream

1. On nonstick pan, toast the cashew nuts for 2 to 3 minutes under a hot broiler, until lightly browned.

2. Cut the apricots into very fine slivers. Mix with cashews, cabbage, and celery. In a small bowl, whisk together the vinegar, horseradish, yogurt and sour cream. Add to cabbage mixture and combine thoroughly.

MAKES 4 SERVINGS.
arginine, tannins, CLA, PQQ, quercetin, isothiocyanates

53 · Tarragon Hamburgers with Pickled Red Onions

FOR THE PICKLED ONIONS
*1 small red onion, cut into very thin rings**
*¼ cup tarragon vinegar**
½ teaspoon salt
¾ cup water

FOR THE HAMBURGERS
½ stick (¼ cup) reduced-calorie margarine, softened
*3 tablespoons minced fresh tarragon leaves**
*1½ teaspoons tarragon vinegar**

salt and pepper to taste
1½ *pounds ground chuck**
salt and pepper to taste
4 *English muffins, split and toasted*

1. To make the pickled onions, combine the onion rings, vinegar, salt, and water in a small saucepan. Bring the liquid to a boil, and simmer the mixture for 4 minutes. Transfer the mixture to a bowl and let it cool.

2. In a food processor or in a bowl with an electric mixer, cream the margarine with the tarragon and blend in the vinegar and salt and pepper to taste. Transfer the mixture to a sheet of waxed paper. Using the wax paper, shape it into a log, and freeze it, wrapped in the wax paper, for 20 minutes, or until it is firm.

3. Handling the chuck as little as possible, divide it into fourths. Shape each fourth into a ball, and with your thumb, make a depression in the center of each ball. Cut the tarragon butter into 4 pieces, insert a piece of butter into each depression, and form the meat around each piece of butter into a 1-inch-thick patty. Season the hamburgers with salt and pepper. Place them on an oiled rack set 5 to 6 inches over glowing coals. Grill for 5 minutes on each side for medium-rare meat. Transfer the hamburgers to the English muffins and top them with the pickled onions, drained.

MAKES 4 SERVINGS.
carnitine, glutamine, inulin and oligofructose, OCs, lignans, quercetin, glutamine, arginine, nucleotides, taurine

54 · Cream Cheese and Pineapple Sandwiches

1 *teaspoon honey*
½ *teaspoon cinammon*
2 *tablespoons low-fat whipped cream cheese*
2 *tablespoons finely chopped fresh or canned pineapple**
2 *teaspoons slivered almonds**
salt and pepper to taste
4 *slices whole wheat bread, toasted*

1. In a bowl, combine the honey, cinnamon, cream cheese, pineapple and almonds into a spreadable paste. Add salt and pepper to taste.

2. Spread equal amounts on the bread slices to make sandwiches.

MAKES 2 SERVINGS.
arginine, CLA, lignans, phytates, phytosterols

55 · Barley and Smoked Turkey Salad

3 cups vegetable stock (see recipe 28 for vegetable stock)
¾ cup pearled barley, rinsed and drained
½ small onion, chopped
2 tablespoons freshly squeezed lemon juice
1 garlic clove, minced
1 teaspoon salt
½ teaspoon pepper
2 tablespoons olive oil
⅓ cup red or white wine vinegar
1 ½ teaspoons Dijon mustard
¼ cup chopped fresh parsley
2 tablespoons chopped fresh tarragon
1 tablespoon chopped chives
5 ounces thickly sliced smoked turkey, cubed*
2 large carrots, grated
1 small cucumber, sliced
½ cup sliced radishes
2 scallions, finely chopped

1. Combine the vegetable stock, barley, onion, lemon juice, garlic, salt, and pepper in a 2-quart saucepan over high heat. Bring to a boil, reduce heat to low, cover and cook 45 to 50 minutes, until barley is tender and the liquid is absorbed. Cool to room temperature in a bowl.

2. Make the dressing by whisking together the olive oil, vinegar, mustard, parsley, tarragon, and chives, in a small bowl.

3. Pour half of the dressing over the cooled barley and mix well. Mix in the turkey, carrots, cucumbers, radishes, and scallions. Add the

remaining dressing and toss again. Taste and adjust seasoning. Refrigerate until 30 minutes before serving.

MAKES 6 TO 8 SERVINGS.
carnitine, tannins, lignans, glutamine, OCs, arginine

56 · Grilled Tempeh Sandwiches

nonstick cooking spray
1 *tablespoon light soy sauce*
8 *ounces tempeh, sliced ¼ inch thick**
*four slices red onion (¼ inch thick)**
8 *slices pumpernickel bread*
2 *tablespoons Dijon mustard*
4 *large leaves green leaf lettuce*
4 *thin slices low-fat Cheddar cheese*
1 *cup canned, strained sauerkraut*
4 *thick tomato slices*

1. Heat a large nonstick skillet over medium heat; spray with nonstick cooking spray. Add the soy sauce, tempeh, and onion; stir the onion and cook the tempeh until lightly browned, about 5 to 6 minutes per side. Remove from heat.
2. For each sandwich, spread a slice of bread with mustard; top with 1 leaf lettuce, 1 slice of cheese, 1 slice tempeh and onion, ¼ cup sauerkraut, and 1 tomato slice. Top each sandwich with another bread slice.
3. Coat the skillet with nonstick cooking spray; heat over medium heat. Heat the sandwiches until the cheese is melted and the bread is golden, about 4 minutes per side.
4. Cut the sandwiches in half and serve warm.

MAKES 4 SERVINGS.
phytoestrogens, glutamine, OCs, lignans, quercetin, arginine, CLA, isocyanates

57 · Japanese Crabmeat Salad

FOR THE SALAD

5–6 *ounces fresh lump crabmeat**
3–4 *red radishes**
1 *cucumber, about 4 inches long*
8 *slices fresh ginger*

FOR THE DRESSING

¼ *cup rice vinegar*
1 *tablespoon light soy sauce*
1 *teaspoon mirin (syrupy rice wine)*
1 *teaspoon lime juice*

1. Pick over the crabmeat to remove all traces of cartilage, and flake the meat.

2. Trim off the top and bottom of each radish, then slice into thin strips. Soak in cold water.

3. Cut the cucumber in half. Slice into thin circular slices.

4. In a small bowl, combine the dressing ingredients. Add the flaked crabmeat to the dressing and allow it to sit for 10 to 15 minutes. Then pour off and reserve the excess dressing.

5. Drain the radish strips and toss them in the reserved dressing. Let the radish sit in the dressing for 5 to 10 minutes, then drain off the excess.

6. Divide the crabmeat into four portions, and place one portion on each of 4 salad bowls. Divide the radish shreds, cucumber slices, and ginger into four portions and scatter them on top of each portion of crab. Cover and chill for 10 minutes (or for up to 2 hours) before serving.

MAKES 4 SERVINGS.
arginine, glutamine, isothiocyanates, pytosterols

58 · Mediterranean Artichokes

FOR THE DRESSING

2 *cups water*
1 *cup dry white wine*
¼ *cup fresh lemon juice*

3 tablespoons wine vinegar
2 tablespoons olive oil
2 garlic cloves
6 black peppercorns
*1 tablespoon coriander seed**
1 bay leaf
4 sprigs parsley
¼ teaspoon dried savory
1 branch fennel, minced
1 stalk celery, minced
½ teaspoon salt
1 large shallot, chopped

FOR THE ARTICHOKES

4–6 large globe artichokes
1 tablespoon chopped fresh parsley or dill

1. Combine all the ingredients for the dressing in a large pot and bring to a simmer. Simmer, covered, for 15 minutes.

2. Cut the stems off the artichoke bottoms. Break off all the leaves and cut off the tops.

3. Cut away all the tough green skin from the bottoms of the artichokes.

4. Drop into the simmering dressing. Simmer, covered, for 30 to 40 minutes or until tender. Remove from the heat and allow to cool in the marinade.

5. Remove the chokes from the artichoke bottoms. Remove the artichoke bottoms from the marinade and carefully pull apart at the center. Return to the marinade and refrigerate for at least 2 hours.

6. Heat the marinade to boiling and reduce to ¾ cup.

7. Place the artichoke bottoms and some of the dressing on a platter or on individual serving plates. Allow to cool or serve warm. Garnish with the parsley or dill, and serve.

MAKES 6 SERVINGS.
inulin, oligofructose, monoterpenes, phytates

59 · Marissa's Favorite Turkey Burgers

¼ *cup low-fat mayonnaise*
1 *tablespoon Dijon mustard*
2 *tablespoons fresh basil leaves, chopped*
10 *black olives, pitted and chopped*
1 *pound ground turkey**
2 *tablespoons chopped dried tomatoes, soaked in boiling water until soft*
¼ *teaspoon chopped fresh thyme leaves*
¼ *teaspoon chopped fresh rosemary leaves*
salt and pepper to taste
4 *sesame buns*
1½ *cups arugula, packed*

1. In a small bowl, stir together mayonnaise, mustard, and basil.

2. In a large bowl, blend together olives, turkey, tomatoes, thyme, rosemary, and salt and pepper to taste.

3. Form mixture into 4 patties and grill. Toast sesame buns. Place burgers on buns and top with basil-mayonnaise and arugula.

MAKES 4 SERVINGS.
carnitine, isothiocyanate, phytosterols

60 · Chicken Salad with Exotic Mushroom Vinaigrette

2 *whole chicken breasts, skinned and boned**
1 *cup water*
1 *tablespoon lemon juice*
¼ *cup dried shiitake mushrooms*
¼ *cup dried cremini mushrooms*
½ *cup red wine vinegar*
¼ *diced sweet red bell pepper*
1 *small onion, thinly sliced*
1 *cucumber, peeled and thinly sliced*
½ *cup olive oil*
1 *tablespoon chopped fresh tarragon*
¼ *teaspoon salt*
⅛ *teaspoon black pepper*

2 cups Bibb lettuce
2 cups lightly packed fresh spinach leaves
1 cup thinly sliced Belgian endive
*2 cups sliced button mushrooms**
4 ripe plum tomatoes, cubed

1. Place chicken, water, and lemon juice in a large, nonstick pan. Heat to simmer; cover and simmer, about 5 to 6 minutes, until center of chicken is no longer pink. Strain. Let chicken cool slightly, then cut into 1½-inch cubes.

2. To prepare dressing, put dried mushrooms and vinegar in a small saucepan. Heat to boiling over medium-low heat. Remove from heat. Let stand, covered, 10 minutes to soak.

3. Put red pepper, onion, and olive oil in a small, nonstick skillet. Cook and stir over medium-low heat for 2 minutes, until softened.

4. Drain mushrooms, reserving liquid. Wash mushrooms briefly under cold water to remove grit. Trim and discard tough ends from mushrooms; chop mushrooms. Add mushrooms, reserved liquid, tarragon, salt and pepper to red pepper mixture. Mix well with fork.

5. To assemble salad, place lettuce and spinach leaves on serving plates. Top with chicken. Arrange Belgian endive, button mushrooms, and cubed tomatoes on salads. Drizzle with wild mushroom dressing.

MAKES 4 SERVINGS.
carnitine, nucleotides, glutamine, arginine, taurine, PQQ

61 · Grapefruit Lime Cooler

*2 cups unsweetened grapefruit juice**
*3 tablespoons lime juice**
4 teaspoons sugar
4 sprigs mint, finely chopped
2 cups seltzer water
4 lime wedges

1. In a 1-quart pitcher, combine the grapefruit juice and lime juice. Set aside.

2. Place 1 teaspoon sugar and ¼ of the chopped mint in each of 4 12-ounce glasses.

3. Combine the grapefruit and lime juices with the seltzer, fill the glasses with ice cubes, and divide the grapefruit juice mixture among them. Stir briskly to mix. Garnish with lime wedges and serve.

MAKES 4 SERVINGS.
glutamine, glutathione, monoterpenes

62 · Tofu Salad and Sprout Sandwiches

*1 pound extra-firm tofu**
¼ cup low-fat mayonnaise
1 tablespoon Dijon mustard
1 tablespoon low-sodium soy sauce
dash salt
⅛ teaspoon ground cumin
⅛ teaspoon ground turmeric
¼ cup chopped zucchini
1 green onion, minced
¼ cup shredded carrot
¼ cup minced celery
2 tablespoons minced green bell pepper
12 slices whole wheat bread
*2 cups alfalfa sprouts**

1. In a medium bowl, crumble tofu with a fork into small pieces. Stir in mayonnaise, mustard, and soy sauce. Add salt, cumin, turmeric, zucchini, green onion, carrot, celery, and green pepper; stir well.

2. For each sandwich, place a mound of salad on a slice of bread, spreading to the edge. Top salad with a layer of sprouts. Place another slice of bread on sprouts.

MAKES 6 SERVINGS.
phytoestrogens, phytates, glutamine, arginine, lignans, phytosterols, PQQ

63 · Vegetable Noodle Soup with Cheddar

1 tablespoon olive oil
½ cup diced carrot

*¼ cup each diced green bell pepper, celery, scallions**
1½ teaspoons all-purpose flour
⅛ teaspoon powdered mustard
dash black pepper
1 cup low-fat milk
½ cup water
1 pack instant chicken broth and seasoning mix
2 ounces vermicelli
2 ounces sharp Cheddar cheese, shredded

1. In medium saucepan, heat oil over medium heat until hot; add vegetables and sauté, stirring occasionally, about 3 to 5 minutes. Reduce heat to medium; cover and let cook until vegetables are soft, about 5 minutes longer.

2. Sprinkle flour, mustard, and pepper over vegetables and stir. Cook, uncovered, stirring constantly, for about 1 minute. Add milk while stirring, and then add water, broth mix, and vermicelli, stirring constantly; bring to just a boil. Reduce heat to low; add cheese and cook, stirring, until cheese is melted and soup is thickened.

MAKES 2 SERVINGS.
glutathione

64 · Tuna Sandwiches with Basil and Tomato

¼ cup red wine vinegar
1 garlic clove, minced
10 black olives, sliced
salt and pepper to taste
2 tablespoons extra virgin olive oil
1 tablespoon Dijon mustard
two 8-inch round loaves of crusty bread
2 cups thinly sliced radish
2 cups loosely packed fresh basil leaves
1 cup minced red onion, soaked in cold water for 10 minutes and drained well
*2 6½-ounce cans tuna packed in water, drained and flaked**
4 tomatoes (about 1½ pounds) sliced thin

1. In a bowl, whisk together vinegar, garlic, olives, mustard, salt and pepper to taste. Add the oil in a stream, whisking, until it is emulsified.

2. Halve the breads horizontally, hollow out the halves, leaving ½-inch-thick shells, and spoon some of the oil and vinegar mixture into each half. On each loaf, layer radish, basil, onion, tuna and tomato. Top with the other half of loaf. Press down on the sandwiches and wrap tightly in plastic wrap; chill them for 1 hour. Serve cut into wedges.

MAKES 6 SERVINGS.
arginine, glutamine, isothiocyanates, lignans

65 · Roasted Garlic and Avocado Crab Sandwiches

*½ pound crabmeat**
¼ cup chives, chopped
½ red onion, cut into ¼-inch dice
1 serrano or jalapeño chili, chopped
2 tablespoons peeled, seeded, and diced cucumber
1 small tomato, finely chopped
1 tablespoon chopped cilantro leaves
2 tablespoons Dijon mustard
juice of 1 orange
juice of 4 limes
1 tablespoon olive oil
salt and pepper to taste
3 heads garlic
¼ cup low-fat mayonnaise
1 mango, sliced
1 teaspoon rosemary, finely minced
1 avocado, pitted, peeled, and thinly sliced
3 ready-made corn muffins, sliced in half and toasted
1 celery heart sliced lengthwise for garnish

1. Preheat oven to 425°F.

2. In a mixing bowl, combine the crabmeat, chives, onion, serrano chili, cucumber, tomato, and cilantro.

3. In a separate bowl, combine the mustard, orange and lime juices, and olive oil and whisk well. Pour over the crabmeat mixture and toss. Season with salt and pepper.

4. Wrap garlic in aluminum foil and place on a baking sheet. Bake for 30 minutes and remove from oven and let cool. Squeeze out the roasted garlic from the cloves. In a small bowl, mix garlic with mayonnaise and rosemary. Refrigerate.

5. Place avocado on muffin half and layer with crabmeat and sliced mangos. Spoon mayonnaise on top of mango and top sandwich with other muffin half. Garnish with celery.

MAKES 3 SERVINGS.
exorphins, OCs, phytosterol, monoterpenes

66 · Grapefruit Cooler

*9 cups (2¼ quarts) fresh red grapefruit juice (from about 6 grapefruits)**
3 cups seltzer or club soda
fresh mint sprigs

1. In a pitcher half-filled with ice cubes, stir together juice and seltzer or soda.

2. Garnish with mint.

MAKES 12 SERVINGS.
glutamine

67 · Fresh Fruit and Cheese Sandwiches

½ tablespoon Dijon mustard
2 teaspoons honey
4 slices whole wheat bread
*2 cups loosely packed Romaine lettuce**
*1 Granny Smith apple, cored and sliced thinly**
1½ ounces crumbled blue cheese

1. Preheat broiler.

2. Stir together mustard and honey.

3. Toast bread and arrange on a baking sheet. Spread toast with honey mustard and top with lettuce. Top with apple and cheese. Broil sandwiches until cheese melts, about 30 seconds.

MAKES 4 SANDWICHES.
PQQ, CLA, tannins, phytates

68 · Ginger Lime Tea

6 teaspoons jasmine tea
1 quart water
1 lime, halved
¼ cup freshly grated ginger
¼ cup honey

1. In a pot, bring the water to a boil; add tea.
2. Juice the lime and add the juice, the squeezed lime rind, and the ginger to the water. Remove from the heat and cover, and let sit for 20 minutes. Stir in the honey.
3. Line a strainer with a thin, wet cloth and strain the tea into a pitcher.
4. Refrigerate until cold. Serve over ice.

MAKES 6 SERVINGS.
monoterpenes, tannins

69 · Turkey and Avocado Tortilla Rolls with Black Bean-Corn Salsa

*½ cup canned black beans, rinsed and drained**
1 large vine-ripened tomato, seeded and chopped
½ cup sweet corn
2 pickled jalapeños, seeded and chopped (wear rubber gloves)
4 teaspoons fresh lime juice
½ teaspoon chili powder
½ tablespoon fresh, chopped oregano, or ½ teaspoon dried
salt to taste
½ ripe California avocado
2 tablespoons low-fat plain yogurt
4 whole wheat tortillas (10-inch)

4 ounces thinly sliced roast turkey breast
1 cup packed fresh coriander sprigs, washed well, spun dry, and chopped coarsely

1. To make the salsa, stir together in a bowl the black beans, tomatoes, corn, jalapeños, 2 teaspoons lime juice, chili powder, oregano, and salt to taste.

2. In a food processor, puree avocado, yogurt, remaining 2 teaspoons lime juice, and salt to taste.

3. Warm tortillas in oven. Spread avocado mixture on tortillas and place turkey over the mixture. Top turkey with salsa and coriander. Roll up tortillas, leaving ends open.

MAKES 4 SERVINGS.
lignans, CLA, saponins, exorphins

70 · Tomato Juice

*4 pounds red, ripe unblemished tomatoes**
¼ cup thinly sliced onion
3 large leaves fresh basil or 1 teaspoon dried
½ cup water
6 sprigs fresh parsley
1 teaspoon sugar

1. Cut the cores from the tomatoes. Cut the unpeeled tomatoes into 1-inch cubes. There should be about 10 cups.

2. Put the tomatoes in a kettle and add the remaining ingredients. Bring to a boil and stir so the tomatoes cook evenly. Cover and cook for 30 minutes.

3. Put the tomato mixture through a food mill, pushing to squeeze the pulp through. There should be about 4 cups. Let cool, then chill.

4. If you wish to can the juice, return it to a kettle and reheat until it is almost but not quite boiling. Pour the juice into 2 pint jars, leaving ¼ inch of heat space. Adjust the caps, turning them to tighten. Process the juice for 10 minutes in a boiling water bath. If you use a quart jar for processing, process the jar for 15 minutes.

MAKES 6 SERVINGS.
PQQ, exorphins

71 · Marinated Green Pepper Hamburgers on Whole Wheat Rolls

1 *green bell pepper, seeded and minced**
1½ *pounds ground beef round*
6 *cloves garlic, minced*
1½ *cups dry white wine*
½ *cup lemon juice*
2 *tablespoons red wine vinegar*
1 *teaspoon parsley*
1 *teaspoon thyme*
1 *tablespoon olive oil*
salt and pepper to taste
6 *whole wheat rolls*

1. In a bowl combine the green peppers with the ground beef and make 6 patties. Place patties in baking pan.

2. In another bowl, stir together the garlic, wine, lemon juice, vinegar, parsley, thyme, and oil and pour over the patties. Sprinkle with salt and pepper to taste. Cover and refrigerate, turning the burgers over frequently. Drain the patties before grilling.

3. Grill or broil 3 to 6 minutes per side. Serve on whole wheat rolls.

MAKES 6 SERVINGS.
PQQ, exorphins, arginine, taurine, carnitine

72 · Honey Darjeeling Iced Tea

8 *cups water*
½ *ounce Darjeeling tea leaves**
6 *or 7 mint leaves*
2 *tablespoons fresh lemon juice**
¼ *cup honey*
ice

1. Bring the water to a boil in a teakettle or pot over high heat.

2. Meanwhile, combine the tea and mint leaves in a paper coffee filter. Twist the filter closed to enclose the contents. Put the filter package in a heat-resistant 2- to 3-quart pitcher.

3. Add the boiling water to the pitcher, pouring it over the filter package. Allow the tea to steep for 5 to 7 minutes. Then remove the filter package. Stir in the lemon juice and honey, and allow the tea to cool to room temperature.

4. Fill tall glasses with ice, and pour the tea into them.

MAKES 8 SERVINGS.
tannins, quercetin, monoterpenes

DINNERS

73 · Shrimp and Fresh Herbs

- 8 *slices of uncured turkey bacon**
- *nonstick cooking spray*
- ½ *cup chopped celery*
- 1 *cup chopped onion*
- ½ *cup chopped green bell pepper*
- 1 *tablespoon all-purpose flour*
- 2 *cups low-fat chicken broth*
- 4 *cups canned tomatoes, drained and chopped, reserving 1 cup of juice*
- 1 *teaspoon sugar*
- 1 *tablespoon fresh basil, chopped*
- 1 *tablespoon fresh parsley, chopped*
- 1 *tablespoon fresh coriander, chopped*
- ¼ *teaspoon cayenne*
- 1½ *pounds medium size shrimp* (about 40), shelled and deveined*
- *salt and pepper to taste*
- 3 *cups steamed long-grain rice such as Carolina or basmati*

1. Microwave bacon until crisp; drain on a paper towel.

2. Coat a large saucepan with cooking spray, cook the celery, onion, and bell pepper over moderately low heat, stirring, until the vegetables are softened. Add the flour, and cook the mixture, stirring, for 3 minutes.

3. Add the chicken broth, tomatoes with the reserved juice, sugar, basil, parsley, coriander and the cayenne. While stirring, bring the mixture to a boil, and simmer for 30 minutes.

4. Add the shrimp and simmer the mixture, stirring, for no longer than 3 to 4 minutes, or until the shrimp are just pink. Add salt and ground black pepper to taste. Do not overcook.

5. Serve shrimp over the rice and top with crumbled pieces of the bacon.

MAKES 6 SERVINGS.
nucleotides, glutamine, inulin and oligofructose, OCs, lignans, PQQ, taurine, arginine

74 · Mediterranean Couscous Salad

- 2¼ *cups water*
- 1½ *cups couscous*
- ½ *teaspoon salt*
- 3 *tablespoons freshly squeezed lemon juice*
- 1 *tablespoon extra virgin olive oil*
- *salt and pepper to taste*
- 1 *small bunch spinach* leaves washed thoroughly, dried, and shredded fine*
- 4 *large scallions, thinly sliced*
- 2 *tablespoons cilantro, finely minced*
- 1 *yellow pepper, stemmed, seeded, and diced*

1. In a saucepan, boil the water and add the couscous and salt. Remove pan from heat, stir, and let couscous stand, covered, for 5 to 6 minutes.

2. Transfer couscous to a bowl. Stir in lemon juice, olive oil, and salt and pepper to taste. Let cool for about 1 hour.

3. Mix spinach, scallions, cilantro, and yellow pepper, and add to couscous. Chill salad, covered, at least 2 hours or overnight.

MAKES 6 SERVINGS.
nucleotides, saponins, protease inhibitors, PQQ, tannins, glutathione, OCs

75 · Lentil Soup

- 2 *garlic cloves, minced*
- 2 *large onions, chopped*
- 2 *cups canned Italian plum tomatoes with their juice, put through a*

food mill to remove seeds
2 *cups dried brown lentils,* washed in several changes of cold water*
2 *quarts cold water*
salt and freshly ground black pepper to taste
1 *head escarole (about 1⅓ pound)*
nonstick cooking spray

1. Coat a large saucepan with nonstick cooking spray and set over medium heat. Add the garlic and cook until it is lightly golden. Add the onions and sauté until they are tender, about 10 minutes. Add the tomatoes and bring to a gentle simmer. Cook, stirring occasionally, for 6 to 8 minutes. Add the lentils and stir well. Add the water, bring to a gentle boil, and season with salt and pepper. Reduce the heat to low and simmer, uncovered, for 20 minutes.

2. While the lentils are cooking, detach the leaves from the root end of the escarole, discarding any that are bruised or wilted. Wash the leaves well under cold running water. Drain and cut into 1-inch strips.

3. Add the escarole to the lentils, cover the pot, and continue cooking at a low simmer until the lentils and escarole are tender, 25 to 30 minutes. Stir the soup from time to time and add a bit more water if it becomes too thick. Turn the heat off and let the soup rest for 20 to 30 minutes.

4. Ladle the soup into individual bowls, and sprinkle with a dash of black pepper. Serve hot.

MAKES 8 SERVINGS.
nucleotides, saponins, phytates, glutamine, tannins, lignans, phytoestrogens, glutamine, PQQ, quercetin

76 · Chocolate Flan

1 *can (14½ ounces) fat-free condensed milk**
1 *can (12 ounces) evaporated milk**
2 *eggs*
6 *egg yolks*
¼ *cup chocolate syrup*
2 *tablespoons dark rum*
1 *cup sugar*

1. Preheat the oven to 375°F.

2. In a food processor with the metal blade running, place the condensed and evaporated milk, eggs, egg yolks, chocolate, and rum. Blend thoroughly.

3. To make the caramel, place the sugar in a heavy-bottomed saucepan and cook over medium heat, stirring constantly, until the sugar is light amber color, about 20 minutes. Pour the caramel into 6 individual 8-ounce baking molds or into a 9" × 4" loaf pan.

4. Pour the flan mixture into the molds or loaf pan on top of the caramel. Place in a water bath and bake uncovered in the oven for 15 minutes. Reduce the heat to 350° and continue baking until set, when a knife inserted comes out clean, about 30 minutes. Remove from the oven and let cool completely.

5. To serve, run a knife around the inside edges of the molds or pan and invert the flans onto a serving platter or individual plates.

MAKES 6 SERVINGS.
arginine, CLA, lignans

77 · Lemon Chicken

1 tablespoon olive oil
2 boneless chicken breasts (about 12 ounces)
salt and pepper to taste
1 small red onion, sliced thin
¾ teaspoon ground coriander
¼ teaspoon paprika
½ teaspoon tarragon
1 tablespoon fresh squeezed lemon juice
2 teaspoons finely grated fresh lemon zest
1½ teaspoons all-purpose flour
1½ cups defatted chicken broth
⅓ cup black olives, pitted and sliced thin
1 tablespoon honey
½ cup canned chickpeas, drained and rinsed*
2 tablespoons chopped fresh parsley sprigs

1. In a 3-quart heavy saucepan, heat oil over moderately high heat until hot.

2. Season chicken with salt and pepper and cook until skin is golden brown. Transfer to a plate and reduce heat to moderate.

3. Add onion to pan and cook, stirring, until softened and not browned.

4. Add coriander, paprika, tarragon, lemon juice and zest, and flour. Cook, stirring, 2 to 3 minutes. Stir in broth, olives, and honey.

5. Return chicken to pan and simmer, uncovered, stirring occasionally, about 10 minutes.

6. Place chicken on 2 plates. Combine chickpeas with sauce. Simmer sauce 3 minutes and season with salt and pepper. Pour sauce over chicken and top with parsley.

MAKES 2 SERVINGS.
saponins, nucleotides, glutamine, exorphins, arginine, taurine, inulin and oligofructose, OCs, lignan

78 · Pea and Mushroom Risotto

2 cups defatted chicken broth
¼ cup finely chopped onion
1 tablespoon olive oil
¾ cup Italian or other short-grain rice
½ cup dry white wine
½ cup chopped fresh mushrooms
1 cup frozen peas, thawed*
½ tablespoon thyme, crumbled
2 tablespoons freshly grated Parmesan cheese
salt and pepper to taste
¼ cup finely grated carrots

1. In a 4-quart saucepan, bring the broth to a simmer; turn heat to low.

2. In a heavy saucepan, cook the onion in the olive oil over moderately low heat, stirring, until it is softened. Add the rice, stirring with a wooden spoon.

3. Pour in the wine and cook the mixture over moderately high heat, stirring, until the wine is absorbed. Add about ½ cup of the simmering broth and cook the mixture, stirring for about 5 minutes.

4. Add the remaining broth in small increments, stirring constantly and letting each portion be absorbed before adding the next.

5. Add the mushrooms, peas, and thyme while stirring. Cook the mixture until the broth disappears and the rice is al dente. Remove the pan from the heat, stir in the Parmesan and salt and pepper to taste. Garnish with carrots.

MAKES 2 SERVINGS.
saponins, glutamine, inulin and oligofructose, OCs, lignans, arginine, CLA, protease inhibitors, PQQ

79 · Asparagus with Parmesan

*1 pound asparagus**
1 quart water, plus 1 tablespoon
2 tablespoons fresh lemon juice
1 teaspoon Dijon mustard
¼ teaspoon sugar
1 teaspoon fresh chives, minced
1 teaspoon fresh dill, minced
¼ teaspoon salt
¼ teaspoon freshly ground pepper
1 tablespoon olive oil
2 paper-thin slices prosciutto, finely chopped
1 tablespoon grated Parmesan cheese

1. Cut 1 inch off end of asparagus stalks. Peel if more than a half inch thick.

2. Boil 1 quart of water. Add asparagus and cook until tender (about 5 minutes). Drain and rinse under cold running water; place in a serving bowl.

3. In a small bowl, combine the lemon juice, mustard, sugar, chives, dill, salt, and pepper with 1 tablespoon water; slowly whisk in the oil. Drizzle the dressing over asparagus; sprinkle with the prosciutto and cheese.

MAKES 4 SERVINGS.
saponins, inulin and oligofructose, glutathione

80 · Crunchy Berries

nonstick cooking spray
¾ *cup rolled oats**
¼ *cup oat bran**
1 *tablespoon firmly packed brown sugar*
½ *teaspoon ground cinnamon*
2 *teaspoons vegetable oil*
2 *tablespoons white grape juice*
1 *cup plain low-fat yogurt*
¼ *cup plus 2 tablespoons fruit-only strawberry jam*
1 *teaspoon maple or rice syrup*
4 *cups sliced or quartered fresh strawberries*
2 *cups blueberries*

1. Preheat oven to 350°F. Spray a nonstick 10" × 15" pan with cooking spray.
2. In a small bowl, combine oats, oat bran, brown sugar, and cinnamon. Mix well. Add oil and white grape juice. Mix until all ingredients are moistened. Spread in prepared pan.
3. Bake 10 to 12 minutes or until lightly browned. Stir several times while baking, breaking up any large lumps with the back of a spoon.
4. Cover pan, place in refrigerator, and cool for at least one hour before serving.
5. Combine yogurt, jam, and syrup in a small bowl. Mix well. Chill several hours or overnight.
6. At serving time, divide strawberries and blueberries evenly into 8 tall-stemmed dessert glasses. Spoon sauce over berries. Sprinkle with oat topping.

MAKES 8 SERVINGS.
saponins, tannins, glutamine, glutathione, lignans, quercetin, phytosterols, nucleotides

81 · Grilled Sesame Chicken Breasts

2 *whole skinless, boneless chicken breasts*
½ *cup sesame dressing (recipe follows)*

1. Place chicken on grill 6 inches from medium-hot coals.

2. Brush with dressing while turning chicken every 2 to 3 minutes. Brush with sauce. Grill until chicken is cooked thoroughly when spread apart with a fork.

MAKES 4 SERVINGS.
phytates, CLA, phytosterols, nucleotides, glutamine, exorphins, arginine, taurine

SESAME DRESSING

*2 tablespoons roasted sesame seeds**
nonstick cooking spray
1 teaspoon minced fresh garlic
2 tablespoons white wine vinegar
dash red pepper flakes
⅛ teaspoon dried oregano
½ teaspoon dried sage
½ teaspoon dried marjoram
¼ teaspoon salt
⅛ teaspoon black pepper
1 tablespoon canola oil
2 tablespoons honey

1. Spread sesame seeds on a large baking pan and cook under broiler until lightly browned.

2. Coat a small saucepan with nonstick cooking spray. Add garlic and brown lightly. Stir in vinegar, red pepper flakes, oregano, sage, marjoram, salt, and pepper and cook 1 to 2 minutes over medium-low heat.

3. Whisk in oil and honey. Add sesame seeds.

82 · Barley, Tomato, and Spinach Pie

3 cups water
1 vegetable bouillon cube
*1½ cups pearled barley**
1 bay leaf
nonstick cooking spray
1 tablespoon olive oil, to drizzle on top
1 large onion, finely chopped

2 garlic cloves, minced
4 ounces sun-dried tomatoes, sliced and reconstituted with 1 cup hot water
10-ounce package frozen chopped spinach, thawed
1 tablespoon balsamic or red wine vinegar
1 teaspoon dried sage
¼ teaspoon grated nutmeg
freshly ground pepper to taste
½ cup bread crumbs plus ½ cup freshly grated Parmesan cheese

1. Preheat oven to 425°F.

2. Boil the water and add the bouillon. Continue to cook while adding the barley and bay leaf.

3. Cover the pan and cook over very low heat for about 25 minutes, until all of the water has absorbed. Remove from the heat and let stand, covered, for at least ½ hour. Stir the grain until it is smooth.

4. Coat a medium-sized casserole dish with nonstick spray.

5. Stir in the onion and sauté over medium-high heat for 7 to 8 minutes, until soft. Stir in the garlic and sauté about 15 seconds more, then stir in the sun-dried tomatoes. Cover the skillet and cook over medium heat for 2 minutes. Mix in the spinach and vinegar.

6. When the spinach is wilted, stir in the sage, nutmeg, and pepper. Mix the spinach mixture with the barley; then turn the grain into the prepared dish. Top with the bread crumbs/cheese. Drizzle the topping with the olive oil to moisten the crumbs, then bake for 25 to 30 minutes, until heated through. Serve hot.

MAKES 8 SERVINGS.
phytates, glutamine, inulin and oligofructose, OCs, lignans, monoterpenes

83 · Asian Eggplant, Green Beans, and Tomatoes with Peanuts

4 teaspoons sugar
2 teaspoons fresh lemon juice
1½ tablespoons Asian fish sauce
½ pound Asian eggplants (about 2)
nonstick cooking spray
½ teaspoon olive oil

½ pound string beans
15 grape tomatoes, halved
2 tablespoons fresh oregano, chopped finely
1 teaspoon allspice
3 tablespoons roasted peanuts, finely chopped*
2 cloves garlic, minced

1. Preheat broiler.
2. In a large bowl, add sugar and lemon juice to the fish sauce. Stir until sugar is dissolved, about 5 minutes.
3. Cut eggplants crosswise into ½-inch-thick slices. Spray a baking pan with nonstick cooking spray and place eggplant slices in pan. Brush eggplant with oil and broil 4 to 5 inches from heat, turning it once, until tender and browned, about 6 minutes.
4. Add eggplant to fish-sauce mixture and toss.
5. Cut beans into 1½-inch lengths. In a saucepan, cook beans in boiling salted water for 2 minutes.
6. Drain beans well, let cool, and add to eggplant mixture.
7. Combine tomatoes, oregano, allspice, 2 tablespoons peanuts, and garlic to eggplant mixture, tossing well.
8. Serve at room temperature sprinkled with remaining peanuts.

MAKES 4 SERVINGS.
phytates, CLA

84 · Cantaloupe Sorbet

1½ cups sugar
½ cup water
9 cups cubed cantaloupe (about 2 medium)
¼ cup unsweetened grape juice
1 waffle cone broken into large pieces

1. Combine sugar and water in a small saucepan. Bring to a boil; cook over medium heat, stirring constantly, until sugar dissolves. Remove from heat and let cool.
2. Using the metal blade of a food processor, process cantaloupe until smooth. Add sugar mixture and grape juice. Pour into a bowl, cover, and chill thoroughly.

3. Transfer to an ice cream maker and follow manufacturer's directions.

4. Scoop sorbet into individual bowls and serve with waffle cone pieces.

MAKES 6 SERVINGS.
glutathione, glutamine, tannins

85 · Zucchini and Smoked Salmon with Linguine in Lemon Cream Sauce

*1 pound zucchini**
2 large shallots, minced
¾ cup half-and-half
1 tablespoon lemon zest
3 tablespoons fresh squeezed lemon
¼ pound sliced smoked salmon, cut into 2-inch strips
1 pound dry fettuccine
salt and pepper to taste

1. Cook zucchini in boiling water until tender, about 5 minutes. Reserve water in pot, over low heat, covered. Drain zucchini.

2. Coat a nonstick skillet with cooking spray and cook shallots over moderately low heat, stirring, until softened, about 5 minutes.

3. Add half-and-half and zest and simmer, stirring occasionally, until slightly thickened, about 12 minutes. Stir in 2 tablespoons lemon juice and remove skillet from heat.

4. Return water in pot to a boil. Cook pasta in boiling water, stirring occasionally, until al dente. Reserve 1 cup pasta water.

5. Drain pasta in a colander and add to sauce with asparagus, ½ cup pasta water, salmon, remaining tablespoon lemon juice, and salt and pepper to taste. Warm over low heat, gently combining pasta with other ingredients.

MAKES 6 SERVINGS.
protease inhibitors, nucleotides, saponins, glutamine, inulin, lignans, carnitine, phytosterols, CLA, arginine

86 · Roasted Cauliflower with Spices

a small head of cauliflower (about 1 pound)*
¼ *teaspoon cumin seeds*
¼ *teaspoon ground coriander*
1 *tablespoon capers*
1 *teaspoons olive oil*
2 *tablespoons bread crumbs as garnish*

1. Preheat oven to 450°F.
2. Cut cauliflower into 1-inch flowerets and place in nonstick roasting pan.
3. Combine cumin, coriander, and capers with oil. Drizzle over cauliflower.
4. Roast mixture in oven 25 minutes, or until cauliflower is just tender.
5. Serve warm, garnish with bread crumbs.

MAKES 2 SERVINGS.
protease inhibitors

87 · Baked Ziti with Eggplant

1 *medium eggplant, peeled and diced*
nonstick cooking spray
3 *tablespoons olive oil*
½ *pound ziti*
6 *garlic* cloves, minced*
¼ *teaspoon crushed red pepper flakes*
1½ *cups canned plum tomatoes,*diced*
2 *tablespoons dry red wine*
½ *teaspoon salt*
¼ *cup chopped fresh parsley*
½ *cup diced red peppers*
4 *tablespoons grated Parmesan cheese**
1½ *cups grated part-skim mozzarella cheese**

1. Preheat oven to 375°F. Bring a large saucepan of water to a boil.
2. Place eggplant on a large cookie sheet sprayed with nonstick

cooking spray. Brush the eggplant with 1 tablespoon of the olive oil. Bake the eggplant until it begins to brown and appears somewhat translucent or shiny. Do not overcook it because additional cooking will be done when it is baked.

3. Remove the eggplant and place it in a shallow 2½-quart baking dish.

4. Drop the ziti in the boiling water and cook until al dente, not mushy. Drain in a colander; put ziti back in the saucepan.

5. Place the remaining 2 tablespoons of oil in the skillet. Add the garlic and red pepper flakes and cook until fragrant. Add the tomatoes, wine, salt, parsley, and red peppers while stirring. Cook no more than 2 minutes and remove from the heat.

6. Stir the ziti into the eggplant and sauce, adding 2 tablespoons of the Parmesan cheese. Place ½ of the mixture in the baking dish. Layer with the mozzarella cheese. Spread the remaining pasta mixture over the mozzarella and sprinkle the remaining 2 tablespoons Parmesan cheese. Cover with foil.

7. Bake until hot and bubbly or about 20 to 30 minutes. Remove the foil and bake 5 more minutes or until cheese is slightly browned.

MAKES 4 SERVINGS.
glutamine, inulin and oligofructose, monoterpenes, OCs, lignans, PQQ, CLA

88 · Spicy Lobster Salad

1 cup Low-Fat Mayonnaise with Fresh Herbs (recipe follows)
½ cup drained capers
½ cup finely chopped celery
¼ cup finely chopped shallots
½ cup finely chopped scallions
2 tablespoons fresh chervil, chopped
1 tablespoon Dijon mustard
3 drops of Tabasco sauce
10 sprigs fresh watercress
salt and black pepper to taste
juice of ½ lime
*1 pound steamed lobster meat**
3 tablespoons chopped fresh parsley or coriander leaves

1. In a small bowl, place the mayonnaise and combine with capers, celery, shallots, scallions, chervil, mustard, Tabasco sauce, watercress, salt and pepper, and lime juice.

2. Add the lobster meat and carefully fold it in, leaving the lumps as large as possible. Sprinkle with the parsley before serving.

MAKES 6 SERVINGS.
glutamine, arginine, glutathione, PQQ

LOW-FAT MAYONNAISE WITH FRESH HERBS

1 cup low-fat mayonnaise
salt and black pepper to taste
2 tablespoons minced scallions
2 tablespoons minced fresh chives
2 tablespoons minced fresh parsley leaves
2 tablespoons minced fresh basil leaves
1 teaspoon minced dill
1 tablespoon finely chopped fresh sage

1. Place mayonnaise in small bowl; stir in the remaining ingredients and blend well.

2. Cover and refrigerate until ready to serve.

MAKES 1 CUP.

89 · Angel Food Cake

*1 cup sifted cake flour**
1½ cups superfine granulated sugar
1½ cups egg whites
1¼ teaspoons cream of tartar
¼ teaspoon salt
1½ teaspoons vanilla extract
¼ teaspoon almond extract

1. Preheat the oven to 325°F.

2. Sift the flour four times with ½ cup of the sugar.

3. To make meringues, beat the egg whites until foamy. Add vanilla and almond extracts. Add the cream of tartar and salt and beat until soft moist peaks form when the beater is withdrawn.

4. Sift about ¼ cup of the flour-sugar mixture at a time over the meringue. Cut and fold it in just until no flour shows.

5. Turn into a nonstick 10" tube pan and bake about one hour. Invert pan and let cake cool one hour.

MAKES 8–10 SERVINGS.
glutamine

90 · Southwest Spicy Pork Skewers

1 tablespoon paprika
1½ teaspoons ground dried red chili powder
1½ teaspoons ground mild to medium-hot dried red chili, such as guajillo or pasilla, or a combination of these
5 tablespoons fennel seeds, crushed
3 tablespoons mustard seeds, crushed
4 cloves garlic, finely minced
1 teaspoon salt
1 teaspoon sugar
1¾ to 2 pounds pork tenderloin, cut into 1-inch cubes*
1 large onion, cut into ⅛-inch sections
1 medium zucchini sliced into ½-inch slices
½ medium red bell pepper, cut into 1-inch squares
12 cherry tomatoes
2 ears of corn, fresh or frozen, husked and cut into 12 rounds about ¾ inch thick
½ medium mild fresh green chili, cut into small pieces
1 tablespoon oil

1. Combine the paprika, chili powder, diced red chilis, fennel, mustard, garlic, salt, and sugar in a small bowl. Toss the pork with the coating and let sit covered at room temperature for about 1 hour.

2. Prepare a grill or preferably a hardwood fire.

3. Divide the pork cubes, onion, zucchini, bell pepper, tomatoes, corn, and green chili chunks in 6 portions and thread them on the skewers. Arrange several pepper and chili pieces together on the skewers, preferably at the ends of the skewers so that they don't dry out before the other ingredients are cooked. Brush the kebobs with the oil.

4. Grill the kebobs for about 15 minutes or until the meat is lightly browned. Serve the kebobs immediately.

MAKES 8 SERVINGS.
exorphins, nucleotides, glutamine, arginine, taurine, CLA, phytates

91 · Green Rice

2¼ cups water
1 cup fresh parsley, chopped
½ teaspoon ground cumin
½ cup fresh cilantro leaves
1 tablespoon vegetable oil
½ medium onion, chopped
1 large garlic clove, minced
1 poblano chili, finely chopped, optional
1 cup long-grain rice
½ teaspoon salt

1. Combine half the water with the parsley, cumin, and cilantro in a blender and blend at high speed until smooth. Reserve ½ and place in a saucepan to simmer at low heat.

2. Heat the oil in a nonstick saucepan over medium heat and add the onion. Stir and cook until just tender, about 3 minutes. Add the garlic, poblano, and rice. Cook, stirring, for 3 to 5 minutes, until the rice is well coated and slightly browned. Pour in the simmering stock and bring to a boil. Cover, reduce the heat, and simmer for 5 minutes until the liquid is absorbed.

3. Add the remaining stock with the blended herbs to the rice, stir the mixture, and bring back to a boil. Reduce the heat again, cover, and continue to simmer until the rice is tender, about 10 minutes. Remove from the heat, cool, and salt as desired.

MAKES 4 TO 6 SERVINGS.
PQQ, glutamine, inulin and oligofructose, monoterpenes, OCs, lignans

92 · Pineapple Parfait

12 ounces pineapple, peeled, cored, cut into 1-inch pieces, and frozen
2 large egg whites

- 1 *tablespoon fresh lemon juice*
- ⅓ *cup sugar*
- 1 *teaspoon honey*
- 1 *tablespoon peach liqueur*

1. With the metal blade of the food processor, finely chop the frozen fruit, scraping down the side of the bowl and top as necessary. The fruit should have a powdery consistency.

2. Using the whisk attachment, add the remaining ingredients to the food processor. Whisk until the mixture is thick and fluffy, about 3 to 5 minutes.

3. Freeze for up to 2 hours before serving.

MAKES 6 SERVINGS.
phytates, glutamine

93 · Indonesian and Chinese Fusion Stir-Fry

- ½ *pound bean sprouts**
- 1 *pound tofu**
- ¾ *cup water*
- 1 *fresh chili pepper, or to taste*
- 2 *teaspoons shrimp paste*
- 2 *cloves garlic*
- ¼ *teaspoon radish, shredded, pickled, and salted*
- 2 *shallots*
- 3 *tablespoons oil*
- *salt*
- ⅓ *cup reduced-fat peanut butter*
- 1 *tablespoon ketchup*
- 2 *tablespoons dark soy sauce*
- 2 *teaspoons sugar*
- 1 *cup steamed rice*

1. Rinse sprouts throughly. Drain the sprouts in a colander. Place tofu in a bowl with ¾ cup water.

2. Seed and slice chili pepper into thin slices. Place pepper with shrimp paste, garlic, radish, and shallots into a food processor and blend until paste-like.

3. Heat 1 tablespoon oil in a wok over high heat. When oil is hot, add sprouts, and stir steadily for 5 minutes. Scoop out and wipe wok.

4. Heat 1 tablespoon oil in wok over high heat and place block of tofu in the wok. Use the tip of a spatula and cut the block into 4 slices. Spread slices out carefully and fry on both sides. Be careful not to disrupt the tofu. Stir-fry for 3 minutes, then remove.

5. Heat 1 tablespoon oil in wok over high heat. When the oil is hot, pour in the paste and turn until the aroma wafts up to your nose. Add peanut butter, ketchup, soy sauce, and sugar. When sauce begins to simmer, pour in the tofu and water. Turn mixture gently, cover, and let sauce simmer for several minutes to allow flavors to penetrate tofu. Add the bean sprouts while carefully turning the tofu. Place a portion of tofu in a dish, top with sprouts and cooking liquid. Serve with steamed rice.

MAKES 4 SERVINGS.
PQQ, glutamine, inulin and oligofructose, monoterpenes, OCs, lignans, saponins, phytates, arginine

94 · Wilted Spinach Salad

2 pounds fresh spinach with stems*
6 cups of water
2 teaspoons olive oil
1 tablespoon minced garlic
10 Kalamata olives, pitted and diced
salt and pepper

1. Remove the stems from the spinach. Wash leaves several times to remove sand. Remove the spinach from final rinse water and place in a colander.

2. Bring the 6 cups of water to a boil. Pour the boiling water over the spinach in the colander, carefully turning the spinach with a set of metal tongs so the water contacts as many leaves as possible. Thoroughly drain by pressing spinach with a large spoon and transfer wilted spinach to a deep bowl.

3. In a large skillet, heat olive oil over medium heat. Add garlic and sauté, stirring constantly until lightly golden, about 1 minute. Stir in spinach and olives, turn heat to high and cook, stirring constantly, until heated through, about 1 minute. Remove from heat, transfer to a serving bowl, season with salt and pepper, and serve.

MAKES 6 SERVINGS.
PQQ, glutamine, inulin and oligofructose, monoterpenes, OCs, lignans

95 · Kiwi Cocktail

2 kiwis, peeled*
2–3 teaspoons lime juice (preferably fresh squeezed)
2–3 teaspoons sugar or honey
1 tablespoon raspberry syrup
½ cup crushed ice
½ cup seltzer or carbonated cold water

1. In a blender, combine the kiwifruit, 2 teaspoons of the lime juice, raspberry syrup, 2 teaspoons of the sugar or honey, ice, and seltzer. Puree until smooth.

2. Taste and add more lime juice and sugar or honey, if desired.

MAKES 1 SERVING.
PQQ

96 · Thai Chicken and Rice Noodles

*½ pound rice noodles**
2 tablespoons vegetable oil
3 cloves garlic, finely chopped
4 red chili peppers, seeded and chopped
¼ pound boneless chicken breast, sliced
1 egg, lightly beaten*
½ pound bean sprouts
1 tablespoon ketchup
1 teaspoon soy sauce
*3 tablespoons coarsely chopped peanuts**
1 teaspoon sugar
3 tablespoons oyster sauce
5 scallions, finely diced

1. Place rice noodles in warm water for 45 minutes; drain. In a wok, sauté garlic and chili peppers until the garlic is light brown. Coat chicken with egg and stir-fry for 3 to 4 minutes. Add rice noodles and half of the bean sprouts; mix well.

2. Stir in ketchup, soy sauce, 2 tablespoons peanuts, sugar, and oyster sauce. Cook for 3 minutes. Add scallions and the remaining bean sprouts; mix well. Serve hot. Sprinkle with extra chopped peanuts.

MAKES 3 TO 4 SERVINGS.
arginine, OCs, lignans, PQQ, nucleotides

97 · New England Baked Apples with Maple Glaze

¼ cup water
¼ cup packed light brown sugar
*1 tablespoon chopped walnuts**
*½ cup chopped pecans**
½ teaspoon nutmeg
½ teaspoon cinnamon
*4 large baking apples (Cortland or McIntosh)**
1 tablespoon reduced-calorie margarine
2 tablespoons maple syrup
cinnamon sticks, to garnish

1. Preheat the oven to 375°F; place ¼ cup water in an 8" square baking dish.

2. In a small bowl, mix the brown sugar, walnuts, pecans, nutmeg, and cinnamon. With an apple corer, remove the core of the apples, but do not cut all the way through the bottoms. Place the apples in the baking dish. Fill each apple with the brown-sugar mixture; dot with the margarine, then drizzle with the maple syrup. Bake, basting the apples occasionally with the pan juices, until just tender, about 40 minutes.

3. With a large spoon, transfer the apples to dessert bowls. Pour the pan juices over the apples. If you like, garnish each apple with a cinnamon stick.

MAKES 4 SERVINGS.
arginine, tannins, phytates

98 · Thai Iced Coffee

¼ cup strong French roast coffee
½ cup boiling water
2 teaspoons sweetened condensed milk
ice cubes

1. Combine coffee, boiling water, and sweetened condensed milk; stir until blended.

2. Pour into 2 tall glasses filled with ice cubes.

MAKES 2 SERVINGS.

99 · Barbecued Tuna with Marinated Arugula Salad

4 tuna steaks, about 8 ounces each
2 tablespoons olive oil, plus 1 tablespoon for grilling
*3 cloves garlic, minced**
salt and pepper to taste
4 cups arugula
1 sweet red pepper
5 ounces asparagus, blanched
4 ounces green beans, blanched
4 celery hearts, cut into 1-inch lengths
3 tablespoons red wine vinegar
2 tablespoons chopped fresh parsley
2 tablespoons chopped fresh tarragon
1 teaspoon Dijon mustard

1. Place tuna in nonstick baking pan. Mix together ¼ cup oil, 2 cloves garlic, and salt and pepper and pour over tuna. Marinate 1 hour, covered, in the refrigerator.

2. Combine arugula, red pepper, asparagus, beans, and celery in bowl. Combine ¼ cup olive oil, vinegar, 1 clove garlic, parsley, tarragon, mustard, and salt and pepper. Pour over vegetables and toss well.

3. Preheat grill, or prepare a charcoal fire; brush with oil to prevent sticking. Cook tuna 4 minutes per side or until fish flakes when tested with a fork. Brush frequently with the marinade.

4. Serve tuna on a bed of the vegetables.

MAKES 4 SERVINGS.
inulin and oligofructose, arginine, taurine, nucleotides, carnitine, PQQ, glutamine

100 · Spring Salad with Dandelion Greens

2½ *pounds dandelion greens**
1 *tablespoon olive oil*
2 *tablespoons chopped chives*
1 *tablespoon chopped parsley*
½ *teaspoon coarse salt*
1 *teaspoon crushed red pepper flakes*
1 *cup water*

1. Cut stems from the dandelion greens and discard. Wash greens thoroughly. After rinsing, place in a large saucepan filled with the water. Cover pot and bring to a boil. Cook dandelion greens until tender, about 5 minutes. Save ⅓ cup of the cooking liquid. Wrap the dandelion greens in a small towel to dry and place in a colander. Let cool. Slice greens into 1½-inch lengths.

2. In a 12-inch nonstick skillet, heat olive oil over medium heat. Remove pan from heat, add chives and parsley and sauté until lightly brown. Add greens and reserved cooking liquid to pan. Cook, covered, stirring frequently, until greens are soft, about 5 minutes. Uncover pan, turn heat to high, and cook, stirring frequently, until liquid is thoroughly absorbed. Season with salt and pepper flakes; remove from heat. Serve immediately.

MAKES 6 SERVINGS.
inulin and oligofructose, glutamine, monoterpenes, OCs, lignans

101 · Chicory with Scallion Oil

8 *cups cold water*
1½ *inch slice fresh ginger, lightly smashed*

1 fennel bulb, cut in small thin strips
1¼ teaspoons baking soda
1¼ teaspoons kosher salt, plus more to taste
2 tablespoons scallion oil (recipe follows)
*2 medium heads chicory, core and outer stalks removed, inner stalks halved crosswise**
1 clove garlic, finely minced

1. Place water, ginger, fennel bulb, baking soda, and 1 teaspoon of the salt in a large pot. Cover and bring to a boil over medium-high heat. Add chicory and blanch until bright green, about 30 seconds. Remove from heat, run cold water into the pot. Drain well and pat dry.

2. In a large, nonstick skillet over high heat, add the scallion oil and ¼ teaspoon of salt. Use a spatula to coat the pan with oil. Sauté garlic for one minute, until brown. When fragrant, add the chicory and toss it in the oil, using a fork separate the leaves if they clump together. Stir-fry for 1½ minutes. Place in a heated dish and serve immediately.

MAKES 4 TO 6 SERVINGS.
inulin and oligofructose, glutathione

SCALLION OIL

1 tablespoon peanut oil
5 scallions, cut into 3-inch pieces, white portions finely minced

1. Heat a wok or heavy skillet over medium heat. Add the oil. When it simmers, add the scallions. Cook until the scallions turn brown, about 3 minutes. Strain through a fine sieve. Pour into a small bowl and refrigerate for no more than two days.

MAKES ¾ CUP.

102 · Nutty Bananas

½ cup water
¼ cup sugar
2 tablespoons slivered almonds
2 tablespoons hazelnuts
*6 green bananas**
low-fat plain yogurt to serve

1. Place the water and sugar in a medium-sized saucepan. Cook on medium heat and stir until the sugar dissolves and becomes syrupy. Add the nuts, turn up the heat, and cook while stirring until the syrup turns to a golden brown. Immediately pour onto a cookie sheet lined with aluminum foil and let cool. When brittle, crush finely.

2. Open up the bananas by making a slit in the peel about 2 inches long. Pull back the skin and add about 1 tablespoon of the nut mixture to each banana. Wrap up tightly in aluminum foil and crimp the top. Cook directly on the grill with medium-hot coals for 8 to 10 minutes or grill in oven over medium heat for 10 to 12 minutes. Rotate bananas every 2 minutes. Serve in the skins, with yogurt.

MAKES 6 SERVINGS.
inulin and oligofructose, phytates, CLA, phytosterols, PQQ, arginine

103 · Angel Hair Pasta with Asparagus and Speck (Italian ham)

2 quarts water
1 pound asparagus, trimmed and cut on the diagonal into ⅛-inch pieces
8 ounces angel hair pasta
1 ounce Parmesan cheese, cut into 2 pieces
2 large garlic cloves, peeled
2 tablespoons fresh lemon juice
1 tablespoon oregano, dried
1 tablespoon basil, dried
½ teaspoon black pepper
salt to taste
½ stick unsalted butter
*¼ pound speck (Italian ham), cut into thin strips**

1. Bring 2 quarts water to a boil in a large saucepan. Add the asparagus and cook for 2 minutes. Drain the asparagus in a colander and set aside.

2. Cook the angel hair pasta according to the manufacturer's directions. Set aside.

3. Drop the Parmesan cheese through the feed tube of a food processor with the metal blade in place and the motor running. Process for 1 minute or until finely chopped. Set aside.

4. Repeat with the garlic, processing until finely chopped, about 10 seconds. Add the lemon juice, oregano, basil, pepper, and salt and process for 5 seconds more.

5. Melt the butter in a large skillet over medium-low heat. Add the speck and stir for 2 minutes. Add the asparagus and the garlic mixture. Add the angel hair pasta and 1 tablespoon of the reserved Parmesan cheese. Toss until well combined and just heated through.

6. Transfer the angel hair pasta to a large serving bowl. Sprinkle with the remaining Parmesan cheese.

MAKES 4 SERVINGS.
taurine, protease inhibitors, nucleotides, saponins, glutamine, inulin and oliogfructose, lignans, carnitine, phytosterols

104 · Collard Soup

2 cups low-fat chicken broth
*1 15-ounce can navy beans, rinsed and drained**
1 14½ can diced tomatoes, drained
1 carrot, peeled and chopped
1 white onion, finely chopped
2 garlic cloves, minced
1 pound collards, cleaned and chopped
*½ pound turkey smoked sausage, chopped**
freshly ground pepper, to taste
4 teaspoons grated Parmesan cheese

1. Bring the chicken broth to a boil. Add beans, tomatoes, carrots, onion, and garlic. Reduce the heat and simmer, covered, until the carrot is tender, about 15 minutes.

2. Stir in the collards and turkey smoked sausage. Cook for 15 minutes, until collards are thicker. Add the salt and pepper to taste. Garnish with cheese.

MAKES 4 SERVINGS.
taurine, saponins, phytates, arginine, CLA

105 · Scallops with Sizzling Herbs

½ cup chopped fresh basil
1 bunch parsley, minced
1 tablespoon olive oil
½ teaspoon salt
1 bunch of scallions, finely sliced
1 fresh hot red pepper, seeded and thinly sliced
1 clove garlic, minced
¼ cup dry white wine
*1 pound scallops**
dash of Tabasco sauce
juice of one lime

1. Combine the basil and parsley in a small bowl.

2. Heat oil and ½ teaspoon salt in a saucepan until it simmers. Add scallions, red pepper, garlic, and wine. Sauté until fragrant. Add scallops and stir-fry quickly until lightly browned. Remove to a serving dish. Reserve liquid in saucepan.

4. In the same saucepan, add the Tabasco, basil, parsley, and lime juice. Cook for 1 minute. Pour over scallops and serve.

MAKES 4 SERVINGS.
taurine, inulin and oligofructose, glutamine, monoterpenes, OCs, lignans

106 · Honeydew Sherbet

3 cups ripe honeydew melon, chopped into cubes
½ cup chopped dates
¼ cup shredded coconut
1 cup unsweetened pineapple juice
1 teaspoon vanilla extract

1. In food processor, combine honeydew melon, dates, and coconut until well combined.

2. Add pineapple juice and vanilla extract. Mix for 10 seconds.

3. Freeze mixture in ice cream maker according to manufacturer's directions.

MAKES 4 SERVINGS.
glutathione

107 · Salmon with Wilted Arugula

⅓ cup olive oil, plus 1 tablespoon for frying
4 8-ounce salmon steaks
salt and freshly ground pepper to taste
*7 ounces arugula (rocket) stems, trimmed, leaves cut in half**
2 cloves garlic, chopped
2 tablespoons fresh parsley, chopped
1 teaspoon tarragon
2 tablespoons lemon juice

1. In a nonstick skillet over medium heat, heat 1 tablespoon oil. Add salmon and cook 3 to 4 minutes per side or until fish begins to flake when tested. Season with salt and pepper. Remove and keep warm.

2. To the same skillet, add ⅓ cup oil, arugula, garlic, parsley, tarragon, and lemon juice. Cook over medium heat until arugula wilts.

3. To serve, place fish on plates and arrange arugula and juices over fish.

MAKES 4 SERVINGS.
arginine, PQQ, quercetin

108 · Baked Endives with Apples and Cloves

4 large Belgian endives, trimmed*
1 tablespoon lemon juice
8 cloves
4 tablespoons unsalted butter
*2 apples, peeled, halved, and thinly sliced**
salt and pepper to taste
½ cup dry white wine
½ cup water

1. Heat the oven to 350°F.

2. Cut each endive in half lengthwise. Stud the core of each half with a clove.

3. Using 1 tablespoon of the butter, generously butter a shallow-lidded casserole dish just the size to hold the endives in a single snug layer. Arrange half the apples in the bottom of the casserole. Fit the endives on top. Push the remaining apple slices into the spaces between the endives. Sprinkle with salt. Pour in the wine, lemon juice, and water. Dot with the remaining 3 tablespoons of butter.

4. Cover with the lid and bake in the preheated oven for 1 hour. Remove the lid and raise the oven temperature to 400°F. Continue baking, uncovered, until the endives are very tender and the juices have reduced, 20 to 30 minutes. Season the endives with pepper. Serve hot.

MAKES 4 SERVINGS.
PQQ, quercetin, phytates, tannins, phytoestrogens, phytosterols

109 · Spinach, Apple, and Potato Salad

1 pound spinach, washed
½ pound potatoes
½ pound crisp eating apples, diced*
2 ounces blue cheese
⅔ cup plain low-fat yogurt
salt and pepper to taste

1. Cook the spinach in a covered pan without adding any extra water for about 6 minutes, until just tender. Chop coarsely.

2. Boil the potatoes until just tender. Drain, peel, and cut into cubes. Leave to cool and mix with the spinach and apple.

3. Mash or blend the blue cheese into the yogurt. Gently mix this dressing into the salad and season to taste.

MAKES 4 SERVINGS.
quercetin, nucleotides, saponins, protease inhibitors, glutamine, PQQ, glutathione, phytates, tannins, phytoestrogens, phytosterols, arginine, monoterpenes, CLA

110 · Apple Harvest Pudding

⅔ cup sugar
1 egg
3 tablespoons margarine
⅓ cup low-fat or skim milk
¾ cup all-purpose flour

1½ teaspoons baking powder
¾ teaspoon cinnamon
*¾ pound Granny Smith apples**
fresh squeezed lemon juice
½ cup red currant jelly

1. Preheat oven to 400°F.

2. Put aside 1½ tablespoons of the sugar. Put the rest of the sugar in a bowl with the egg and beat until thick. Heat the margarine and milk in a saucepan, stirring constantly, and bring to a boil. Pour into the egg and sugar mixture, whisking. Sift together the flour, baking powder, and cinnamon, and fold into the egg mixture. Pour the batter into a greased and lightly floured 8-by-8-inch baking pan.

3. Peel and core the apples and cut into slices. Arrange on top of the batter, covering it thoroughly. Sprinkle with lemon juice and then with the reserved sugar. Brush lightly with the jelly. Bake about 40 minutes or until lightly browned. Refrigerate before serving.

MAKES 4–6 SERVINGS.
quercetin, nucleotides, arginine, CLA, lignans

111 · Spaghetti with Tempeh Tomato Sauce

*1 10-ounce cake tempeh**
2 tablespoons olive oil
1 medium onion, finely chopped
2 garlic cloves, minced
1 cup water
1 tablespoon tamari or soy sauce
1 28-ounce can diced, peeled tomatoes
½ cup sun-dried tomatoes
1 ounce dried porcini mushrooms
1 bell pepper, quartered and thinly sliced
2 tablespoons chopped fresh basil or 2 teaspoons dried
3 tablespoons chopped fresh parsley
2 teaspoons dried oregano
salt and pepper to taste
*1 pound dried whole wheat spaghetti**

1. Break up the tempeh into small pieces and place in a bowl. Set aside. Heat the oil in a large nonstick saucepan or skillet. Stir in the onion and sauté over medium-high heat for 7 minutes, stirring often. Stir in the garlic, sauté 15 more seconds, then stir in the tempeh, water, and tamari.

2. Bring the water to a boil, cover, and reduce the heat slightly. Simmer the tempeh for 8 minutes. Then remove the cover and continue to cook until the water is absorbed.

3. Stir the tomatoes, mushrooms, bell pepper, basil, parsley, and oregano into the tempeh. Cover and simmer for 10 minutes, correcting the seasoning as it simmers. Meanwhile, bring a large pot of salted water to a boil. Cook the spaghetti al dente, then drain and serve with the hot sauce.

MAKES 4–5 SERVINGS.
phytoestrogens, glutamine, inulin and oligofructose, OCs, lignans, monoterpenes, PQQ

112 · The Very-Berry Tofu Smoothie

4 cups fresh or frozen blueberries or blackberries (boysenberries), thawed
*¼ cup lite soy milk**
½ cup unsweetened apple juice
1 teaspoon maple syrup
½ teaspoon ground cinammon
*½ pound soft tofu**

1. Puree all ingredients in a food processor or blender until smooth.

2. Freeze in ice cream maker according to manufacturer's instructions.

MAKES 4 SERVINGS.
phytoestrogens, taurine, tannins, phytosterols

113 · Barbecued Halibut with Bean Salad

*½ cup aduki or pinto beans**
4 cups of water, plus 1 tablespoon water for salad
*1 onion, thinly sliced**
1 tablespoon chopped capers

1 teaspoon chopped fresh oregano or ½ teaspoon dried
1 teaspoon chopped fresh chives or ½ teaspoon dried
⅓ cup olive oil, plus 1 tablespoon for fish
1 tablespoon water
salt and pepper to taste
1 pound halibut or other white-fleshed fish fillets, skinned
fresh green leaf lettuce

1. Soak beans in 4 cups water overnight. Drain. Place in large saucepan with the water and bring to a boil. Simmer until beans are tender, 1 to 1½ hours. Drain and cool.

2. Combine cooked beans with onion, capers, oregano, chives, ⅓ cup oil, and 1 tablespoon water. Season with salt and pepper. Mix well.

3. Preheat grill or broiler or prepare a charcoal fire. Brush fillets with 1 tablespoon oil and season with salt and pepper. Cook 2 to 3 minutes per side or until fish flakes when tested with a fork.

4. Place beans on lettuce and serve with fish.

MAKES 4 SERVINGS.
lignans, phytates, glutamine, phytoestrogens, nucleotides

114 · Stuffed Summer Squash

4 large yellow summer squash (about 3 pounds), scrubbed*
4 quarts water, plus 2 cups
*1 cup peeled minced carrots**
½ cup quick-cooking couscous
⅓ cup thinly sliced scallions
2 celery stalks, chopped
1 teaspoon miso
½ teaspoon ground cinnamon
1 tablespoon finely grated lemon zest
½ teaspoon coarse salt
½ teaspoon white pepper
¼ cup minced fresh parsley
1 egg, lightly beaten
nonstick cooking spray
¼ cup strained fresh lemon juice

1. Adjust oven rack to upper third of oven and preheat to 375°F.

2. Cook squash for about 5 minutes in 4 quarts boiling water or until barely tender. Place in a colander and drain thoroughly. Let squash cool, trim an inch from each end and slice each squash in half lengthwise. Scoop out and discard seeds, leaving flesh intact.

3. In a large saucepan, bring 2 cups water to a boil over moderate high heat. Add carrots and cook until barely tender, about 5 minutes. Add couscous and stir vigorously until almost all the water is absorbed, about 1 minute. Stir in scallions and celery. Remove pan from heat and let couscous mixture stand, covered, for about 10 minutes. Transfer to a bowl and add miso, cinnamon, lemon zest, salt, pepper, and parsley. Let stand and cool to room temperature. Stir in egg and mix well to combine.

4. Lightly spray a large baking pan with cooking spray. Spoon equal amounts of filling into squash halves. Place squash in pan and drizzle ½ tablespoon lemon juice over each stuffed squash half.

5. Bake in preheated oven until squash are tender and the tops are lightly browned, about 25 minutes. Remove from oven and let stand on cooling rack for 15 minutes. Transfer to platter and serve warm.

MAKES 4 SERVINGS.
lignans, protease inhibitors, PQQ, glutathione, OCs, monoterpenes

115 · Pear Delight

6 *medium firm Bartlett pears,* peeled and cored with stems left intact*
1 *cup dry red wine*
½ *cup sugar*
1 *tablespoon honey*
¼ *cup crème de cassis*
2 *tablespoons fresh lemon juice*
6 *strips orange rind, removed with a vegetable peeler*
½ *teaspoon pure vanilla extract*
½ *teaspoon ground cloves*

1. Place the pears in a pan large enough to hold all of them on their sides. Add all of the remaining ingredients and stir over moderate heat until the sugar has dissolved. Lay the pears in the wine mixture, turning frequently to coat them. Bring just to a boil, cover, reduce the

heat, and simmer gently for 30 minutes, turning the pears after 15 minutes.

2. Remove the pan from the heat. With a slotted spoon, lift the pears from the pan and stand them in a shallow serving dish. Pour the wine mixture over them. Set aside to cool completely, basting often with the liquid.

3. Cover and refrigerate them overnight. Baste again with the liquid just before serving.

MAKES 6 SERVINGS.
lignans, tannins, glutathione

116 · Herbed Lamb Chops

2 tablespoons dried marjoram
2 tablespoons dried cumin
1 tablespoon dried savory
2 teaspoons dried rosemary
1 teaspoon dried tarragon
1 teaspoon dried lavender
1 teaspoon dried fennel
¼ cup extra virgin olive oil
4 New Zealand lamb chops (about 1 ¼ to 1 ½ inches thick), trimmed*

1. Place the marjoram, cumin, savory, rosemary, tarragon, lavender, and fennel in a small bowl and mix until combined.

2. Prepare a charcoal grill. On a cutting board, brush olive oil on both sides of chops. Sprinkle 2 tablespoons herbs and rub seasonings into both sides of chops.

3. Grill over medium heat, 3 minutes per side, until well done and the surfaces are seared. Transfer to a platter and sprinkle immediately with remaining herbs.

MAKES 4 SERVINGS.
CLA, arginine, phytosterols

117 · Baked Cheese Polenta with Escarole

1 tablespoon olive oil
6 garlic cloves, minced

8–10 cups escarole, washed and chopped
3½ cups water, plus 3 tablespoons for escarole
½ teaspoon salt
1 cup cornmeal
*3 tablespoons grated Parmesan cheese**
1 tablespoon butter
*¾ cup grated part-skim mozzarella cheese**
*⅓ cup low-fat sour cream**

1. Heat the oil in a large skillet over medium heat. Add the garlic and cook 30 seconds, then stir in the escarole. Pour in a few tablespoons of water and cover the pan. Cook the escarole for 3 minutes. Cover the pan and cook until the leaves wilt, about 3 minutes. Toss occasionally. Remove the pan from the heat and let cool, uncovered.
2. To make the polenta, preheat the oven to 375°F.
3. Combine the 3½ cups water and salt in a medium-sized nonstick saucepan. Bring to a boil. Reduce the heat to medium and add the cornmeal by the handful in a constant stream. Stir constantly to prevent lumps from forming. Continue to simmer and whisk for about 5 minutes until the mixture is consistent and pulls away effortlessly from the side of the pot. Whisk in 2 tablespoons of the Parmesan cheese, the butter, and the mozzarella cheese.
4. Spread half of the polenta in a 9-by-13-inch baking dish. Layer with the escarole, followed by the sour cream, and topped evenly by the remaining polenta. Sprinkle with the remaining tablespoon Parmesan cheese.
5. Bake for 20 to 25 minutes until golden brown. Do not overcook.

MAKES 8 SERVINGS.
CLA, inulin and oligofructose, glutamine, monoterpenes, OCs, lignans, arginine, protease inhibitors

118 · Flounder with Lemon Champagne Beurre Blanc

salt and pepper to taste
1½ pounds flounder
2 tablespoons butter, melted

1½ cups dry champagne
1 tablespoon lemon juice
*2 teaspoons Dijon mustard**
¼ teaspoon dill
1 tablespoon fresh chives, chopped
1 tablespoon fresh thyme, chopped
4 tablespoons unsalted cold butter

1. Preheat oven to 375°F.

2. Salt and pepper the fish. Then brush fish with melted butter, and bake in preheated oven for 15 to 20 minutes.

3. In a nonstick saucepan over high heat, mix champagne and lemon juice, simmer, and reduce to about ¾ cup. Add mustard, dill, chives, and thyme. Reduce heat. Over very low heat, whisk in 1 tablespoon cold butter until melted. Repeat with each tablespoon of butter. Continue cooking until sauce thickens and becomes creamy.

4. Pour sauce over fish and serve.

MAKES 4 SERVINGS.
isothiocyanates, glutamine, arginine, taurine

119 · Broccoli with Squash and Corn

2 tablespoons olive oil
2 medium onions, chopped
2 garlic cloves, minced
⅛ teaspoon cayenne
6 ounces mushrooms
2 cups water
1 teaspoon dried oregano
½ teaspoon salt, plus salt to taste
*1 to 1½ pounds broccoli florets**
1 medium butternut squash, peeled and cut into bite-size chunks
1½ cups fresh corn off the cob or frozen corn
½ cup coarsely chopped fresh or canned tomatoes
black pepper to taste

1. Heat the oil in a large nonstick soup pot. Stir in the onions and sauté over medium heat, stirring often, for 8 to 9 minutes or until browned. Stir in the garlic and cayenne and sauté another minute.

2. Add the mushrooms, water, oregano, and salt. Bring to a boil, cover and simmer 10 minutes. Stir in the broccoli, squash, and corn. Cover and simmer 10 minutes more, until the squash begins to lose its firmness. Stir in the chopped tomatoes and simmer 5 minutes more. Salt and pepper to taste.

MAKES 6 SERVINGS.
isothiocyanates, glutamine, inulin and oligofructose, OCs, lignans, monoterpenes, nucleotides

120 · Baked Red Cabbage

1 small head red cabbage, cored and cut to fit the feed tube of a food processor*
½ stick low-fat margarine, cut into 4 pieces
1 cup water
4 small garlic cloves, minced
1 teaspoon dried sage
¼ teaspoon cayenne pepper
½ teaspoon salt

1. Preheat the oven to 350°F.

2. Shred the cabbage with the slicing disc of a food processor. Put the sliced cabbage in a baking dish with a cover. Bake in the center of the preheated oven until the cabbage is just wilted, about 20 to 25 minutes.

3. In a saucepan, melt the margarine in the water. Stir in the chopped garlic, sage, cayenne pepper, and salt. Boil the liquid, then pour it over the cabbage. Toss and serve.

MAKES 8 SERVINGS.
isothiocyanates, PQQ, lignans, glutamine, inulin, monoterpenes, OCs, lignans

121 · Honeydew Granite

¼ cup sugar
¼ cup water
½ medium, ripe honeydew melon, peeled, seeded, and cut into ½-inch cubes (about 4 cups)

3 tablespoons fresh lemon juice
2 tablespoons sparkling wine
¼ teaspoon freshly ground pepper

1. In a saucepan over medium high heat, combine sugar and water. Bring to a boil, reduce heat and simmer for 5 minutes. Set aside until cool.

2. Process the melon, sugar syrup, and lemon juice in a blender until smooth. Add the sparkling wine and pepper, then blend until well mixed.

3. Pour the mixture into a large, nonreactive pie plate and place in the freezer. Stir every 30 minutes until frozen. Scrape up the granite, divide among 4 dishes, and serve.

MAKES 4 SERVINGS.
glutathione

122 · Herbed Chicken with Wine

2 whole chicken breasts (4 halves), skinned and boned*
1 tablespoon olive oil
½ cup dry white wine
2 tablespoons water
2 teaspoons fresh tarragon or ½ teaspoon dried
1 bunch of fresh chervil, finely chopped
4 fresh sprigs of marjoram, finely chopped
2 peeled shallots, diced
4 white peppercorns, crushed
juice of one lemon
¼ teaspoon salt

1. Pound chicken to ¼-inch thick.

2. Put the olive oil, white wine, water, tarragon, chervil, marjoram, shallots, peppercorns, lemon juice, and salt into a large, nonstick skillet. Heat to simmer while stirring. Put in chicken and cover; simmer over medium-low heat for 8 to10 minutes. Remove chicken to a serving dish. Continue to simmer juices for another minute and pour over chicken.

MAKES 4 SERVINGS.
carnitine, nucleotides, arginine, glutamine, exorphins, taurine

123 · Tennessee Banana Pudding

nonstick cooking spray
1 *box vanilla wafers*
1 *envelope (4 ½-cup servings) reduced-calorie vanilla pudding mix*
2 *cups low-fat (1%) milk*
½ *teaspoon vanilla extract*
1 *medium banana, sliced*
2 *large egg whites*
2 *tablespoons granulated sugar*

1. Preheat oven to 350°F. Spray a 1½-quart casserole with nonstick cooking spray; set aside.
2. Cover bottom of casserole dish with 1 layer of vanilla wafers.
3. Prepare vanilla pudding with low-fat milk according to package directions. Stir in vanilla.
4. Layer half the banana slices over wafers. Cover with pudding mixture. Repeat layering with remaining wafers, banana, and pudding.
5. In medium bowl, with electric mixer on high speed, beat egg whites 1 minute, until foamy. Gradually add sugar; continue beating on high speed until egg whites are stiff but not dry. Using a rubber spatula, spoon meringue over ingredients in casserole dish. Bake until golden brown, about 5 minutes.

MAKES 4 SERVINGS.

124 · Beef and Basil

2 *hot red peppers,* or to taste*
4 *shallots*
4 *cloves garlic*
1 *tablespoon shrimp paste*
2 *cups packed fresh basil**
8 *ounces flank steak*
2 *teaspoons fish sauce*
2 *teaspoons sherry*
1 *tablespoon olive oil*

1. Seed the peppers, and slice them and the shallots. Place peppers and shallots in a blender or food processor along with the garlic and shrimp paste. Puree until you have a paste.

2. Wash the basil and pinch off individual leaves and leaf clusters, removing them from the central stalk. Discard the stalks. Cut steak across the grain into thin slices, about 1⁄16 inch thick and to the scale of the basil leaves.

3. Pour the fish sauce and sherry over the beef slices. Mix thoroughly.

4. Heat oil in wok over high heat. Stir-fry the paste first. When heated and the aroma fills the air, add the beef. Toss and stir vigorously. When the meat has lost almost all its redness, add the basil leaves. Toss moderately and then serve immediately, with a great deal of plain rice.

MAKES 2 SERVINGS.
phytosterols, glutamine, OCs, inulin and oligofructose, glutamine, monoterpenes, lignans, nucleotides, exorphins, arginine, carnitine

125 · Sweet Glazed Carrots with Sesame Seeds

1 pound carrots, scraped and peeled*
1 1⁄4 cups water
2 tablespoons butter or margarine
2 tablespoons honey
pinch of salt
2 tablespoons sesame seeds, toasted*

1. Cut the carrots into sticks and put them in a medium pan with the water. Boil uncovered until tender, about 7 minutes.

2. In a nonstick skillet, add the carrots, butter, honey, and salt. Cook over low heat while turning carrots over until they are lightly browned and glazed. Remove from heat and top with sesame seeds.

MAKES 4 SERVINGS.
phytosterols, protease inhibitors, PQQ, glutathione, phytates

126 · Asparagus with Lemon and Sage

*2½ pounds medium-size asparagus**
½ teaspoon salt
½ teaspoon black pepper
2 tablespoons strained fresh lemon juice
1½ tablespoons extra virgin olive oil
*1 tablespoon minced fresh sage or 1 teaspoon dried sage**
1 tablespoon finely grated lemon zest, for garnish

1. Rinse asparagus to remove soil and cut stalks on the bias. Peel the stalks about 2 inches up from the ends. Stalks should be all the same length.

2. In a steamer set over a large saucepan, steam the asparagus until tender, about 6 minutes. Remove from steamer, reserve liquid, and with a pair of tongs align asparagus in a 2-inch-deep serving dish. Spoon out 3 tablespoons of liquid from bottom of saucepan for the dressing.

3. In a small bowl, whisk the cooking liquid, salt, pepper, lemon juice, olive oil, and sage. Drizzle dressing over asparagus, garnish with grated lemon zest, and serve warm.

MAKES 6 SERVINGS.
phytosterols, nucleotides, saponins, protease inhibitors, glutamine, monoterpenes

127 · Honeyed Figs

3 cups water
¾ cup honey
¾ cup sugar
½ teaspoon cinnamon
*1 pound dried figs, stemmed**

1. In a large saucepan, add water, honey, sugar, and cinnamon. Bring to a boil.

2. Add figs and cook until softened, about 10 minutes.

3. Remove figs, set aside.

4. Continue to boil mixture until liquid is reduced to 1 cup.

5. Let liquid cool to room temperature
6. Serve over figs.

MAKES 4 SERVINGS.
phytosterols

128 · Scallops with Limes

2 tablespoons reduced-fat margarine
2 tablespoons olive oil
1 green pepper, cored, seeded, and cut into julienne strips
2 tablespoons drained capers
6 scallions, trimmed and cut into 1-inch-long pieces
1 tablespoon dry white wine
1 pound bay scallops
2 tablespoons Pernod
2 tablespoons fresh lime juice
1 tablespoon lime zest
salt and pepper to taste

1. Over medium heat in a nonstick frying pan, combine 1 tablespoon of the butter and 1 tablespoon of the olive oil. Saute for 10 minutes while adding the peppers, capers, and the scallions. After 5 minutes, add the wine, stirring.

2. In a separate pan, heat the remaining 1 tablespoon of butter and 2 tablespoons of the olive oil. Add the scallops, Pernod, lime juice, and lime zest. Cook for about 1 minute, shaking the pan. Add the contents of this pan to the other pan and cook for 2 minutes over medium heat. Serve immediately.

MAKES 3 SERVINGS.
nucleotides, taurine

129 · Cranberries and Rice

3 cups water
1½ cups long-grain rice
*¼ cup red wine**
*½ cup dried cranberries**
⅓ cup olive oil
2 tablespoons balsamic vinegar

1 tablespoon rosemary, chopped
¼ teaspoon salt
6 scallions, white and light green parts coarsely chopped
2 large ripe pears, such as Bartlett, cored, peeled, and diced*
⅓ cup coarsely chopped almonds

1. In a saucepan, cook the rice with 3 cups boiling water for 25 to 30 minutes or until the rice becomes tender but is firm. Drain the rice well of any excess water.

2. Combine the wine and the cranberries and marinate until the cranberries enlarge.

3. For the dressing, combine the oil, vinegar, rosemary, and salt together in a small bowl.

4. Place the cooked rice in a large bowl and mix in the scallions, dressing, pears, and cranberries along with their soaking wine. The salad can be prepared a day ahead. Sprinkle the almonds on top before serving.

MAKES 4 SERVINGS.
tannins, glutathione, lignans, OCs

130 · Green Tea Ice Cream

2 cups whipping cream
1 cup milk
1 cup raw sugar
½ teaspoon ground ginger
1 teaspoon vanilla
*1 heaping teaspoon green tea, ground to powder**
water for tea

1. Combine cream, milk, sugar, ginger and vanilla in large bowl. Mix until sugar dissolves.

2. Place ground green tea in measuring cup and add enough lukewarm water to measure ¾ cup. Mix tea and water, then combine with cream mixture.

3. Pour into ice cream maker and follow manufacturer's directions.

4. Serve in bowls.

MAKES 6 SERVINGS.
tannins, CLA

131 · Orange Grilled Chicken with Spicy Salsa

4 boneless, skinless chicken breast halves
salt and pepper to taste
*½ cup orange juice**
*2 tablespoons lime juice**
*2 tablespoons zest from one orange**
2 garlic cloves, minced
4 fat-free flour tortillas (8-inch diameter)
4 sprigs fresh cilantro
Roasted Corn and Pepper Salsa (recipe follows)

1. Arrange chicken breasts in a standard-sized glass baking dish and season with salt and pepper.

2. In a small bowl, mix the orange juice, lime juice, orange zest, and garlic. Pour ingredients over the chicken. Cover, let stand at room temperature for 10 minutes, and marinate in the refrigerator for 1 hour.

3. Just before serving, preheat the grill or make a charcoal fire. Grill the chicken or broil 4 inches from the heat for 2 minutes per side, or until no longer pink in the center. Warm the tortillas on the grill or under the broiler for 10 to 20 seconds per side.

4. Spoon one-quarter of the salsa on each of 4 plates. Place a grilled chicken breast in the center of each and garnish with a cilantro sprig. Serve with the tortillas.

MAKES 4 SERVINGS.
monoterpenes, taurine, nucleotides, glutamine, exorphins, arginine, glutathione, inulin and oligofructose, OCs, lignans, PQQ

ROASTED CORN AND PEPPER SALSA

1 canned chipotle chili pepper, seeded and minced
1 ear fresh corn, blanched, roasted and kernels removed
1 red bell pepper, roasted, peeled, seeded, and cut into ½-inch dice
1 yellow bell pepper, roasted, peeled, seeded, and cut into ½-inch dice
1 green bell pepper, roasted, peeled, seeded, and cut into ½-inch dice
½ tablespoon chopped fresh oregano leaves
1 tomato, seeded and cut into ½-inch dice
¾ teaspoon sugar

¼ cup olive oil
1½ tablespoons cider vinegar
salt and pepper to taste

1. Combine all of the ingredients in a mixing bowl.
2. Refrigerate for up to 2 days.

MAKES 2 CUPS.

132 · Corn with Chipotle Lime Vinaigrette

3½ quarts salted water, plus ¼ cup water
fresh corn kernels cut from 7 large ears of corn (about 6½ cups)
1 small zucchini, diced
3 large ripe tomatoes, diced
4 scallions, white part and 4 inches of green, cut into ⅛-inch slices
3 tablespoons olive oil
1 chipotle pepper (smoked jalapeño; available in most supermatkets)
*juice of 2 limes**
*zest of one lime**
3 tablespoons minced dried cumin
salt and pepper to taste

1. In a large saucepan, boil 3½ quarts of salted water. Add the corn kernels, cover, and cook for 2 minutes until the corn is tender. Add the zucchini and cook for 1 minute. Drain. Place in a bowl, then add the tomatoes and the scallions. Combine using two large forks.

2. Heat the olive oil in a medium pot over medium-high heat. Add the chipotle pepper. Cook the pepper for 3 minutes, turning frequently with tongs, to coat with the oil. Add the ¼ cup of water and raise the heat to high.

3. When the water comes to a boil, stir once, then remove from the heat. Let the mixture cool for about 5 minutes, or until the pepper is cool enough to handle. Remove the stem from the pepper and discard. Chop the pepper finely. Return the chopped pepper and its juices to the pot. Stir in the lime juice, lime zest, and cumin. Pour the dress-

ing over the corn salad and toss thoroughly, using two spoons. Salt and pepper to taste. Serve at room temperature or chilled.

MAKES 8 SERVINGS.
monoterpenes, phytates, glutamine, lignans, phytosterols

133 · Tangerine Ice

- ¼ *cup water*
- 1¼ *cups sugar*
- *zest of 5 medium lemons**
- 1½ *cups fresh tangerine juice,* strained*
- 1 *cup ice water*
- 2 *tablespoons fresh lemon juice**
- *zest of three medium tangerines**
- *mint leaves,* for garnish*

1. Boil the water, and add the sugar and lemon zest. Boil for 2 minutes over moderate heat. Reduce the heat and simmer, uncovered, stirring frequently.
2. Refrigerate the syrup for at least 3 hours.
3. Strain the syrup into a large bowl and discard the lemon zest. Stir in the tangerine juice, ice water, lemon juice, and grated tangerine zest.
4. Use an ice cream maker, following the manufacturer's directions, to make the ice.
5. Garnish each scoop with mint leaves.

MAKES 4–6 SERVINGS.
monoterpenes, tannins

134 · Savory Shrimp Stir-Fry

- 2 *tablespoons oil*
- 5 *scallions,* chopped*
- 3 *cloves garlic,* minced*
- 1 *tablespoon minced gingerroot*
- 1 *pound shrimp, deveined and shelled*
- 1 *cup straw mushrooms*
- 3 *tablespoons dark soy sauce*

3 teaspoons light soy sauce
1 tablespoon sherry
1 teaspoon cider vinegar
1 teaspoon sugar
⅓ cup water

1. Heat oil in wok. When oil is hot, add scallions, garlic, and ginger. When the scallions are softened, add the shrimp and mushrooms. Stir-fry about 2 minutes until the shrimp change color. Do not overcook.

2. Add the soy sauces, sherry, vinegar, sugar, and water. Cover and let mixture come to a boil, then reduce heat to simmer for about 3 minutes. Uncover, stir mixture, and bring back to a rapid boil. Let liquid simmer and stir until liquid reduces and concentrates in color, about 2 minutes.

3. Serve over steamed rice.

MAKES 2–4 SERVINGS.
OCs, taurine, inulin and oligofructose, glutamine, monoterpenes, lignans

135 · Snow Peas

1 tablespoon vegetable oil
4 cloves garlic, chopped finely*
4 hot chili peppers
¼ cup oyster sauce
½ pound snow peas, trimmed
¼ cups fresh peanuts

1. To a wok, add the oil and garlic and stir-fry for 1 minute over medium heat.

2. Add snow peas, peanuts, chili peppers, and oyster sauce, and stir-fry for 3 to 4 minutes until the snow peas turn bright green.

MAKES 2–4 SERVINGS.
OCs, inulin and oligofructose, monoterpenes, lignans, tannins, phytates, CLA

136 · Marinated London Broil

1 cup soy sauce
8 cloves garlic, minced
¼ cup olive oil
1 cup red wine
*½ teaspoon dried basil**
*½ teaspoon dried thyme**
½ teaspoon coriander seeds, crushed finely
8 black peppercorns, crushed
zest of one orange
1 well-trimmed 2- to 3-pound 1½-inch-thick London broil or sirloin steak

1. To prepare the marinade, combine the soy sauce, garlic, olive oil, wine, basil, thyme, coriander, peppercorns, and orange zest in a glass cooking dish or nonstick pan. Add the London broil, cover, and refrigerate for at least 4 hours or preferably overnight. Remove from the refrigerator at least 1 hour before grilling.

2. Preheat the grill or prepare a charcoal or hardwood fire.

3. Remove the meat from the marinade. Grill over high heat for 1 to 2 minutes on each side to sear the meat. Move the meat away from the hottest part of the grill and cook on each side for 5 minutes or until cooked the way desired.

4. Place the meat on a serving platter and slice after it has stopped sizzling. Cut the London broil against the grain into ½-inch slices.

MAKES 6–8 SERVINGS.
glutathione, glutamine, monoterpenes, lignans, tannins

137 · Squash Baked with Leeks

nonstick cooking spray
2 tablespoons olive oil
1 pound acorn or butternut squash, peeled, seeded, and cubed*
1 pound leeks, white part, and 2 inches of pale green, coarsely chopped
4 cloves garlic, chopped finely
¼ teaspoon salt

¼ teaspoon pepper
1 tablespoon tarragon leaves, minced

1. Preheat oven to 425°F.

2. Spray a large deep dish skillet with nonstick cooking spray. Add the olive oil and heat over medium heat. Add the squash, leeks, and garlic, and sauté over medium heat for 5 to 6 minutes. Season to taste with salt and pepper.

3. Put the vegetables in a medium baking dish and add the tarragon. Cover with foil and bake for about 20 minutes, until the vegetables are tender.

MAKES 4 SERVINGS.
glutathione, lignans, inulin and oligofructose

138 · Seasoned Baked Potatoes

1 teaspoon parsley, minced
1 teaspoon basil, minced
1 teaspoon oregano, minced
2 baking potatoes (5 ounces each)*
2 teaspoons olive oil
2 tablespoons finely chopped red bell pepper
2 tablespoons grated Parmesan cheese

1. In a small bowl, thoroughly combine parsley, basil, and oregano.

2. Wash potatoes, and prick with a fork. In a microwave oven, cook potatoes at high speed until soft. Let cool and cut each potato lengthwise and spread open.

3. In a small nonstick skillet, heat 1 teaspoon oil; add pepper and cook over medium-high heat, stirring frequently, until tender-crisp, about 30 seconds. Remove from heat, stir in parsley, basil, and oregano and the cheese.

4. Brush each potato half with ½ teaspoon oil, and sprinkle each with ¼ teaspoon of the seasoning.

MAKES 2 SERVINGS.
glutathione, protease inhibitors, glutamine, PQQ, arginine, CLA

139 · Peach Crisp

FOR THE PEACHES

*2 pounds ripe peaches**
3 tablespoons sugar
zest of two lemons
1 tablespoon fresh lemon juice

FOR THE DOUGH

1¼ cups all-purpose flour
pinch of salt
2 tablespoons sugar
1 teaspoon baking powder
3 tablespoons margarine
1 large egg, beaten
2–4 tablespoons skim milk

1. Preheat oven to 400°F.

2. Put peaches in a large bowl and cover with boiling water for about 2 minutes. Remove and let cool. Pierce the skin with a sharp knife and lift off skin.

2. Remove pits, slice and place in the bottom of an 8-by-8-inch nonstick baking dish. Sprinkle with the sugar and lemon zest. Drizzle with the lemon juice.

4. In a food processor, with the metal blade running, combine the flour, salt, sugar, and baking powder. Add the margarine and pulse for a few seconds until it resembles fine bread crumbs. Add the egg and pour in milk; process until a dough forms in the processor. Add extra flour or milk depending on the dough's consistency. Remove the dough, and on a floured cutting board, roll it out.

5. Cover the peaches completely with the dough. Bake until the topping is golden brown, 25 to 30 minutes.

6. Serve warm.

MAKES 6 SERVINGS.
glutathione, arginine, monoterpene

140 · Spice-Rubbed Filets Mignons

FOR THE STEAKS

1 tablespoon chili powder
1 teaspoon dried marjoram
1 teaspoon freshly ground black pepper
⅛ teaspoon ground allspice
½ teaspoon sugar
1 tablespoon olive oil
1 tablespoon lemon juice
1½ teaspoons finely chopped garlic, minced into a paste
2 7-ounce filets mignons (about 2 inches thick)*

FOR THE SAUCE

1¼ cups water
1½ tablespoons Worcestershire sauce
½ teaspoon tomato paste
2 tablespoons shallots, minced
1 dried chili pepper, crushed
½ Italian pepper, minced

1. Preheat oven to 450°F.

2. In a small bowl, stir together chili powder, marjoram, black pepper, allspice, sugar, olive oil, lemon juice, and garlic. Rub spice mixture on all sides of each steak. Marinate steaks in a baking dish or nonstick pan covered and chilled at least one hour or overnight.

3. Place pan in oven and bake for 30 to 35 minutes for medium done.

4. While steaks are cooking, prepare sauce. In a saucepan set over medium heat, add water, Worcestershire sauce, tomato paste, shallots, chili pepper, Italian pepper, and garlic. Cook until shallots turn brown and liquid is reduced to about ⅓ cup, about 15 minutes.

5. Remove steak from oven and reserve juices.

6. Pour sauce into reserved juices in baking pan and deglaze pan over moderate heat, stirring and scraping up any brown bits in pan until the mixture is uniform.

7. Halve the steaks and place on separate plates. Pour some sauce onto each steak.

MAKES 4 SERVINGS.
carnitine, exorphins, nucleotides, glutamine, PQQ, lignans, glutamine, OCs

141 · French Country Potatoes

nonstick cooking spray
¼ *chopped onion**
¼ *cup sliced mushrooms**
4 *medium potatoes, peeled and thinly sliced**
⅛ *teaspoon dried thyme, crushed**
¼ *teaspoon dried nutmeg**
⅛ *teaspoon freshly ground pepper*
¼ *cup low-fat sour cream**
2 *ounces reduced-fat Cheddar cheese, shredded**
3 *tablespoons Parmesan cheese**
⅓ *cup water*

1. Preheat oven to 425°F.
2. Spray 1-quart casserole or large skillet with nonstick cooking spray.
3. In medium nonstick skillet, over medium heat, cook onions and mushrooms for about 2 minutes or until onions are translucent. Stir in potatoes, thyme, nutmeg, and pepper; transfer to casserole dish.
4. In a small bowl combine sour cream, Cheddar cheese, Parmesan cheese, and water. Pour evenly over the top of the potatoes.
5. Bake, uncovered, until cheese is a golden brown and the potatoes are tender, about 30 minutes.

MAKES 2 SERVINGS.
phytosterols, PQQ, protease inhibitors, glutamine, tannins, glutathione, quercetin

142 · Green Beans with Almonds

½ *pound green beans, trimmed**
nonstick cooking spray
1 *garlic clove, minced*
¼ *cup blanched whole almonds, finely ground**

½ *teaspoon ground ginger*
salt and pepper to taste

1. Steam beans over a large pot of water until crisp-tender.

2. Spray a nonstick skillet and set over moderate heat. Sauté garlic until golden, about 1 minute. Add almonds and ginger and cook for 2 to 3 minutes, until almonds color slightly. Add beans and cook until heated through, about 2 minutes. Season with salt and pepper.

MAKES 2 SERVINGS.
arginine, saponins

143 · Berry Yogurt Parfaits

4 *ounces whipped light cream cheese**
10 *ounces nonfat lemon yogurt**
2 *tablespoons honey*
1 *teaspoon vanilla extract**
1 ¼*-ounce envelope unflavored gelatin*
¾ *cup water, divided use*
8 *graham crackers, crumbled*
1 *cup raspberries**
4 *tablespoons raspberry jam, melted**

1. In a medium bowl, beat the cream cheese until smooth. Stir in the yogurt, honey, and vanilla.

2. Sprinkle the gelatin over ¼ cup of the water in a saucepan; let soften 1 minute.

3. Place saucepan on medium heat and stir until gelatin is dissolved. Add the remaining ½ cup water and combine with the cheese mixture. Chill until cool.

4. In tall dessert glasses, place a spoonful of graham cracker crumbs, then a portion of the filling, followed by a layer of berries. Repeat the layers and then drizzle with melted jam. Cover and refrigerate overnight.

MAKES 4 SERVINGS.
CLA, glutamine, tannins, glutathione, lignans, quercetin

144 · Salt-Crusted Breast of Chicken with Artichokes

1 *large fennel bulb*
2¾ *cups all-purpose flour*
4 *ounces kosher salt*
1 *egg*
⅔ *cup water*
1 *tablespoon olive oil*
2 *skinless chicken breasts**
8 *oz. Jerusalem artichokes, peeled**
2 *medium potatoes*
2 *cups low-fat milk*
salt and freshly ground pepper
2 *medium leeks, sliced lengthwise*
nonstick cooking spray
salt and pepper to taste

1. Preheat oven to 400°F.

2. Chop finely the stalk and stems of the fennel. Combine with the flour and salt. Add egg and water. Knead together to form a ball of dough and set aside in the refrigerator.

3. Heat the olive oil in a nonstick skillet and sear the chicken until golden brown on both sides. Set aside to cool.

4. To make the artichoke puree, roughly chop the artichokes and potatoes. (See recipe #33 for preparing artichokes). Place in a medium-size nonstick pan, add the milk, and cook for about 30 minutes, or until soft. Drain well, puree in a food processor, and return to the saucepan. Cook over low heat to thicken the puree. Keep warm.

5. Roll the dough out on a well-floured cutting board. Divide the crust in two and place one chicken breast in the center of one-half of the crust. Gently fold the crust over and around the chicken breast so it is completely wrapped. Repeat for the other breast. Place breasts on a nonstick baking sheet sprayed with cooking spray. Bake in the oven for 12 to 15 minutes. Remove the sheet from the oven and set aside for 5 minutes.

6. Place the leeks in a nonstick skillet sprayed with cooking spray. Sauté until translucent.

7. To serve, slice each chicken breast diagonally into 3 or 4 pieces.

Heat the puree and season to taste with salt and pepper. Spoon the puree onto the center of each serving plate, and place the chicken breast over each serving. Place the leeks around the perimeter of the chicken.

MAKES 2 SERVINGS.
exorphins, phytosterols, inulin and oligofructose, OCs, lignans, phytates, saponins, quercetin, nucleotides

145 · Rice Topped with Tomato Sauce

- *1 cup uncooked long-grain white rice**
- *1¾ cups water*
- *1 teaspoon salt*
- *2 cups diced ripe tomatoes*
- *1 roasted red bell pepper, chopped (see recipe #28 for roasting red peppers)*
- *1 tablespoon olive oil*
- *½ tablespoon chopped fresh oregano*
- *1 small clove garlic, crushed*
- *⅓ cup grated Monterey Jack cheese**

1. Cook the rice in a rice cooker with water and ½ teaspoon salt.
2. Combine the tomatoes, red peppers, olive oil, oregano, remaining salt, and garlic. Toss to blend and set aside.
3. Spoon the rice into serving bowl. Sprinkle with the cheese. Spoon the tomato mixture over the top, and fluff with a spoon and a fork just to blend. Serve immediately.

MAKES 6 SERVINGS.
arginine, glutamine, CLA, inulin and oligofructose, monoterpenes, OCs, lignans

146 · Lime Blackberry Pudding

- *2 pints blackberries*
- *½ cup sugar, plus 2 tablespoons*
- *1 tablespoon almond extract*
- *1 tablespoon honey*

4 eggs, separated
2 teaspoons lime zest
½ cup fresh lime juice
3 tablespoons flour
¼ teaspoon kosher salt
2 tablespoons melted reduced-fat margarine, cooled
1 cup skim milk
1 tablespoon tapioca
confectioners sugar for garnish

1. Preheat the oven to 350°F.

2. In a bowl, toss blackberries with 2 tablespoons sugar, almond extract, and honey. Let stand for 30 minutes.

3. Whisk together the egg yolks, lime zest, and lime juice in a large bowl. While whisking, add the flour, salt, and 1 cup sugar and blend until smooth. Add the butter and milk. In another bowl, beat the egg whites until stiff and peaks form, but not dry. Using a spatula, fold the whites into the batter.

4. Sprinkle the tapioca over the blackberries and toss until well coated. Place berries into a shallow baking dish and bake until the top is lightly browned, about 40 to 45 minutes. Serve warm or at room temperature, dusted with confectioners sugar.

MAKES 6 SERVINGS.
CLA, tannins, monoterpenes, arginine

147 · Orange-Flavored Poached Salmon

zests of 1 orange
2 tablespoons chopped fresh dill
½ cup fresh squeezed orange juice
1 teaspoon allspice
¼ cup honey
¼ cup dry white wine
4 salmon steaks (8 ounces each)

1. Combine zest, dill, juice, allspice, honey, and wine in a large nonstick skillet. Set over medium heat and bring to a boil, until ingredients are combined. Add the salmon and cook over low heat for 15 minutes until the fish is tender. Remove fish with slotted spoon, and place on a serving plate. Reserve liquid.

2. Simmer liquid while stirring over high heat and cook until slightly reduced and thickened. Spoon over fish and serve.

MAKES 4 SERVINGS.
arginine, glutamine, lignans, tannins, gluathione, phytosterols

148 · Country Asparagus Soup

*2 pounds trimmed fresh asparagus**
1 tablespoon olive oil
1 cup leeks, chopped
1 clove garlic, minced
½ teaspoon nutmeg
2 cups russet potatoes, peeled and diced
½ cup dried mushrooms
5 cups low-fat chicken stock
1 cup half-and-half
salt and freshly ground white pepper to taste

1. Steam asparagus until tender. Remove asparagus and plunge into cold water. Drain and cut into 1-inch pieces. Set some aside for garnish.

2. Heat the olive oil in a large nonstick saucepan. Add the leeks, garlic, and nutmeg, and cook over moderate heat until the onions begin to brown, about 6 to 7 minutes. Add the asparagus, potatoes, and mushrooms and cook until the asparagus turns bright green. Pour in the chicken stock and bring to a boil. Reduce the heat and simmer for 15 minutes, or until the mushrooms, potatoes, and asparagus are tender.

3. Using the metal blade of the food processor, process asparagus, potatoes, and mushrooms until smooth. Pour into a saucepan and simmer. Add half-and-half to the desired thickness and heat, but do not boil. Add salt and pepper to taste. Garnish with asparagus and serve.

MAKES 6 SERVINGS.
phytosterols, inulin and oligofructose, saponins, protease inhibitors, glutamine, lignans

149 · Kiwi-Mango Sherbet

- 2 *pounds kiwifruit, peeled and quartered**
- ½ *mango, peeled and sliced*
- ½ *cup sugar*
- 1 *tablespoon honey*
- 1 *teaspoon fresh squeezed lemon juice*

1. In a food processor with the metal blade running, process all ingredients until finely pureed.

2. Spread the puree in a cake pan and freeze it for 1 hour. Return to food processor and process again until fluffy.

3. Place sherbet in a plastic container and freeze for at least 2 hours, or until frozen.

MAKES 3–4 SERVINGS.
PQQ, tannins

150 · Flounder Fillets Coated with Pine Nuts

- 2 *tablespoons olive oil*
- 1 *tablespoon finely chopped garlic*
- 3 *ripe tomatoes (about 1 pound), cored, seeded, peeled, and cut into small cubes*
- 2 *tablespoons chopped fresh parsley leaves*
- ¼ *cup dry white wine*
- *salt and freshly ground black pepper to taste*
- ¼ *cup fresh squeezed lime juice*
- 4 *tablespoons pine nuts*
- 1½ *pounds skinless flounder fillets**
- 4 *lime wedges*

1. Heat 1 tablespoon of the olive oil in a nonstick saucepan. Add the garlic and cook briefly. Add the tomatoes, parsley, wine, lime juice, salt, and pepper, and sauté over high heat, stirring, for 5 minutes. Remove the sauce from the heat and keep warm.

2. In a food processor with the metal blade running, process the pine nuts into fine pieces. Season the fillets with salt and pepper. Coat the fillets with the pine nuts.

3. Heat the remaining oil in a large nonstick frying pan and cook the flounder over medium heat until the fillets are golden brown on both sides. The time will vary, depending on the thickness of the fillets.

4. Place the fish on a plate, and pour the sauce around the fish. Garnish with lime wedges.

MAKES 4 SERVINGS
arginine, glutamine, inulin and oligofructose, monoterpenes, OCs, lignans

151 · Carrot Salad with Cilantro Dressing

*1 pound carrots, peeled and cut into 2-inch pieces**
½ cup tightly packed fresh cilantro, coarsely chopped
⅓ cup light soy sauce
¼ teaspoon salt
1 tablespoon sugar
3 tablespoons clear rice vinegar
1 tablespoon rice wine, such as sake
*2 tablespoons sesame oil**

1. In a food processor, using the medium shredding disk, shred the carrots. Transfer the carrots to a large bowl and add the cilantro.

2. To make the dressing, process the remaining ingredients with the metal blade for about 20 seconds or until the sugar has dissolved. Pour over the carrots and cilantro and toss to coat. Cover and refrigerate for 1 hour. With a slotted spoon, transfer to a serving bowl.

MAKES 6 SERVINGS.
phytosterols, lignans, glutathione, PQQ, protease inhibitors

152 · Cinnamon Baked Bananas

*4 medium unpeeled bananas**
4 teaspoons honey
¼ teaspoon cinnamon
1 large lemon, quartered

1. Preheat oven to 350°F.
2. Line baking pan with foil. Place bananas in pan, spacing evenly.

Bake until skins are golden brown and soft, about 20 to 30 minutes. Let cool 10 minutes.

3. Cut bananas lengthwise through skin, opening skin slightly. Mix honey with cinnamon; drizzle 1 teaspoon of the mixture over each banana. Then squeeze one lemon wedge over each and serve.

MAKES 4 SERVINGS.
PQQ, inulin and oligofructose, tannins, phytosterols

153 · Roast Pork with Spice Crust

- 2 *tablespoons mustard seed*
- 1 *tablespoon coriander seed*
- 1 *tablespoon coarse salt*
- 1 *teaspoon ground cardamom*
- 1 *teaspoon ground ginger*
- ⅓ *teaspoon ground cloves*
- 2 *diced jalapeño chilis*
- 2 *tablespoons black pepper*
- 1 *well-trimmed, 3- to 4-pound boneless pork loin,* * *tied*
- 3 *cloves garlic, cut in slivers*
- *nonstick cooking spray*
- 1 *carrot, chopped*
- 1 *onion, chopped*
- 1 *stalk celery, chopped*
- 1½ *cups white wine*

1. Preheat the oven to 375°F.

2. To make the spice rub, toast the mustard and coriander seeds in a pan over medium-high heat, stirring frequently, until fragrant, 2 to 3 minutes. Cool the seeds. Combine them with the salt, cardamom, ginger, cloves, jalapeño chilis, and pepper. Crush to a coarse texture.

3. Make 1-inch-deep holes in the pork with a small sharp knife, and insert the slivers of garlic. Rub the pork with the spice rub, pushing some of it in with the garlic. Set aside for 45 minutes.

4. With nonstick spray, coat the bottom of a roasting pan. Place the pork in the skillet and brown over medium-high heat on top of the stove, 3 to 4 minutes each side. Add the carrot, onion, and celery, and

cook them for a few minutes. Add 1 cup of the white wine, cover, and roast in the oven for 1 hour.

5. Remove the cover and continue to roast until the pan juices run clear or until a meat thermometer reads 155°F, about 30 minutes more. Remove the meat to a serving platter and allow it to stand for 30 minutes before slicing.

6. Pour off the excess fat from the roasting pan. Heat the roasting pan on top of the stove over high heat and deglaze it with the remaining ½ cup of wine, scraping up any bits of meat that are stuck to the bottom of the pan. Pour the pan juices through a strainer into a saucepan and discard the vegetables. Bring the juices to a boil and cook until reduced by half, about 5 minutes. Drizzle the roast with the sauce.

MAKES 10 SERVINGS.
carnitine, nucleotides, glutamine, exorphins, arginine, taurine, CLA

154 · Rice with Lemon and Cilantro

2 teaspoons unsalted margarine
¼ cup green onion, chopped fine
*¾ cup basmati rice**
1 ¼ cups low-sodium chicken broth
1 tablespoon grated lemon rind
1 tablespoon lemon juice
¼ teaspoon dried turmeric
⅛ teaspoon black pepper
2 tablespoons fresh chopped cilantro
nonstick cooking spray

1. Preheat the oven to 350°F.

2. Spray a nonstick pan with cooking spray and place over medium heat; add the onion and cook uncovered, until soft, about 5 minutes. Mix the rice, chicken broth, lemon rind, lemon juice, turmeric, and pepper, and bring to a simmer.

3. Cover the pan; transfer to the oven and bake for 20 minutes or until the rice is tender.

4. Add the cilantro and serve.

MAKES 4 SERVINGS.
arginine, glutamine, lignans, quercetin

155 · Papaya Ice

- 2 *cups low-fat milk*
- ⅓ *cup granulated sugar*
- 1 *teaspoon gelatin*
- ½ *teaspoon vanilla*
- 1 *ripe papaya**
- ¼ *cup sugar*
- 2–3 *tablespoons fresh orange juice (if needed)*

1. Bring the milk to a boil. Meanwhile, place the granulated sugar and gelatin in a food processor with a metal blade. With the machine running, pour 1 cup of the boiling milk and then the vanilla through the feed tube. By hand, stir in the remaining milk and pour the milk into an ice cube tray. Freeze at least 24 hours or until quite solid.

2. Peel, seed, and cut the ripe papaya into chunks about the size of ice cubes. Sprinkle with ¼ cup sugar. Freeze papaya overnight or 2 hours. Separate the papaya chunks, but do not let either the fruit or milk-sugar cubes thaw. Place both mixtures in the processor fitted with the metal blade and pulse until very finely chopped and resembling snow. Then run the machine continuously, until an ice cream-like texture is achieved. Stop the machine and scrape sides of the bowl several times. Depending on the moisture content of the fruit, it may be necessary to add 2 to 3 tablespoons of orange juice to make a creamy texture.

4. This can be served at once or refrozen for 3 to 4 hours. After that, it becomes quite hard.

MAKES 4 SERVINGS.
PQQ

156 · Dandelion Green Salad

- 1 *pound dandelion greens, stems trimmed, and torn into 2-inch pieces, washed and dried (about 10 cups)**
- 3 *tablespoons pine nuts*
- 1 *tablespoon olive oil*
- 2 *tablespoons red wine vinegar, or to taste*
- 1½ *teaspoons paprika*
- *coarse salt and pepper to taste*

1. Place the dandelion greens in a large salad bowl.

2. In a small nonstick skillet, cook the pine nuts in the oil over moderate heat, stirring, until they are golden. Sprinkle the pine nuts over the greens. Drizzle the hot oil over the greens until wilted, tossing the mixture. Sprinkle it with the vinegar, paprika, and salt and pepper to taste. Toss it well.

MAKES 6 SERVINGS.
inulin and oligofructose, arginine, phytosterols

157 · Salmon with Mediterranean Sauce

salt to taste if desired
freshly ground black pepper
*4 salmon steaks, each about 1 inch thick (a total of about 2 pounds)**
1 tablespoon grated fresh gingerroot
1 tablespoon Dijon mustard
1 tablespoon fresh lemon juice
1 tablespoon olive oil
Mediterranean Sauce (recipe follows)

1. Preheat broiler to high, or preheat outdoor grill.

2. Salt and pepper the salmon. Combine ginger, mustard, lemon juice, and olive oil in a small bowl. Rub the mixture on both sides of the salmon. Cover with aluminum foil.

3. If broiling, place the steaks on a rack and place under the broiler about 6 inches from the heat. Broil 5 minutes on each side with the oven door slightly open.

4. If grilling, put the steaks on the hot grill and cover. Let cook 5 minutes on each side. Serve with Mediterranean Sauce on the side.

MAKES 4 SERVINGS.
arginine, glutamine, inulin and oligofructose, OCs, monoterpenes

MEDITERRANEAN SAUCE

1 ripe tomato
2 tablespoons balsamic vinegar
2 tablespoons olive oil
*¼ cup finely chopped leeks**

1 teaspoon finely minced garlic
1 tablespoon finely minced sage
¼ cup finely chopped fresh parsley
½ teaspoon grated lemon rind
salt to taste if desired
black pepper to taste

1. Put the tomato in boiling water for about 10 seconds. Pull away the skin and core the tomato. Cut the tomato in half crosswise, discarding the seeds. Cut into small cubes.

2. Put the vinegar in a small bowl and add the oil, leeks, garlic, sage, parsley, and tomato. Add the lemon rind, salt, and pepper. Blend well with a whisk.

MAKES ABOUT 1 CUP.

158 · Broiled Apples with Maple Syrup

*4 Fuji or Royal Gala apples, peeled, cored and each cut into 16 wedges**
¼ cup fresh lemon juice
4 tablespoons sugar
⅓ cup pure maple syrup
2 tablespoons Calvados

1. Preheat broiler.

2. Toss apples with lemon juice and 2 tablespoons sugar. Coat a shallow nonstick pan with cooking spray. Arrange apples in 1 layer in pan. Broil apples 6 inches from heat until edges are pale golden and apples are just tender, 8 to 10 minutes. Sprinkle remaining 2 tablespoons sugar over apples and broil until sugar is melted, 1 to 2 minutes.

3. While apples are broiling, boil maple syrup and Calvados 2 minutes.

4. Serve apples topped with sauce.

MAKES 4 SERVINGS.
PQQ, tannins, phytosterols

159 · Lemon Shrimp and Asparagus Fettuccine

1 pound fresh or frozen medium shrimp, peeled and deveined*
⅔ cup water
1 teaspoon finely shredded lemon peel
3 tablespoons lemon juice
2 tablespoons brown sugar
1 tablespoon cornstarch
2 tablespoons sherry
1 tablespoon olive oil
2 teaspoons grated gingerroot
2 cloves garlic, minced
*1 pound fresh asparagus, woody ends trimmed, and bias-cut into 1-inch pieces (3 cups)**
½ cup finely chopped red bell pepper
4 scallions, sliced
1 teaspoon fresh thyme
8 ounces hot cooked fettuccine

1. Thaw shrimp, if frozen. Set aside.

2. For sauce, in a small bowl stir together water, lemon peel, lemon juice, brown sugar, cornstarch, and sherry. Set aside.

3. Pour oil into a wok. Preheat over medium-high heat. Stir-fry ginger and garlic for 15 seconds. Add asparagus and red bell pepper; stir-fry for 1 to 2 minutes.

4. Add shrimp to hot wok. Stir-fry for 2 to 3 minutes or until shrimp turn pink.

5. Add sauce to center of wok. Cook and stir until thickened. Add scallions and thyme. Stir to coat with sauce. Cook and stir about 1 minute more or until heated through. Serve immediately over hot fettuccine.

MAKES 6 SERVINGS.
inulin and oligofructose, glutamine, tannins, monoterpenes, nucleotides, saponins

160 · Papaya Salad with Lime Vinaigrette

FOR THE SALAD

*1 pound green papaya, peeled, seeded, and finely julienned**
3 small green chilies, seeded and finely chopped
1 small red onion, peeled and finely sliced
1 small bunch fresh cilantro, minced
*3 kiwifruit, peeled and sliced**

FOR THE DRESSING

5 tablespoons lime juice
1 teaspoon sugar
2 trimmed inner hearts lemongrass, very finely sliced
2 teaspoons Thai fish sauce
2 teaspoons crushed fresh ginger
1 tablespoon lime zest
1 teaspoon dijon mustard

1. In a bowl, toss the papaya and kiwifruit with the chilies, red onion, and cilantro.

2. To make the dressing, stir all the ingredients in a small bowl.

3. To serve, pour the dressing over the salad and toss well.

MAKES 4 SERVINGS.
PQQ, inulin and oligofructose

161 · Apple, Pear, and Cranberry Gratin

1 large orange
4 cups water
1½ cups granulated sugar
1 teaspoon unsalted butter
zest of 1 lemon
*6 Granny Smith apples, peeled, cored, and cut into large chunks**
6 pears, peeled, cored, and cut into large chunks
*2 cups fresh cranberries**
nonstick cooking spray
6 medium biscotti

½ *cup packed light brown sugar*
nonfat vanilla yogurt (optional)

1. Remove the zest from the orange in long, thin strips and place in a large nonstick saucepan. Remove and discard the outer white pith from the orange. Section the orange, removing the membranes between sections. Set the sections aside.

2. Add the water, granulated sugar, butter, and lemon zest to the saucepan. Bring to a boil over high heat. Reduce the heat to medium and simmer for 3 minutes.

3. Add the apples and simmer for 8 minutes, or until the apples are tender but still firm. Using a slotted spoon, lift the apples from the syrup and transfer to a large bowl.

4. Add the pears to the simmering syrup and cook for 4 minutes, or until the pears are tender but still firm. Using a slotted spoon, lift the pears from the syrup and add to the apples.

5. Remove the syrup from the heat. Using a slotted spoon, remove half of the orange zest from the syrup. Using a sharp knife, finely chop it. Transfer to a medium nonstick sauté pan.

6. Measure ⅓ cup of the syrup and add to the sauté pan. Add the cranberries. Bring to a boil over medium-high heat. Reduce the heat to medium and simmer for 2 minutes, or until the berries pop. Remove from the heat.

7. Lightly coat an 11-by-7-inch baking dish with nonstick spray. Evenly spread the apple mixture in the dish. Spoon the cranberry mixture over the top.

8. Preheat the broiler.

9. Place the biscotti and brown sugar in a blender or food processor fitted with the metal blade. Process until finely ground. Evenly sprinkle over the fruit. Broil for 3 minutes, or until golden. Serve warm, garnished with the reserved orange sections and a dollop of nonfat vanilla yogurt, if desired.

MAKES 12 SERVINGS.
phytosterols, tannins, glutathione, phytates, PQQ, quercetin, phytoestrogens

162 · Jasmine Iced Tea

*¼ cup jasmine tea leaves**
2 cups boiling water
2 teaspoons half-and-half
2 tablespoons sugar, or to taste
ice cubes

1. Combine tea, boiling water, half-and-half, and sugar; stir until blended.

2. Pour into 2 tall glasses filled with ice cubes.

MAKES 2 SERVINGS.
tannins

163 · Steamed Dover Sole in Olive and Pine Nut Sauce

nonstick cooking spray
2 shallots, chopped
2 cloves garlic, chopped
2 large tomatoes, peeled and chopped
2 tablespoons tomato paste
¼ cup sun-dried tomatoes, soaked in boiling water until soft
3 tablespoons chopped fresh basil
⅓ cup Kalamata olives
¼ cup pine nuts
2 tablespoons capers
1 pound Dover sole fillets, scaled and cleaned

1. Spray a nonstick pan with cooking spray and set over medium heat.

2. Add shallots and cook 2 to 3 minutes or until tender. Add garlic and sauté 1 minute until lightly browned. Pour in tomatoes, tomato paste, sun-dried tomatoes, and basil. Cover and cook 15 minutes.

3. Add olives, nuts, capers, and fish, cover, and simmer 20 minutes or until fish is opaque and beginning to flake. Serve hot.

MAKES 4 SERVINGS.
arginine, nucleotides, glutamine, inulin and oligofructose, OCs, phytosterols

164 · Artichokes with Roman Vinaigrette

*3 artichokes (1 pound each)**
2 lemons
1 teaspoon coriander seeds
1 teaspoon peppercorns
1 hard-boiled large egg
1 teaspoon drained capers
1 leek, sliced
¼ teaspoon dried thyme
¾ tablespoon minced fresh basil or ¾ teaspoon dried
3 tablespoons balsamic vinegar
1 teaspoon Dijon-style mustard
1 garlic clove, sliced
salt to taste
2 tablespoons olive oil

1. Trim the artichokes by breaking off the stems and tough outer leaves. Cut off the top half of each artichoke, snap off any remaining sharp tips from the leaves with scissors. Trim the bases and drop the artichokes into a bowl of cold water containing the juice of one of the lemons.

2. In a saucepan of boiling salted water, combine the artichokes, drained, with the juice of the other lemon, the coriander seeds, and the peppercorns, and simmer them for 40 minutes, or until the bottoms are tender. Remove the artichokes and let them drain upside down on a rack until they are cool enough to handle.

3. Reduce the cooking liquid to about 2 cups and strain it, reserving 2 tablespoons of the liquid and spice mixture.

4. Cut the artichokes in half lengthwise and remove the inside leaves and the chokes. Cut each half into 3 wedges and arrange the wedges cut sides up on a platter.

5. Mash the egg with a fork and sprinkle it and the capers over the artichokes.

6. In a food processor or blender, blend the reserved cooking liquid and spice mixture, the leek, thyme, basil, vinegar, mustard, garlic, and salt to taste, until the mixture is smooth. With the motor running, add the olive oil in a stream and blend the dressing until it is emulsified. Pour the dressing around the artichoke wedges.

MAKES 3 SERVINGS.
phytates, phytosterols, monoterpenes, arginine, CLA, OCs, lignans

165 · Honey Apple Sorbet

½ cup honey
½ cup water
½ cup light corn syrup
juice of 2 limes
10 apples, peeled, cored, and cut into 1-inch cubes*

1. In a mixing bowl, mix together the honey, water, corn syrup, and lime juice.
2. Juice the apple cubes in a juicer and stir the juice into the honey mixture.
3. Pour into the container of an ice cream machine and freeze according to the manufacturer's directions.

MAKES 8 SERVINGS.
PQQ, phytates, tannins, quercetin, phytoestrogens, phytosterols

166 · Sun Salad

1 green pepper
1 red pepper
*1 onion**
*1 head romaine lettuce**
4 cucumbers
1 stalk of celery
10 green olives
½ cup balsamic vinegar
salt and black pepper to taste

1. Chop peppers, onion, lettuce, cucumbers, and celery in ¼ inch slices. Combine with olives and vinegar. Salt and pepper to taste.
2. Cover bowl and place in the sun for 2 hours.

MAKES 4 SERVINGS.
phytoestrogens, glutamine, lignans, quercetin, protease inhibitors

167 · Sesame and Ginger Asparagus

1 *pound fresh asparagus spears**
1 *tablespoon sesame oil*
2 *tablespoons low-sodium soy sauce*
2 *teaspoons sesame seeds, toasted**
1 *teaspoon gingerroot, peeled and minced*
1 *clove garlic, minced*
dash of pepper
2 *teaspoons grated lemon rind*

1. Remove tough ends of asparagus, peeling to remove scales as well. Cut spears into 2-inch pieces.

2. In a saucepan, heat oil over medium-low heat until hot. Add asparagus, soy sauce, sesame seeds, gingerroot, garlic, and pepper. Cook, stirring, for 5 minutes, or until asparagus is crisp-tender. Transfer to a serving bowl, and sprinkle with lemon rind. Serve immediately.

MAKES 4 SERVINGS.
inulin and oligofructose, nucleotides, saponins, protease inhibitors, glutamine, taurine, lignans

168 · Roast Chicken with Mushroom and Pecan Stuffing

1 *onion, finely chopped*
1 *cup chopped button mushrooms*
1 *cup minced celery*
1 *cup coarsely grated carrots*
¼ *cup chopped pecans**
1 *tablespoon chopped fresh thyme or 1 teaspoon dried*
1 *tablespoon chopped fresh sage or 1 teaspoon dried*
1 *cup fresh white bread crumbs*
1 *egg, beaten*
salt and pepper to taste
1 *chicken (3½ pounds)**
¼ *cup water*
⅔ *cup marsala*
nonstick cooking spray

1. Preheat oven to 375°F.

2. Coat a large nonstick suacepan with cooking spray. Add onion and sauté until softened. Add mushrooms, celery, and carrots; cook, stirring, 5 minutes. Remove from heat; stir in pecans, thyme, sage, bread crumbs, egg, and salt and pepper.

3. Stuff chicken with the stuffing mixture. Place, breast down, in a roasting pan; add ¼ cup water. Roast 45 minutes; turn chicken breast. Roast about 45 minutes more or until a meat thermometer inserted in thickest part of thigh (not touching bone) registers 185°F. Transfer to a platter; keep warm.

4. Discard fat from roasting pan; to make gravy, add marsala to remaining cooking juices, stirring to scrape up any browned bits. Boil over high heat 1 minute to reduce.

5. Carve chicken and serve with stuffing, gravy, and seasonal vegetables.

MAKES 4 SERVINGS.
arginine, nucleotides, glutamine, exorphins, taurine

169 · Orange Almond Iced Tea

*¾ cup unsweetened orange juice**
⅓ cup sugar
½ teaspoon ground nutmeg
2 (3-inch) sticks cinnamon
*8 almond-flavored tea bags**
5½ cups boiling water

1. Combine juice, sugar, nutmeg, and cinnamon in a large pitcher; add tea bags. Add boiling water; cover and steep 10 minutes.

2. Remove and discard tea bags and cinnamon sticks; let cool. Serve over ice.

MAKES 8 SERVINGS.
PQQ, glutamine, monoterpenes, tannins

170 · New Potatoes with Chicory

1 tablespoon walnut oil
3 large cloves garlic, cut into thick slices

*1 pound tiny new potatoes, sliced in half**
1 rib celery, cut into thin slices
1 small bulb fennel, trimmed and cut into thick wedges
1 tablespoon thyme
*2 large heads chicory (about 2 pounds), bottom 2 inches trimmed off, cut into 2-inch pieces**
salt and pepper to taste
½ cup water
3 tablespoons fresh lemon juice

1. Heat the oil in a large nonstick pot over medium-low heat. Add the garlic, potatoes, celery, fennel, thyme, chicory, salt, and pepper. Combine the ingredients with the oil. Cover and cook, stirring frequently, for 6 to 8 minutes, or until the chicory is wilted.

2. Add the water, stirring well to mix. Cover and continue cooking, stirring occasionally, for about 15 minutes or until the potatoes are tender. Stir in the lemon juice.

MAKES 8 SERVINGS.
inulin and oligofructose, glutamine, monoterpenes, OCs, lignans, tannins, phytosterols

171 · Herbed Grilled Lamb Chops

6 lean lamb loin chops (6 ounces each), 1-inch thick, trimmed of all fat*
¼ cup white wine
2 tablespoons water
2 tablespoons fresh rosemary, minced
2 tablespoons fresh thyme, minced
2 tablespoons fresh flat-leaf parsley, chopped
1 tablespoon lemon juice
1 tablespoon Worcestershire sauce
2 cloves garlic, minced
vegetable cooking spray

1. Place chops in a large shallow dish. Combine wine, water, herbs, lemon juice, Worcestershire sauce, and garlic in a small bowl; stir well. Pour over chops; cover and refrigerate 2 hours, turning occasionally.

2. Remove chops from marinade, reserving marinade. Coat grill with cooking spray. Grill chops 5 to 6 inches over medium coals for 35 minutes or until desired degree of doneness. Turn chops over and baste frequently with reserved marinade.

MAKES 6 SERVINGS.
arginine, exorphins, carnitine, nucleotides

172 · Swiss Vegetable Soup

*1 ounce Canadian bacon, cubed**
1 tablespoon olive oil
*2 leeks, white parts only, thinly sliced**
1 carrot, cubed
1 rib celery, sliced
2 ounces cabbage leaves, cut into thin strips
6 cups water
salt to taste
1 large potato, peeled and cubed
1 medium turnip, peeled and cubed
black pepper to taste
*1 ounce fresh green peas**
1 ounce fresh sweet corn
2 ounces reduced-fat Swiss cheese, shredded

1. Bring a small pot of water to a boil. Add bacon and cook for 5 minutes. Drain and pat dry.

2. Warm oil in a large saucepan over low heat. Add bacon and cook slowly for 3 minutes. Stir in the leeks, carrots, and celery; cook slowly for 10 minutes. Stir in the cabbage and add the water. Season with the salt, then bring to a simmer over medium heat. Cook for 10 minutes. Add the potatoes and turnips. Simmer for 10 minutes or until vegetables are tender. Season with pepper. Add peas and corn and simmer for 5 minutes more.

3. Serve in warm soup bowls. Top each with cheese.

MAKES 4 SERVINGS.
arginine, inulin and oligofructose, phytates, phytoestrogens

173 · Cannelloni and Cauliflower Sauté

FOR THE PASTA

2 ¼ *cups all-purpose flour*
3 *eggs*
1 *tablespoon olive oil*

THE FILLING AND SAUTÉ

1 ¼ *pounds spinach, stemmed**
¾ *pound mesclun*
¼ *pound arugula, stemmed*
1 *ounce dried porcini mushroom, soaked in 1 cup of water for 15 minutes*
2 *tablespoons olive oil*
1 *clove garlic*
2 *egg yolks*
⅛ *teaspoon ground nutmeg*
¼ *teaspoon saffron*
2 *teaspoons salt*
freshly ground pepper to taste
½ *cup reduced-fat ricotta cheese*
½ *cup freshly grated Parmesan cheese*
nonstick cooking spray
1 *cup low-fat chicken broth*
1 *small head cauliflower, broken into florets**

1. To make the pasta, place the flour, eggs, and olive oil in a food processor and process until well combined. Turn the mixture out on a work surface and knead until smooth. Cover with a damp towel and let stand for 1 hour.

2. Meanwhile, to make the filling, toss together the spinach, mesclun, and arugula. Coat a nonstick skillet with nonstick cooking spray. Sauté the garlic in oil for 1 minute. Add two-thirds of the greens to the skillet and set the rest aside. Stir the greens until wilted (about 5 minutes) and remove from heat. When cool enough to handle, press the excess moisture from the greens. Place in a food processor with the egg yolks, nutmeg, saffron, 1 teaspoon of salt, pepper to taste, 1 tablespoon of olive oil, and ¼ cup of Parmesan and ¼ cup ricotta. Process until smooth. Scrape into a bowl and refrigerate until ready to use.

3. Uncover pasta and place on well-floured cutting board. Pound pasta into a circle while continuing to flour the cutting board. With a rolling pin, roll out pasta into a rectangle, about 12 by 14 inches, as thin as possible. Cut pasta into 3-by-4-inch rectangles. Repeat with the remaining dough. Bring a large pot of water to a boil. Gently drop 3 pieces of pasta in the water. Wait 15 seconds and remove with spatula or tongs. Lay the pieces flat on towels to drain. Repeat with the remaining pasta.

4. Preheat the oven to 350°F. Spray a medium-sized heatproof dish with cooking spray. For each pasta rectangle, use 2 tablespoons of filling, spread evenly in line, crosswise in the center of the rectangle. Roll the pasta up with the filling into a small tube. Repeat for all pasta rectangles. Arrange the cannelloni in the dish and pour the chicken broth over them.

5. Bake the pasta for 10 minutes. Heat 1 tablespoon of olive oil in a large skillet over medium heat. Add cauliflower florets and sauté, stirring, for 5 minutes. Add the remaining greens and sauté until florets are tender, about 5 minutes longer. Season with 1 teaspoon of salt and pepper to taste and keep warm.

6. Sprinkle the remaining cheese over the pasta and place under the broiler until lightly browned, about 3 minutes. Divide the cauliflower mixture among 4 plates, top each with 3 cannelloni, and serve immediately.

MAKES 6 SERVINGS.
lignans, saponins

174 · Curly Chicory and Red-Leaf Lettuce Salad

6 tablespoons tarragon vinegar
1 teaspoon Dijon mustard
1½ tablespoons minced fresh tarragon or 1 teaspoon dried and crumbled
salt and pepper to taste
1 tablespoon olive oil
8 cups torn curly chicory, rinsed and spun dry
4 cups torn red-leaf lettuce, rinsed and spun dry

1. In a bowl, whisk together the vinegar, mustard, tarragon, and salt and pepper to taste. Add the oil in a stream, and whisk the dressing until it is emulsified.

2. In a large bowl, toss the curly chicory and the red-leaf lettuce with the dressing.

MAKES 8 TO 10 SERVINGS.
inulin and oligofructose, protease inhibitors, lignans, quercetin, phytoestrogens, phytosterols

175 · Chocolate Almond Mousse with Raspberries

- ½ *cup sugar, plus ⅓ cup sugar*
- ¼ *cup cornstarch*
- ¼ *cup unsweetened cocoa*
- 1 *teaspoon unflavored gelatin*
- 3 *cups low-fat milk*
- 1 *teaspoon almond extract*
- 1 *teaspoon vanilla extract*
- 3 *egg whites*
- *dash of cream of tartar*
- 2½ *tablespoons water*
- 2 *cups fresh raspberries*

1. Combine ½ cup sugar, cornstarch, cocoa, and gelatin in a large pot. Gradually stir in milk, stirring until smooth. Cook over medium heat, stirring, until mixture comes to a boil. Reduce the heat, and simmer, stirring for 2 minutes. Remove from heat; stir in vanilla and almond extracts. Cover with plastic wrap. Let cool.

2. Beat egg whites and cream of tartar with an electric mixer on high speed until stiff.

3. Combine ⅓ cup sugar and water in a small saucepan. Bring mixture to a boil; cook, without stirring, until candy thermometer registers 238°F (about 7 to 8 minutes).

4. Gradually pour sugar mixture into beaten egg whites while beating constantly at high speed. Continue to beat until egg white mixture is cool and set.

5. Fold chocolate mixture into egg white mixture. Spoon into individual dessert glasses and cover with plastic wrap; chill 4 hours. To serve, top with raspberries.

MAKES 10 SERVINGS.
inulin and oligofructose, tannins

176 · Green Beans with Pine Nuts

*1 pound fresh green beans, washed and ends trimmed**
1 tablespoon olive oil
2 tablespoons soy sauce
juice from ½ lemon
salt and freshly ground pepper to taste
*2 tablespoons toasted pine nuts**

1. Steam the beans in a large pot of rapidly boiling water. Drain under cold running water.

2. In a large skillet, heat the oil over medium-high heat. Add the beans and stir. Add the soy sauce and lemon juice and cook, stirring constantly, for 2 minutes.

3. Remove from the heat. Season with salt and pepper and sprinkle with pine nuts.

MAKES 4 SERVINGS.
arginine, lignans, monoterpenes

177 · Honey Glazed Carrots

½ cup water
1 tablespoon unsalted butter
2 tablespoons honey
1 tablespoon fresh ginger, finely minced
1¼ teaspoons kosher salt
ground pepper
1 pound peeled baby carrots

1. Combine the water, butter, honey, ginger, salt, and pepper in a medium skillet. Add the carrots and place over medium high heat.

2. Cook, stirring occasionally, until all of the water has evaporated and the carrots are tender, about twenty minutes.

MAKES 4 SERVINGS.
protease inhibitors, PQQ, glutathione, lignans

178 · Oyster and Romano Soufflé

2 tablespoons reduced-calorie margarine
1½ tablespoons all-purpose flour
½ cup low-fat milk
1 teaspoon Dijon mustard
salt and pepper to taste
2 tablespoons Romano cheese
2 tablespoons chopped scallions
2 eggs, separated
*24 freshly shucked oysters on the half shell**

1. Melt butter in a small pan over medium heat. Add flour and cook 1 minute, stirring. Remove from heat and stir in milk. Return to heat and stir until sauce boils. Remove from heat again and add mustard, salt and pepper to taste, Romano, scallions, and egg yolks. Cool slightly.

2. Preheat broiler. Place oysters on baking pan. Beat egg whites in a large bowl until soft peaks form. Fold into cheese mixture until well combined. Place a spoonful of the mixture on each oyster and broil until puffy and golden. Serve hot.

MAKES 6 SERVINGS.
arginine, glutamine, CLA, inulin and oligofructose

179 · Pineapple and Grape Sorbet

1 large, fresh pineapple
1 cup granulated sugar
juice of 1 lemon
¼ cup white grape juice
¼ cup honey

1. Remove the skin and core of the pineapple and cut it into small pieces. Puree in a food processor or blender. Pour the fruit into a bowl, add the sugar and honey, and stir until completely dissolved. Add the lemon and grape juices.

2. Pour the sorbet mixture into ice trays and allow it to set until firm, but not rock-hard.

3. Serve in tall glasses.

MAKES 6 SERVINGS.
monoterpenes, glutamine, protease inhibitors

180 · Roasted Red Snapper with Potatoes and Red Wine

*1 red snapper, about 3 pounds, cleaned and scaled with skin on**
1 teaspoon salt
12 small red-skin potatoes, cut in half
3 tomatoes, halved and sliced
1 cup pitted black olives
1 teaspoon chopped oregano leaves
2 tablespoons olive oil
4 cloves garlic, sliced
1 cup pearl onions
¼ cup dry red wine
salt and pepper to taste

1. Preheat oven to 450°F.

2. Slit the fish along each side its length, about 3 inches apart. Rub with salt and place in a deep nonstick baking dish.

3. Combine the potatoes, tomatoes, olives, oregano, olive oil, garlic, pearl onions, and wine in a bowl. Mix well. Pour around the fish. Salt and pepper to taste.

4. Bake until the fish flakes when a fork is inserted, about 30 to 35 minutes. Remove the dish from the oven and serve immediately.

MAKES 6 SERVINGS.
PQQ, tannins, OCs

181 · Stirred Rice with Spinach

1 tablespoon olive oil
2 cups chopped onion
1 small clove garlic, minced
1 cup uncooked long-grain white rice
1¾ cups water or half water and half chicken broth
salt to taste (optional)
1 package (10 ounces) fresh spinach, rinsed, trimmed, and torn into 1-inch pieces

2 tablespoons freshly grated Parmigiano-Reggiano cheese
2 tablespoons pignoli (pine nuts), lightly toasted in a skillet

1. Heat the oil over low heat in a large heavy saucepan. Add the onion and garlic and sauté, stirring occasionally, until golden, about 10 minutes. Stir in the rice and turn the heat to medium-low. Sauté, stirring constantly, about 2 minutes.

2. Stir in the water (or broth and water) and salt, if using, and heat to simmer. Cook, covered, over low heat for 12 minutes. Add the spinach and cheese to the saucepan, stirring once or twice just to blend. Cover and cook over medium-low heat for 3 minutes, or until the spinach is wilted.

3. Spoon into a serving dish and sprinkle with toasted pignoli. Serve at once.

MAKES 4 SERVINGS.
glutamine, inulin and oligofructose, OCs, monoterpenes, nucleotides, saponins, protease inhibitors

182 · Warm Goat Cheese Salad with Dried Cherries and Pancetta Vinaigrette

8 cups mesclun (mixed baby greens), washed and dried
*4 ounces dried cherries (about 1 cup)**
*6 ounces soft mild goat cheese**
¼ teaspoon black pepper, or to taste
½-pound piece pancetta (Italian unsmoked cured bacon), cut into strips about ⅛ inch thick and 1 inch long
1 tablespoon olive oil
1 tablespoon finely chopped garlic
1 tablespoon finely chopped fresh thyme leaves
6 tablespoons sherry vinegar

1. In a large serving bowl, combine mesclun and dried cherries. Crumble goat cheese on top and sprinkle with pepper.

2. In a large nonstick skillet coated with cooking spray, cook pancetta in oil over moderate heat, stirring, until lightly browned. Add garlic and sauté mixture, stirring, until garlic is golden. Carefully add

thyme and vinegar. Increase heat to moderately high and boil mixture 1 minute.

3. Add hot vinaigrette to salad and toss. Serve salad immediately.

MAKES 4 GENEROUS SERVINGS.
CLA, phytosterols, monoterpenes, arginine

183 · Chocolate Walnut Angel Cookies

3 egg whites
⅛ teaspoon cream of tartar
¾ cup granulated sugar
1 teaspoon vanilla
3 tablespoons unsweetened cocoa powder
*¼ cup unsalted chopped walnuts**
nonstick cooking spray
¼ cup confectioners' sugar

1. Preheat oven to 375°F.
2. In a medium bowl, beat egg whites and cream of tartar with an electric mixer on medium speed, until soft peaks form. Beat in the granulated sugar and vanilla on high speed until the whites are stiff.
3. Fold the cocoa and walnuts in until blended.
4. Drop spoonfuls of batter onto baking sheets coated with nonstick spray, 1 inch apart. Bake for 30 minutes, or until dry. Cool on a wire rack and sprinkle with confectioners' sugar.

MAKES 24 COOKIES (12 SERVINGS).
arginine

184 · Black and White Salad

*¼ cup dried hijiki (black sea vegetable)**
½ tablespoon vegetable oil
1 carrot sliced finely
¾ cup Dashi (basic sea stock, recipe follows)
1 tablespoon sake (Japanese rice wine)
¼ tablespoon sugar

3 tablespoons soy sauce
*½ cake tofu (bean curd), about 2 ounces**
2 tablespoons sesame seeds
1 teaspoon mirin (syrupy rice wine)
*1 teaspoon usukuchi shoyu (light soy sauce)**
1 teaspoon rice vinegar
salt to taste

TOPPINGS:
2 sprigs parsley
1 scallion, green part only, chopped finely

1. Place the dried hijiki in pan with warm water for 20 to 30 minutes. Drain, and set aside.

2. Place the oil in nonstick skillet set on medium heat. Add the hijiki and carrot. Sauté while stirring for 3 to 4 minutes. Lower the heat, add ¼ cup of the sea stock and the sake, and simmer for 8 minutes.

3. Add the sugar and soy sauce to the skillet. Simmer while stirring for 7 to 8 minutes, or until the liquid is completely reduced and the sea vegetable looks glossy. If it seems tough, add a teaspoon of stock and simmer for an additional 3 to 5 minutes. Remove the skillet from the heat, and let cool to room temperature.

4. To make the dressing, place the tofu in boiling water for 1 minute and then drain. Let cool and place in a fine meshed cloth. Squeeze out all the moisture, mashing the bean curd to a smooth paste. Transfer to a bowl.

5. Place the sesame seeds on a foil-lined baking sheet and toast under the broiler until the seeds start to change color, about 30 seconds. Transfer the seeds to a cutting board, and crush them. Add the seeds to the tofu paste.

6. Combine well the mirin, usukuchi shoyu, vinegar, and a pinch of salt with the bean curd. Drain the sea vegetables thoroughly and toss in the dressing. Mix well. Serve in small mounds, at room temperature or chilled.

MAKES 4 TO 6 SERVINGS.
phytoestrogens, lignans, phytosterols

DASHI

4½ *cups cold water*
20 *square inches dashi kombu (kelp for stock making)*
1 *packet or ⅓ cup loosely packed katsuo bushi (dried bonito flakes)*

1. Add the water to a large saucepan and add the kombu. Bring the water to a boil.

2. Turn the heat off and add the katsuo bushi. Let the broth stand for 2 to 3 minutes, until the flakes combine.

3. Remove the kombu with tongs or a spatula, and strain the broth immediately through a fine mesh colander.

MAKES 1 QUART.

185 · Glaze-Grilled Swordfish

4 *tablespoons soy sauce*
3 *tablespoons mirin (syrupy rice wine)*
1 *tablespoon honey*
2 *cloves garlic, minced*
4 *pieces swordfish, each about 4–5 ounces and at least ½ inch thick**
3 *tablespoons sake (Japanese rice wine)*
¼ *teaspoon salt*
2 *tablespoons sesame seeds**
2 *teaspoons vegetable oil*

1. In a small saucepan set over low heat, combine the soy sauce, mirin, honey, and garlic, stirring constantly. Cook the sauce for three minutes until bubbly. Pour the sauce into a small bowl, and let it sit until cool.

2. When you are ready to cook, place the pieces of swordfish in a flat-bottomed glass dish and sprinkle the sake over them. Let the fish sit for five minutes. Just before cooking, sprinkle salt and sesame seeds on each piece of fish.

3. Heat the oil in a heavy skillet over high heat. Sear the fish for 1½ minutes on each side. Remove the fish and set aside. Lower the heat slightly and add half the soy glaze to the empty pan, cooking it until bubbly. Return 2 pieces of fish to the pan and cook for 2 minutes.

Flip the fish, raise the heat to high, and continue cooking for another minute. Transfer the glazed fish to serving plates and pour any remaining pan juices over fish; keep these pieces warm. Rinse out pan and repeat with the remaining soy glaze and seared fish.

MAKES 4 SERVINGS.
CLA, arginine

186 · Berries in Meringue Baskets

2 large egg whites
½ teaspoon lemon juice
½ cup sugar
Marinated Berries (recipe follows)
4 whole strawberries
light whipped topping to serve

1. Preheat oven to 200°F.

2. Place egg whites and lemon juice in a large bowl. Beat with an electric mixer on medium speed until soft peaks form. Gradually add sugar and beat on high until the whites are shiny and stiff.

3. Using a pastry bag with a fluted tip, fill bag with egg white mixture. Onto a nonstick baking sheet, squeeze out 4 3-inch-diameter circles by forming a spiral, working from the inside out to form the meringue base. Pipe around the edge of the base, forming a 2-inch-high cup.

4. Bake the meringues for 3 hours, until they are dry and a dark cream color. Remove from the oven and cool. Place each shell on a dessert plate, fill with marinated berries. Top with whipped topping and whole strawberries.

MAKES 4 SERVINGS.
tannins, glutamine

MARINATED BERRIES

½ cup Port
2 tablespoons orange juice
1 teaspoon honey
½ teaspoon grated orange zest

- 1 *cup strawberries, hulled and quartered**
- ½ *cup blueberries**
- ½ *cup raspberries**

1. In a small bowl whisk together Port, juice, honey, and orange zest.
2. Pour over berries and combine well.
3. Cover and refrigerate for 2 hours, stirring occasionally.

187 · Pasta with Pine Nuts and Broccoli

- 2 *bunches broccoli (about 1 pound each), ends trimmed off, cut into individual florets*
- 1 *pound rigatoni*
- 1 *tablespoon olive oil*
- 5 *tablespoons pine nuts*
- 6 *cloves garlic, finely minced*
- 4 *tablespoons water*
- ½ *teaspoon paprika*
- 1 *tablespoon fresh lemon juice*
- 2 *teaspoons salt, plus more to taste*
- *Freshly ground pepper to taste*
- *Parmesan cheese as a garnish*

1. To a large pot of boiling water add the broccoli and cook for about 2 minutes or until blanched. Drain in a colander. To another pot of salted boiling water add the rigatoni and cook until al dente, about 12 minutes.
2. Heat the olive oil in a large nonstick skillet over medium heat. Add the garlic and sauté for about 1 minute. Add the pine nuts and cook, while stirring for about 3 minutes or until lightly browned. Add the water, broccoli, and paprika and cook for about 5 minutes or until tender.
3. Combine the pasta and broccoli. Add the lemon juice, toss and season with salt and pepper to taste. Toss to combine. Sprinkle with Parmesan cheese.

MAKES 6 SERVINGS.

lignans, isothicyanates, glutamine, arginine, phytosterols, monoterpenes

REFERENCES

PQQ

Steinberg, F.M., Gershwin, M.E. & Rucker, R.B. Dietary pyrroloquinoline quinone: growth and immune response in BALB/c mice. J. Nutr. 124: 744–753, 1994.

Smidt, C.R., Unkefer, C.J., Houck, D.R. & Rucker, R.B. Intestinal absorption and tissue distribution of [^{14}C]pyrroloquinoline quinone in mice. Proc Soc Expl Biol Med. 97: 19–26, 1991.

Saponins

Higashitani, A., Tabata, S., Hayashi, T. & Hotta, Y. Plant saponins can affect DNA recombination in cultured mammalian cells. Cell Structure and Function 14: 617–624, 1989.

Chavali, S.R., Francis,T. & Campbell, J.B. An in vitro study of immodulatory effects of some saponins. Int. J. Immunopharmac. 9: 675–683, 1987.

Phytates

Ohlrogge, J.B., & Kerman, T.P. Oxygen-dependent aging of seeds. Plant Physiol. 70: 791–794, 1982.

Berridge, M.J. & Irvine, R.F. Inositol phosphates and cell signaling. Nature 341: 197–204, 1989.

Carnosine

Decker, E.A. & Faraji, H. Inhibition of lipid oxidation by carnosine. J. Am. Oil Chem. Soc. 67: 650–652, 1990.

Egorov, S.Y., Kurella, E.G., Boldyrev, A.A. & Krasnovsky Jr., A.A. Quenching of singlet molecular oxygen by carnosine and related antioxidants. Biochem. Molec. Biol. Int. 41: 687–694, 1997.

Phytosterols

Awad, A.B., Tagle Hernandez, A.Y., Fink, C.S. & Mendel, S.L. Effect of dietary phytosterols on cell proliferation and protein kinase C activity in rat colonic mucosa. Nutr. Cancer 27: 210–215, 1989.

Cerqueira, M.T., McMurry Fry, M. & Connor, W.E. The food and nutrient intakes of the Tarahumara Indians in Mexico. Am. J. Clin. Nutr. 32: 905–915, 1979.

Isothiocyanates

Kolm, R.H., Danielson, H., Zhang, Y., Talalay, P. & Mannervik, B. Isothiocyanates as substrates for human glutathione transferases: structure-activity studies. Biochem. J. 311: 453–459, 1995.

Tawfiq, N., Heaney, R.K., Plumb, J.A., Fenwick, G.R., Musk S.R.R. & Williamson, G. Dietary glucosinolates as blocking agents against carcinogenesis: glucosinolate breakdown products assessed by induction of quinone reductase activity in murine hepalclc7 cells. Carcinogenesis 16: 1191–1194, 1995.

Taurine

Odle, J., Roach, M. & Baker, D.H. Taurine utilization by cats. J. Nutr. 123: 1932–1933, 1993.

Welty, J.D. & McBroom, M.J. Effects of verapamil and taurine administration on heart taurine and calcium in BIO 14.6 cardiomyopathic hamsters. Res. Comm. Chem. Pathol. Pharmacol. 49: 141–144, 1985.

Monoterpenes

He, L., Mo, H., Hadisusilo, S., Qureshi, A.A. & Elson, C.E. Isoprenoids suppress the growth of murine B16 melanomas in vitro and in vivo. J. Nutr. 127: 668–674, 1997.

Elson, C.E. Suppression of mevalonate pathway activities by dietary isprenoids: protective roles in cancer and cardiovascular disease. J. Nutr. 125: 1666S–1672S, 1995.

Elegbede, J.A., Maltzman, T.H., Elson, C.E. & Gould, M.N. Effects of anticarcinogenic monoterpenes on phase II hepatic metabolizing enzymes. Carcinogenesis: 14: 1221–1223, 1993.

Carnitine

Hagen, T.M., Ingersoll, R.T., Wehr, C.M., Lykkesfeldt, J., Vinarsky, V., Bartholomew, J.C., Song, M. & Ames, B.N. Acetyl-L-carnitine fed to old rats partially restores mitochondrial function and ambulatory activity. Proc. Natl. Acad. Sci. 95: 9562–9566, 1998.

De Angelis, C., Scarfo, C., Falcinelli, M., Perna, E., Reda, E., Ramacci, M.T. & Angelucci, L. Acetly-L-carnitine prevents age-dependent structural alterations in rat peripheral nerves and promotes regeneration following sciatic nerve injury in young and senescent rats. Exp. Neurology. 128: 103–114, 1994.

Shigenaga, M.K., Hagen, T.M. & Ames, B.N. Oxidative damage and mitochondrial decay in aging. Proc. Natl. Acad. Sci. 91: 10771–10778, 1994.

Lignans

Adlercreutz, H., Fotsis, T., Bannwart, C., Wahala, K., Makela, T., Brunow, G. & Hase, T. Determination of urinary lignans and phytoestrogen metabolites, potential antiestrogens and anticarcinogens, in urine of women on various habitual diets. J. Steroid Biochem. 25: 791–797, 1986.

Wahg, C., Makela, T., Hase, T., Adlercreutz, H. & Kurzer, M.S. Lignans and flavonoids inhibit aromatase enzyme in human preadipocytes. J. Steroid Biochem. Molec. Biol. 50: 205–212, 1994.

OCs

Sigounas, G., Hooker, J., Anagnostou, A. & Steiner, M. S-allylmercaptocysteine inhibits cell proliferation and reduces the viability of erythroleukemia, breast, and prostate cancer cell lines. Nutr. Cancer 27: 186–191, 1997.

Burk, R.F. & Hill, K.E. Selenoprotein P. A selenium-rich extracellular glycoprotein. J. Nutr. 124: 1891–1897, 1994.

Gudi, V.A., Singh, S.V. Effect of diallyl sulfide, a naturally occurring anti-carcinogen, on glutathione-dependent detoxification enzymes of female CD-1 mouse tissues. Biochem. Pharmac. 42: 1261–1265, 1991.

Tannins

Miyamoto, K., Muramya, T., Nomura, M., Hatano, T., Yoshida, T., Furukawa, T., Koshiura, R. & Okuda, T. Antitumor activity and interleukin-1 induction by tannins. Anticancer Research 13: 37–42, 1993.

Klaunig, J.E., Xu,Y., Han, C., Kamendulis, L.M., Chen, J., Heiser, C., Gordon, M.S., Mohler III, E.R. The effect of tea consumption on oxidative stress in smokers and nonsmokers. P.S.E.B.M. 220: 249–254, 1999.

Polya, G.M., Wang, B.H., Foo, L.Y. Inhibition of signal-regulated protein kinases by plant-derived hydrolysable tannins. Phytochemistry 38: 307–314, 1995.

Glutathione

Lang, C.A., Naryshkin, S., Schneider, D.L., Mills, B.J., Lindeman, R.D. Low blood glucose levels in healthy aging adults. J. Lab. Clin. Med. 120: 720–725, 1992.

Chen, T.S., Richie Jr., J.P., Lang, C.A. Life span profiles of glutathione and acetaminophen detoxification. Drug Metabolism and Disposition 18: 882–887, 1990.

Chen, T.S., Richie Jr., J.P. & Lang, C.A. The effect of aging on glutathione and cysteine levels in different regions of the mouse brain. P.S.E.B.M. 190: 399–402, 1989.

Inulin & Oligofructose

Gibson, G.R., Beatty, E.R., Wang, X. & Cummings, J.H. Selective stimulation of bifidobacteria in the human colon by oligofructose and inulin. Gastroenterology 108: 975–982, 1995.

Moshfegh, A.J., Friday, J.E., Goldman, J.P. & Chug Ahuja, J.K. Presence of inulin and oligofructose in the diets of Americans. J. Nutr. 129: 1407S–1411S, 1999.

Clausen, M.R. Production and oxidation of short-chain fatty acids in the human colon: implications for antibiotic-associated diarrhea, ulcerative colitis, colonic cancer, and hepatic encephalopathy. Danish Medical Bulletin 45: 53–76, 1998.

Protease Inhibitors

Ghibelli, L., Maresca, V., Coppola, S. & Gualandi, G. Protease inhibitors block apoptosis at intermediate stages: a compared analysis of DNA fragmentation and apoptopic nuclear morphology. F.E.B.S 377: 9–14, 1995.

Billings, P.C., Brandon, D.L. & Habres, J.M. Internationalization of the Bowman-Birk protease inhibitor by intestinal epithelial cells. Eur. J. Cancer 27: 903–908, 1991.

CLA

Van den Berg, J.J.M., Cook, N.E. & Tribble, D.L. Reinvestigation of the antioxidant properties of conjugated linoleic acid. Lipids 30: 599–605, 1995.

Park, Y., Albright, K.J., Liu, W., Storkson, J.M., Cook, M.E., Pariza, M.W. Effect of conjugated linoleic acid on body composition in mice. Lipids 32: 853–858, 1997.

Sugano, M., Tsujita, A., Yamasaki, M., Yamada, K., Ikeda, I. & Kritchevsy, D. Lymphatic recovery, tissue distribution, and metabolic effects of conjugated linoleic acid in rats. J. Nutr. Biochem. 8: 38–43, 1997.

Phytoestrogens

Anderson, J.J.B. & Garner, S.C. The effects of phytoestrogens on bone. Nutr. Research 17: 1617–1632, 1997.

Martin, M.E., Haourigui, M., Pelissero, C., Benassayag, C. & Nunez, E.A. Interactions between phytoestrogens and human sex steroid binding protein. Life Sciences 58: 429–436, 1996.

Record, I.R., Dreosti, I.E. & McInerney, J.K. The antioxidant activity of genistein in vitro. Nutr. Biochem. 6: 481–485, 1995.

Arginine

Reckelhoff, K.F., Kellum Jr., J.A., Racusen, L.C., Hildebrandt, D.A. Long-term dietary supplementation with L-arginine prevents age-related reduction in renal function. Am. J. Physiol. 272: R1768–R1774, 1997.

Kirk, S.J., Hurson, M., Regan, M.C., Holt, D.R., Wasserkrug, H.L., Barbul, A. Arginine stimulates wound healing and immune function in elderly human beings. Surgery 114: 155–160, 1993.

Chauhan, A., More, R.S., Mullins, P.A., Taylor, G., Petch, M.C.,

Schofield, P.M. Aging-associated endothelial dysfunction in humans is reversed by L-arginine. J. Am. Coll. Cardiol. 28:1796–1804, 1996.

Reckelhoff, J.F., Kellum, J. A., Blanchard, E.J., Bacon, E.E., Wesley, A. J. & Kruckeburg, W.C. Changes in nitric oxide precursor, L-arginine, and metabolites, nitrate and nitrite, with aging. Life Sciences 55: 1895–1902, 1994.

Glutamine

Amores-Sanchez, M.I. & Medina, M.A. Glutamine, as a precursor of glutathione, and oxidative stress. Molec. Gen. Metab. 67: 100–105, 1999.

Newsholme, E.A., Crabtree, B. & Ardaw, S.M. Glutamine metabolism in lymphocytes: its biochemical, physiological and clinical importance. Quart. J. Exp. Physiol. 70: 473–489, 1985.

Van Acker, B.A.C., von Meyenfeldt, M.F., van der Hulst, R.R.W.J., Hulsewe, K.W.E., Wagenmakers, A.J.M., Deutz, N.E.P., de Blaauw, I., Dejong, G.H.C., van Kreel, B.K. & Soeters, P.B. Glutamine: the pivot of our nitrogen economy? J. Parent. Ent. Nutr. 23: S45–S48, 1999.

Newsholme, E.A. & Calder, P.C. The proposed role of glutamine in some cells of the immune system and speculative consequences for the whole animal. Nutrition 13: 728–730, 1997.

Nucleotides

Lopez-Navarro, A.T., Bueno, J.D., Gil, A. & Sanchez-Pozo, A. Morphological changes in hepatocytes of rats deprived of dietary nucleotides. Brit. J. Nutr. 76: 579–589, 1996.

Berthold, H.K., Crain, P.F., Gouni, I., Reeds, P.J. & Klein, P.D. Evidence for incorporation of intact dietary pyrimidine (but not purine) nucleosides into hepatic RNA. Proc. Natl. Acad. Sci. 92: 10123–10127, 1995.

Sanderson, I.R. & He, Y. Nucleotide uptake and metabolism by intestinal epithelial cells. I Nutr. 124: 131S–137S, 1994.

Jyonouchi, H. Nucleotide actions on humoral immnune responses. J. Nutr. 124: 138S–143S, 1994.

Quercetin

Duthie, S.J., Collins, A.R., Duthie, G.G. & Dobson, V.L. Quercetin and myricetin protect against hydrogen peroxide-induced DNA damage (strand breaks and oxidised pyrimidines) in human lymphocytes). Mutation Research 393: 223–231, 1997.

Hollman, P.C.H., van Trijp, J.M.P., Buysman, M.N.C.P., v.d. Gaag, M.S., Mengelers, M.J.B., deVries, J.H.M. & Katan, M.B. Relative bioavailability of the antioxidant flavonoid quercetin from various foods in man. FEBS Letters 418: 152–156, 1997.

Ferrali, M., Signorini, C., Caciotti, B., Sugherini, L., Ciccoli, L., Giachetti, D. & Comporti, M. Protection against oxidative damage of erythrocyte membrane by the flavonoid quercetin and its relation to iron chelating activity. FEBS Letters 416: 123–129, 1997.

Aging

Pawelec, G., Wagner, W., Adibzadeh, M. & Engel, A. T cell immunosenescence in vitro and in vivo. Exp. Gerontol. 34: 419–429, 1999.

Song, H., Price, P.W. & Cerny, J. Age-related changes in antibody repertoire: contribution from T cells. Immunological Reviews 160: 55–62, 1997.

Morrison, J.H. & Hof, P.R. Life and death of neurons in the aging brain. Science 278: 412–418, 1997.

Harman, D. The aging process: major risk factor for disease and death. Proc. Natl. Acad. Sci. 88: 5360–5363, 1991.

Bohr, V.A. & Anson, R.M. DNA damage, mutation and fine structure DNA repair in aging. Mutation Research 338: 25–34, 1995.

Wang, P. S., Lo, M. & Kau, M. Glucocorticoids and aging. J. Formos. Med. Assoc. 96: 792–801, 1997.

Vahl, N., Jorgensen, J.O.L., Jurik, A.G. & Christiansen, J.S. Abdominal adiposity and physical fitness are major determinants of the age associated decline in stimulated GH secretion in healthy adults. J. Clin. Endocrinol. Metab. 81: 2209–2215, 1996.

Jensen, M.D. Health consequences of fat distribution. Horm. Res. 48: 89–92, 1997.

Lazarus, R., Sparrow, D. & Weiss, S. Temporal relations between obesity and insulin: longitudinal data from the normative aging study. Am. J. Epidemiol. 147, 173–179, 1998.

Neumann, D.A. Joint deformity and dysfunction: a basic review of underlying mechanisms. Arthritis Care and Research 12: 139–151, 1999.

Bailey, A.J., Paul, R.G. & Knott, L. Mechanisms of maturation and ageing of collagen. Mechanisms of ageing and development 106: 1–56, 1998.

Perez, R., Lopez, M. & de Quiroga, G.B. Aging and lung antioxidant enzymes, glutathione, and lipid peroxidation in the rat. Free Radical Biology & Medicine 10: 35–39, 1991.

Robert, L. & Peterszegi, G. Aging and matrix biology. Path. Biol 46: 491–495, 1998.

Meyer, K.C., Ershler, W., Rosenthal, N.S., Lu X. & Peterson, K. Immune dysregulation in the aging human lung. Am. J. Respir. Crit. Care Med. 153: 1072–1079, 1996.

Guyton, K.Z., Gorospe, M., Wang, X., Mock, Y.D., Kokkonen, G.C., Liu, Y., Roth, G.S. & Holbrook, N.J. Age-related changes in activation of mitogen-activated protein kinase cascades by oxidative stress. J. Investigative Dermatol. Symposium Proceedings #: 23–27, 1998.

Wei, Q. Effect of aging on DNA repair and skin carcinogenesis: a minireview of population-based studies. J. Investigative Dermatol. Symposium Proceedings 3: 19–22, 1998.

Uitto, J. & Bernstein, E.F. Molecular mechanisms of cutaneous aging: connective tissue alterations in the dermis. J. Investigative Dermatol. Symposium Proceedings 3: 41–44, 1998.

Yaar, M. Skin aging: observations at the cellular and molecular levels. Isr. J. Med. Sci. 32: 1053–1058, 1996.

Vissers, M.C.M. & Winterbourn, C.C. The effect of oxidants on neutrophil-mediated degradation of glomerular basement membrane collagen. Biochemica et Biophysica Acta 889: 277–286, 1986.

Makita, Z., Radoff, S., Rayfield, E.J., Yang, Z., Skolnik, E., Delaney, V., Friedman, E.A., Cerami, A. & Vlassara, H. Advanced glycosylation end products in patients with diabetic nephropathy. N. Engl. J. Med. 325: 836–842, 1991.

Vlassara, H. Protein glycation in the kidney: role in diabetes and aging. Kidney Intl. 49: 1796–1804, 1996.

Stio, M. Iantomasi, T., Favilli, F., Marraccini, P., Lunghi, B., Vincenzini, M.T. & Treves, C. Glutathione metabolism in heart and liver of the aging rat. Biochem. Cell Biol. 72: 58–61, 1994.

Horbach, G.J.M.J., van Asten, J.G., Rietjens, I.M.C.M., Kremers, P. & van Bezooijen, C.F.A. The effect of aging on inducibility of various types of rat liver cytochrome P-450. Xenobiotica 22: 515–522, 1992.

Sastre, J. Pallardo, F.V., Pla, R., Pellin, A., Juan, G., O'Connor, J.E., Estrela, J.M., Miguel, J. & Vina, J. Aging of the liver: age-associated mitochondrial damage in intact hepatocytes. Hepatol. 24: 1199–1205, 1996.

Pardridge, W.M. Blood-brain barrier carrier-mediated transport and brain metabolism of amino acids. Neurochem. Res. 23: 635–644, 1998.

Morrison, J.H. & Hof, P.R. Life and death of neurons in the aging brain. Science 278:412–419, 1997.

Carney, J.M. & Carney, A.M. Role of oxidation in aging and in age-associated neurodegenerative diseases. Life Sciences 55: 2097–2103, 1994.

Manolagas, S.C. Cellular and molecular mechanisms of osteoporosis. Aging Clin. Exp. Res. 10: 182–190, 1998.

Seeman, E. Osteoporosis in men. Osteoporosis Int. 2: S97–S110, 1999.

Lakatta, E.G. &Yin, F.C.P. Myocardial aging: functional alterations and related cellular mechanisms. Am. J. Physiol. 242: H927–H941, 1982.

Harrison, D.G. Endothelial control of vasomotion and nitric oxide production. Cardiology Clinics 14: 1–15, 1996.

Fiatarone, M.A., Marks, E.C., Ryan, N.D., Meredith, C.N., Lipsitz, L.A. & Evans, W.J. High-intensity strength training in nonagenarians. JAMA: 263: 3029–3034, 1990.

Brown, M. & Hasser, E.M. Complexity of age-related change in skeletal muscle. J. Gerontol. 51A: B117–B123, 1996.

Smith, J.A. Exercise immunology and neutrophils. Int. J. Sports Med. 18: S46–S55, 1997.

Eriksson, J., Taimela, S. & Koivisto, V.A. Exercise and the metabolic syndrome. Diabetologia: 125–135, 1997.

Borst, S.E. & Lowenthal, D.T. Role of IGF-I in muscular atrophy in aging. Endocrine 7: 61–63, 1997.

Short, K.R. & Nair, K.S. Mechanisms of sarcopenia of aging. J. Endocrinol. 22: 95–105, 1999.

Bartke, A. Growth hormone and aging. Endocrine 8: 103–108, 1998.

Gooren, L.J.G. Endocrine aspects of ageing in the male. Molec. Cellular Endocrinol. 145: 153–159, 1998.

Vermeulen, A. & Kaufman, J.M. Ageing of the hypothalamo-pituitary-testicular axis in men. Horm. Res. 43: 25–28, 1995.

Rossmanith, W.G. Gonadotropin secretion during aging in women: review article. Exp. Gerontol. 30: 369–381, 1995.

Schwenke, D.C. Aging, menopause, and free radicals. Seminars in reproductive endocrinology 16: 281–308, 1998.

Skafar, D.F., Xu, R., Morales, J., Ram, J. & Sowers, J.R. Female sex hormones and cardiovascular disease in women. J. Clin. Endocrinol. Metab. 82: 3913–3918, 1997.

Yen, S.S.C. & Laughlin, G.A. Aging and the adrenal cortex. Exp. Gerontol. 33: 897–910, 1998.

Masoro, E.J. Glucocortcoids and aging. Aging Clin. Exp. Res. 7: 407–413, 1995.

Sapolsky, R.M. Glucocorticoids, stress, and their adverse neurological effects: relevance to aging. Exp. Gerontol. 34: 721–732, 1999.